DIAGNOSTIC MUSCULOSKELETAL IMAGING

DIAGNOSTIC MUSCULOSKELETAL IMAGING

Editors

Theodore T. Miller, MD

Associate Professor of Radiology
New York University School of Medicine
New York, New York
Chief, Division of Musculoskeletal Imaging
Department of Radiology
North Shore-Long Island Jewish Health System
Manhasset, New York

Mark E. Schweitzer, MD

Professor of Radiology and Orthopaedic Surgery
New York University Medical Center
New York, New York
Chief, Department of Radiology
Hospital for Joint Diseases Orthopaedic Institute
Director of Musculoskeletal Radiology NYU/Tisch Medical Center
New York, New York

Forewords by Donald Resnick, MD and Jeremy J. Kaye, MD

McGraw-Hill
Medical Publishing Division
New York   Chicago   San Francisco   Lisbon   London   Madrid   Mexico City   Milan   New Delhi
San Juan   Seoul   Singapore   Sydney   Toronto

DIAGNOSTIC MUSCULOSKELETAL IMAGING

Copyright © 2005 by the **McGraw-Hill Companies, Inc.** All rights reserved. Printed in the United States of America. Except as permitted under the United States Copyright Act of 1976, no part of this publication may be reproduced or distributed in any form or by any means, or stored in a data base or retrieval system, without the prior written permission of the publisher.

1234567890 KGP/KGP 0987654

ISBN 0-07-143962-5

This book was set in Times Roman by Tech Books.
The editors were Andrea Seils and Nicky Fernando.
The production supervisor was Catherine H. Saggese.
The cover designer was John Vairo, Jr.
The index was prepared by Jerry Ralya.
Quebecor/Kingsport was the printer and binder.

This book is printed on acid-free paper.

Library of Congress Cataloging-in-Publication Data

Miller, Theodore T.
    Diagnostic musculoskeletal imaging / Theodore T. Miller,
        Mark E. Schweitzer.
        p. ; cm.
    ISBN 0-07-143962-5
        1. Musculoskeletal system—Imaging.   2. Musculoskeletal
    system—Diseases—Diagnosis.
    I. Schweitzer, Mark E., MD.   II. Title.
        [DNLM: 1. Musculoskeletal Diseases—diagnosis.   2. Athletic
    Injuries—diagnosis.   3. Diagnostic Imaging—methods.
    4. Musculoskeletal System—injuries. WE 141 M651d 2004]
    RC925.7.M556 2004
    616.7'0754—dc22   2004042557

To my wife and children, without whom all this is meaningless.
To my parents, who have always been supportive of me.

Theodore T. Miller

To my beautiful wife, Sheryl, and my wonderful children, Shira
and Daniel, for challenging and encouraging me.
To the memory of my mother who continues to inspire me.

Mark E. Schweitzer

CONTENTS

CONTRIBUTORS

John Carrino, MD
Assistant Professor of Radiology
Department of Radiology
Harvard Medical School
Brigham and Women's Hospital
Boston, Massachusetts
Chapter 3

Kathleen Finzel, MD
Assistant Professor of Radiology
Weill Medical College of Cornell University
New York, New York
Associate Attending Radiologist
Department of Radiology and Imaging
Hospital for Special Surgery
New York, New York
Chapter 19

Bernard Ghelman, MD
Associate Professor of Radiology
Weill Medical College of Cornell University
New York, New York
Attending Radiologist
Department of Radiology and Imaging
Hospital for Special Surgery
New York, New York
Chapter 19

Nogah Haramati, MD
Professor of Clinical Radiology & Surgery
Albert Einstein College of Medicine
Bronx, New York
Chief of Service
Department of Radiology
Jack D. Weiler Hospital of the Albert Einstein College
    of Medicine
Bronx, New York
Chapter 9

Richard Katzberg, MD
Professor
Department of Radiology
University of California, Medical Center
Sacramento, California
Chapter 16

Terry L. Levin, MD
Clinical Associate Professor of Radiology
Albert Einstein College of Medicine
Montefiore Medical Center
Bronx, New York
Chapters 8 & 12

James Manzione, MD
Associate Professor of Clinical Radiology and
    Neurological Surgery
Chief, Neuro Interventional Radiology
Department of Radiology
SUNY at Stonybrook
Stonybrook, New York
Chapter 16

Theodore T. Miller, MD
Associate Professor of Radiology
New York University School of Medicine
New York, New York
Chief, Division of Musculoskeletal Imaging
Department of Radiology
North Shore-Long Island Jewish Health System
Manhasset, New York
Chapters 1, 5, 8, 10, 12, 13 & 18

William Morrison, MD
Associate Professor of Radiology
Jefferson Medical College of Thomas Jefferson
    University
Philadelphia, Pennsylvania
Director
Division of Musculoskeletal and General Diagnostic
    Imaging
Department of Radiology
Thomas Jefferson University Hospital
Philadelphia, Pennsylvania
Chapter 3

Robert Schneider, MD
Associate Professor Clinical Radiology
Weill Medical College of Cornell University
New York, New York
Attending Radiologist
Chief of Nuclear Medicine
Department of Radiology and Imaging
Hopital for Special Surgery
New York, New York
Chapter 2

Elizabeth Schultz, MD
Chief of Musculoskeletal Radiology
BAB Radiology
Bayshore, New York
Chapters 4 & 7

Mark E. Schweitzer, MD

Professor of Radiology and Orthorpaedic Surgery
New York University Medical Center
New York, New York
Chief, Department of Radiology
Hospital for Joint Diseases Orthopaedic Institute
Director of Musculoskeletal Radiology New York
    University/Tisch Medical Center
New York, New York
Chapters 6, 11, 14 & 15

Ronald B. Staron, MD

Associate Professor of Clinical Radiology
Columbia University College of
    Physicians and Surgeons
New York, New York
Department of Radiology
Columbia-Presbyterian Medical Center
New York, New York
Chapter 18

Hillary Umans, MD

Associate Clinical Professor of Radiology & Orthopaedic
    Surgery
Albert Einstein College of Medicine
Bronx, New York
Director of Musculoskeletal Radiology
Jacobi Medical Center
Bronx, New York
Chapter 9

Lawrence M. White, MD

Associate Professor of Radiology
University of Toronto
Toronto, Ontario, Canada
Head, Division of Musculoskeletal Imaging
Department of Medical Imaging
Mount Sinai Hospital and the University Health Network
Toronto, Ontario, Canada
Chapter 17

FOREWORD

In the pages that follow, two prominent bone radiologists, Drs. Theodore Miller and Mark Schweitzer, both of New York, provide an up-to-date text dealing with the imaging findings related to disorders of the musculoskeletal system. At a time when conventional and advanced imaging studies are being applied more frequently to the assessment of such disorders and when the results of these studies are having a greater and greater influence on diagnostic and management issues, this text is both needed and welcome.

It's organization follows the traditional and successful technique of addressing in order specific categories of disease and subsequently individual sites of involvement. Additional chapters address such issues as bone densitometry and interventional techniques. The text is concise and well-written, the illustrations superb, and the material current and pertinent. Along with skilled contributors, the two editors provide a readable and organized account of the imaging findings that accompany both common and a few not so common diseases. These findings are displayed with a spectrum of imaging methods that range from conventional radiography through MR imaging, sonography, CT scanning, and bone scintigraphy. Selected references await the interested reader who would like to seek additional information on any topic.

Having written texts myself, I know full well the dedication and hard work that went into the production of this work. If their experience was similar to my own, I suspect that there were times when their enthusiasm was tested a bit and even that the ultimate goal seemed far away and perhaps unobtainable. That is why we, the readers, owe them a great deal of gratitude, for it is we who will truly benefit from their efforts. Whether a resident or fully trained or a radiologist, orthopedic surgeon, internist, sport medicine physician, or some other specialist, there is a lot to be learned here. This is not a text to be left unused on the shelf but one to be handled on a regular basis.

Writing a Foreword for a text is always a great honor. Writing one for a work as good as this is even a greater honor. To Ted and Mark, I offer my congratulations. Simply, you have done an outstanding job. Now we who read your book will benefit from your efforts and, remarkably, enjoy the experience.

Donald Resnick, MD
Professor of Radiology
University of California San Diego
VA Medical Center
Department of Radiology
San Diego, California

"Let such teach others who themselves excel."
ALEXANDER POPE
Essay on Criticism

In *Diagnostic Musculoskeletal Imaging,* Drs. Miller and Schweitzer and their contributors clearly follow the advice of Alexander Pope; they should be able and capable of teaching us, since they all write in their areas of expertise. The text uses a combination of approaches: disease, region and technique. Although not a comprehensive work, as the authors freely admit, its role is intended as a book to be used primarily by radiology residents and by others seeking an approach to musculoskeletal radiology.

Musculoskeletal radiology is not rocket science; the material is not intrinsically overly difficult. It's just that there is so much of it! In a way, it is just like medical school all over again, and musculoskeletal radiology is just one (arguably the most important and interesting) of the various subspecialties in the discipline of diagnostic radiology. Complicating matters further, the last decade has seen an explosion in technology, much of which has applications in the study of musculoskeletal disorders. Where is the first-year radiology resident to turn to find an introduction to this extensive, seemingly overwhelming knowledge base? Moreover, where should senior residents and practitioners turn to refresh their knowledge?

There has long been a perceived need for an introductory textbook in musculoskeletal radiology, and the goal of the authors in providing one is admirable. The textual materials are all very readable and the illustrations clear; tables are used effectively to present information concisely. Rather than providing an extensive bibliography, the authors have given the reader selected recommended reading. Especially considering the intended audience, this seems a most appropriate choice.

In radiology, book authors usually choose a disease oriented approach, or one that focuses on techniques, or one that examines regions. In this work, the authors have effectively used all three approaches. Moreover, they have done so without undue duplication and repetition of text and illustrations. Correlation of imaging techniques is often difficult in musculoskeletal radiology. The authors have done an excellent job of giving the right amount of emphasis to those techniques which will be most useful.

In summary, *Diagnostic Musculoskeletal Imaging* really gives radiology residents and radiologists an excellent way to approach complex material. Basic diseases, sports injuries, information on the radiographic appearances of orthopedic hardware, and some special techniques that are utilized in musculoskeletal radiology are all covered.

As someone who has spent a career in teaching radiology residents and fellows, I really look forward to having this text available to recommend to students of a complex (but not inherently difficult) subject.

Jeremy J. Kaye, MD
Professor and Vice-Chairman
Department of Radiology & Radiological Sciences
Vanderbilt University Medical Center
Nashville, Tennessee

PREFACE

This project has been long coming. When the idea for this book was first proposed in 1997, the musculoskeletal imaging textbook market was wide open. There were standard texts on musculoskeletal radiology, mostly dealing with plain radiographs and there were a few modality-specific texts and teaching files, but a book dealing with a multi-modality approach to musculoskeletal imaging had not yet been written. In the interim, however, several such texts have appeared, and our book now joins this crowded field. However, each of these books has its own style, strengths, and weaknesses, and we hope that readers will find our work useful and its shortcomings not too distracting.

This text is meant to be an introduction to musculoskeletal imaging, targeted to radiology residents as a first exposure to musculoskeletal imaging, and to senior residents and general radiologists as an overview to refresh their memories. In all of the chapters, we have tried to take a multi-modality, correlative imaging approach. It is not meant to be an in-depth, reference text, and thus a "suggested reading" list is given at the conclusion of each chapter rather than a reference list.

We have organized the book into three major sections. The first section deals with general disease topics such as infection, trauma, arthritis, etc., including a chapter on musculoskeletal manifestations of AIDS. The second section discusses regional sports injuries as well as diseases of the lumbar spine and temporomandibular joint. The third section deals with miscellaneous topics that we thought were important for residents to know, but which are not usually found in general texts, such as bone densitometry, imaging of orthopedic instrumentation, and musculoskeletal interventional procedures.

As with any introductory text, there is debate over what topics to include and what the depth of discussion of each topic should be. As we read the galley proofs we were occasionally gripped by pangs of anxiety realizing that some subjects had been left out unintentionally or feeling that we did not explain a particular topic well. There is also the disappointment of finding a beautiful example of a particular abnormality after the book has already gone into production and being unable to include it.

We view this text as a work in progress. We know that there are some redundancies in the text, some deficiencies in our discussion of topics, some topics omitted, and some illustrations of which we wish we had better examples. Undoubtedly, more deficiencies will be pointed out to us by our residents and other users of this book. We hope that this text will nonetheless be popular enough to allow us to correct these shortcomings in a second edition.

Lastly, many authors contributed to this text, but we have tried to homogenize the writing style to maintain an informal teaching tone. We hope that readers enjoy reading it as much as learning from it.

Theodore T. Miller, MD
Mark E. Schweitzer, MD
September 2004

ACKNOWLEDGMENTS

No project of this size can be completed without the help and contributions of many people. We thank all of the authors who contributed chapters. Many other colleagues were kind enough to lend us illustrations, and although they are acknowledged in the captions, we would like to mention them here: Dr. Frieda Feldman, Dr. Henry Pritzker, Dr. James Nadich, Dr. Christopher Palestro, Dr. Rolando Singson, Dr. Kathleen Finzel, Dr. Bernard Ghelman, Dr. Marcia Blacksin, Dr. Susan Cushin, Dr. Jerald Zimmer, and Dr. Timothy Sanders.

We must thank Marc Strauss of McGraw-Hill for believing in this project and helping us to stay on schedule to finally complete it. We also thank Andrea Seils, Marsha Loeb, and Nicky Fernando of McGraw-Hill for their help in the production of the text. Thank you to our secretaries Lorraine White, Diane Byard, and Kimberly Lucas for their help transcribing our chapters and for keeping track of everything.

Lastly, we must thank our families for giving us the time in the evenings and on weekends to write our chapters and edit the book. Their support is deeply and lovingly appreciated.

DIAGNOSTIC MUSCULOSKELETAL IMAGING

PART I

DISEASES

CHAPTER 1

MUSCULOSKELETAL INFECTIONS

THEODORE T. MILLER

Evaluation of clinically suspected infection is a common imaging task. Many factors have to be taken into consideration, such as the pathogen (eg, bacteria, mycobacteria, fungus, or virus), the location of the suspected infection (eg, bone, soft tissue, joint, or disc space), the age of the patient (eg, infant, child, adult), the time course of the infection (eg, acute, subacute, or chronic), and whether there are any underlying complicating factors such as infarct or other bone disease, joint replacement in the area of clinical concern, or diabetic arthropathy. Radiography, computed tomography (CT), sonography, scintigraphy, and magnetic resonance imaging (MRI) have roles and different degrees of usefulness in the imaging evaluation.

ACUTE OSTEOMYELITIS

Pyogenic

Osteomyelitis is infection of the medullary cavity of bone and may occur as a result of hematogenous spread, contiguous spread from an adjacent site of infection, or direct inoculation such as iatrogenic or traumatic (including penetrating trauma such as bullets and open fractures). The most common pathway is hematogenous spread, and in children and adults the most common site of infection in a long bone is the metaphysis because of sluggish flow in the end arterioles in this region allowing the deposition of organisms. In babies and children up to approximately 18 months of age, the most common site in a long bone is the epiphysis because transphyseal vessels allow the bloodborne organisms to cross the growth plate from the metaphysis into the epiphysis.

Plain radiographs should be the starting point for any imaging evaluation of suspected infection. The earliest radiographic changes are soft tissue swelling and blurring of adjacent fat planes, which may take several days to become apparent after the onset of infection. Approximately 10 days after the onset of infection, the radiographs may demonstrate lysis of the medullary trabeculae, focal loss of cortex, and periosteal reaction (Figure 1-1). If the radiographs are normal or equivocal, more advanced imaging may be required, and the two most commonly

used modalities are MRI and nuclear scintigraphy. General advantages of MRI over scintigraphy are its superb anatomic detail, including the ability to evaluate bone and adjacent soft tissue, and its quicker performance. A disadvantage of both modalities is that young children may need to be sedated to prevent blurring due to patient motion.

When performing MRI, a coil appropriate to the body part being imaged should be used, and a field of view should be selected that covers the area of concern without being too large. Similarly, slice thickness appropriate to the area of clinical concern can increase anatomic resolution and decrease misinterpretation due to partial volume averaging. Standard sequences that should be used are T_1-weighted spin-echo and fat-suppressed T_2-weighted fast spin-echo. If the fast spin-echo T_2-weighted sequences are not fat suppressed, the high signal intensity of marrow edema may be masked by the high signal intensity of the marrow fat. Fat suppression can be achieved by using frequency-selective presaturation or inversion recovery techniques. Frequency selection uses the difference in precessional frequencies between fat and water protons to presaturate the fat protons; a prescan sequence determines the maximum frequency peak of water protons and then produces a frequency pulse that is 220 MHz higher (on a 1.5-T scanner) to suppress fat protons. Frequency-selective presaturation cannot be performed on low field strength magnets (0.3 T) because the difference in precessional frequency between fat and water protons is proportional to the field strength of the magnet, and the precessional frequencies are too close to each other to resolve at low field strength. In the inversion recovery technique, all protons are flipped 180°, and scanning begins after some chosen "inversion time" near the null point of the fat signal. A disadvantage of the frequency-selective technique is that it is sensitive to field inhomogeneity resulting in uneven fat suppression, and a disadvantage of inversion recovery is that it may have poor signal-to-noise ratio. Moreover, depending on the inversion time selected, even gadolinium contrast enhancement can be suppressed. Conventional dual-echo spin-echo sequences can be used but take more time than a fast spin-echo sequence. If the patient is being imaged on a high field strength magnet (eg, 1.5 T), then gradient echo imaging should not be used because the local dephasing effects of the trabeculae may mask marrow

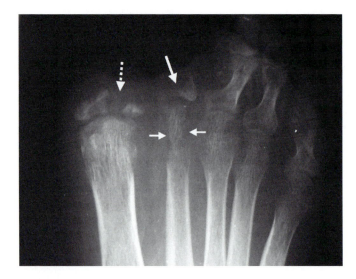

FIGURE 1-1. Osteomyelitis. Radiograph of the toes in a patient who has undergone amputation of the first and second toes shows lysis of the surgical stump of the second proximal phalanx (large white arrow) and trabecular and cortical losses involving the second metatarsal head and neck (small white arrows). There is also involvement of the stump of the first proximal phalanx (dashed arrow) and possibly of the first metatarsal neck and head.

edema; such local dephasing is not a concern at low field strengths. Other technical factors that can lead to uneven signal intensity across the field are imaging of a body part that is off center within the magnet and poor coil placement, which can lead to *coil burnout* (high signal intensity in regions next to the coil) or *coil drop-off* (loss of signal at regions away from the coil). The normal fatty marrow signal intensity of T_1-weighted images is a useful internal check for coil burnout and drop off (Figure 1-2).

The earliest finding of acute osteomyelitis on MRI is alteration of normal marrow signal intensity, which can be seen as soon as 1 to 2 days after the onset of infection. The signal intensity of the normal medullary cavity is high on T_1-weighted images in an adult due to fatty marrow, intermediate (isointense to muscle) in children and infants due to red marrow, and intermediate to low on fat-suppressed fast T_2-weighted sequences in all age groups. Normal cortex shows low signal intensity in all age groups on all pulse sequences, and muscle has intermediate signal intensity in all age groups on T_1- and fat-suppressed T_2-weighted sequences. Due to the inflammatory edema that is the hallmark of acute infection, the signal intensity of marrow becomes low to intermediate on T_1-weighted sequences and high on fat-suppressed T_2-weighted sequences, reflecting the free water content of the inflammatory exudate. The margins of the abnormal signal intensity are usually ill-defined. Periosteal reaction and adjacent soft tissue edema subsequently occur and will become apparent sooner on MRI than on radiography (Figure 1-3).

MRI has 100% negative predictive value for excluding osteomyelitis; ie, if the marrow is completely normal on all pulse sequences, then infection can be reliably excluded. Its positive predictive value, ie, its accuracy for determining osteomyelitis if abnormal signal intensity is present in the marrow, is not as good because of other causes of edema such as neuropathic arthropathy (see below) and reactive marrow edema. Reactive marrow edema is non-infectious edema occurring in marrow adjacent to a site of soft tissue infection or even adjacent to another site of osteomyelitis. Its exact pathogenesis is unknown,

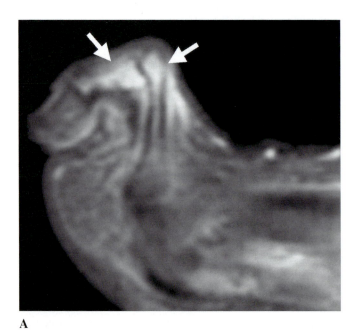

A

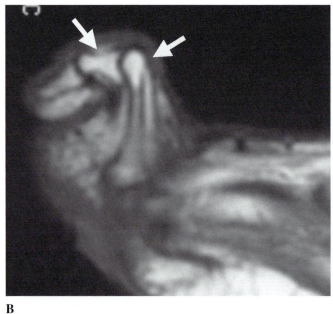

B

FIGURE 1-2. Coil burnout. *(A)* Sagittal fat-suppressed fast spin-echo T_2-weighted image shows high signal intensity in the head of the proximal phalanx and middle phalanx (arrows), mimicking marrow edema. *(B)* The corresponding sagittal T_1-weighted image shows high signal intensity fatty marrow within these same regions. Because of the flexion deformity of the toe, these portions of the toe are closer to the coil and thus produce artifactual high signal intensity.

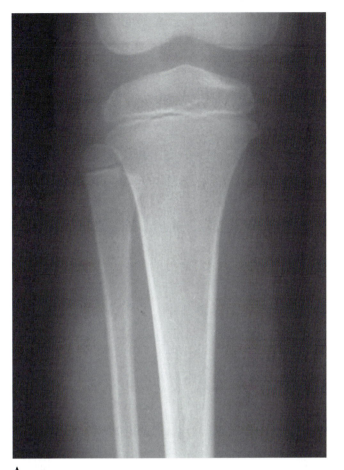

A

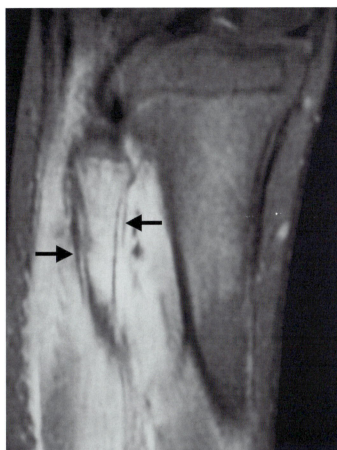

B

FIGURE 1-3. Osteomyelitis of the proximal fibula. *(A)* Frontal radiograph shows no abnormality. *(B)* Corresponding fat-suppressed T$_2$-weighted magnetic resonance image shows high signal intensity marrow edema within the fibula, periosteal reaction (arrows), and surrounding soft-tissue inflammatory edema.

but it is thought to represent a type of vasogenic hyperemia. The signal intensity of reactive marrow edema can mimic that of osteomyelitis, and it can enhance with gadolinium contrast agents, similar to osteomyelitis, thus causing false-positive interpretations (Figure 1-4).

Different scintigraphic methods using different radiopharmaceuticals are also available for the evaluation of osteomyelitis. The traditional method of scintigraphic evaluation has been the 3-phase bone scan using technetium Tc 99m methylene diphosphonate (MDP). A positive examination will show increased uptake in all 3 phases but will appear most intense in the bone phase at 4 hours (the third phase) and in 24-hour delayed bone phase images (Figure 1-5). An advantage of this method over MRI is its ability to image the entire body in cases of suspected multifocal osteomyelitis. Disadvantages include exposure to ionizing radiation, lack of anatomic detail, and false-positive studies due to uptake by other bone abnormalities (Table 1-1). False-negative bone scans can result from poor blood supply to the infected site or bony lysis without a compensatory bone reaction. To increase the accuracy of bone scanning, it has been combined with gallium Ga 67 scanning because Ga 67 is also a bone agent; decreased gallium uptake relative to technetium mitigates against

osteomyelitis, whereas increased gallium uptake suggests infection. Another scintigraphic method is white cell imaging, in which neutrophils are linked to In 111 or to Tc 99m. A disadvantage of this technique is that it requires that blood be drawn from the patient, labeled ex vivo, and then reinjected, with imaging performed approximately 24 hours after injection. Another disadvantage is that the white cell tracer will accumulate in areas of normal red marrow in addition to areas of neutrophil uptake. Therefore, to improve the accuracy of the technique, it has been combined with Tc 99m sulfur colloid scanning, in which a positive scan is demonstrated by spatial incongruence of uptake of white cell tracer without uptake of sulfur colloid. White cell studies may not be feasible if the patient is leukopenic because there may not be enough white cells to label and is not useful in nonbacterial or chronic infections because the inflammatory response is not neutrophilic. Other techniques have focused on the use of radiolabeled monoclonal antibodies, which have the advantages of in vivo labeling and more rapid time to imaging, but has no better accuracy or anatomic detail than labeled white cells.

CT and sonography also can evaluate acute osteomyelitis but are not first-choice imaging modalities. Features of acute osteomyelitis on CT are increased density of the normal fatty

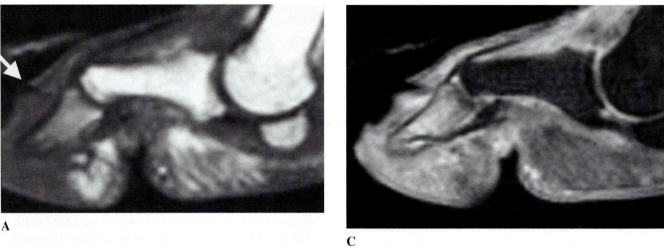

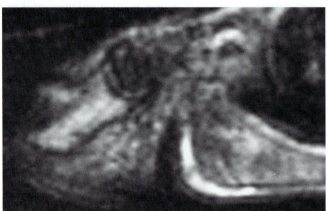

FIGURE 1-4.   Reactive marrow edema. *(A)* Sagittal T_1-weighted magnetic resonance image shows low signal intensity in the distal phalanx of the first toe. Note the surrounding soft tissue edema and the ulcer over the dorsal aspect of the distal toe (arrow). *(B)* Corresponding sagittal fat-suppressed fast spin-echo T_2-weighted image shows high signal intensity in the distal phalanx and surrounding soft tissue. *(C)* Corresponding fat-suppressed T_1-weighted image after intravenous administration of gadolinium contrast shows enhancement of the distal phalanx and surrounding soft tissue. The toe was amputated and showed staphylococcal infection of the soft tissues with normal underlying bone. *(Courtesy of Dr. Susan Cushin.)*

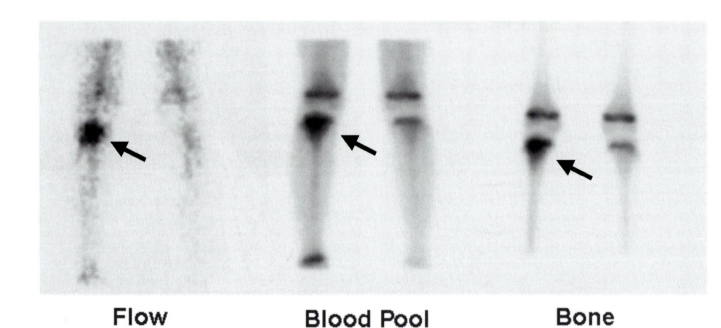

FIGURE 1-5.   Three-phase bone scan of a child with osteomyelitis of the proximal right tibia shows increased radiotracer uptake in all phases of the study (arrows). *(Courtesy of Dr. Christopher Palestro.)*

TABLE 1-1

Increased Uptake on Bone Scan

Osteomyelitis
Bone infarction, healing avascular necrosis
Fracture, stress reaction and stress fracture
Arthritis
Most metastatic diseases, primary malignant bone tumors
Osteoid osteoma
Paget disease, fibrous dysplasia

medullary canal as it is replaced by the infectious edema, blurring of fat planes, and eventually periosteal reaction and loss of cortex. Although CT may show these changes sooner than plain radiographs, the modality is less preferable than MRI because of decreased soft tissue contrast and exposure to ionizing radiation in children.

Sonography is used in many places in the world that do not have immediate access to MRI. The sonographic criterion for acute osteomyelitis is the presence of a subperiosteal abscess (Figure 1-6). Advantages of sonography are that it is rapidly performed, does not use ionizing radiation, and does not require sedation of small children. Disadvantages are that it is operator-dependent and can produce false-negative and false-positive results. Sonography cannot image past the cortex of a bone; therefore, early osteomyelitis that has not yet produced a subperiosteal abscess may be falsely interpreted as normal. Conversely, a soft tissue abscess that is adjacent to bone but is not truly subperiosteal may be falsely interpreted as positive. In addition, complicated anatomic regions such as the wrist or foot may be difficult to evaluate. Power Doppler sonography eventually will show hyperemia around the periosteal abscess but may not do so in the first several days of abscess formation.

Sonography also can be helpful in regions that are complicated by orthopedic instrumentation or in patients who have a contraindication to MRI.

Tuberculosis

Tuberculous osteomyelitis has a much more prolonged and insidious time course than pyogenic infection, running on the order of months. It is hematogenous in etiology, but only about one third of patients have concurrent pulmonary involvement.

Radiographically, the tuberculous lesion of long bones is lytic with minimal, if any, periosteal reaction, and these lesions occur at the end of the bone or in the metaphyseal region (Figure 1-7). Tuberculosis of the short tubular bones of the hands and feet (tuberculous dactylitis) has a different appearance, the so-called *spina ventosa*, consisting of bony expansion and prominent periosteal reaction. Spina ventosa is more common in children than in adults and may have multifocal involvement in up to one third of cases.

There may be an associated abscess, typically larger than that associated with pyogenic infections; the tuberculous abscess is considered "cold" because it is usually well defined and lacks

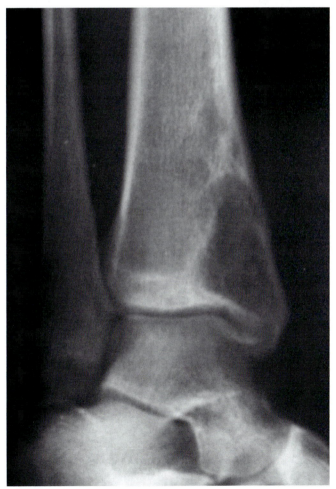

FIGURE 1-7. Oblique radiograph of the ankle shows a focus of tuberculous osteomyelitis involving the distal aspect of the tibia. Note that there is no adjacent periosteal reaction.

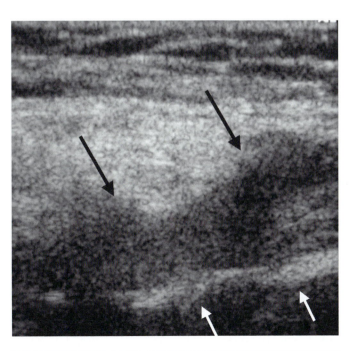

FIGURE 1-6. Ultrasound of osteomyelitis. Longitudinal sonogram shows a hypoechoic sub-periosteal abscess (black arrows) adjacent to an irregularly thickened cortex of the femur (white arrows).

the surrounding inflammatory edema of pyogenic abscesses that blurs the adjacent soft tissue planes. CT and MRI can show the bony involvement and cold abscess. Bone scan is falsely negative in as many as 33% of cases because of the lack of bony response to the infection, and white cell imaging is not helpful because the inflammatory response is histiocytic, not neutrophilic.

Fungus

Fungal osteomyelitis due to such organisms as histoplasmosis, blastomycosis, and coccidioidomycosis has a variable appearance that can mimic pyogenic or tuberculous infection. It also has a predilection for ends of bone.

CHRONIC RECURRENT MULTIFOCAL OSTEOMYELITIS

Chronic recurrent multifocal osteomyelitis (CRMO), despite its name, is a noninfectious inflammatory disorder of bone. Its etiology is unknown but may be a post-infectious autoimmune response. It has some features in common with the synovitis, acne, pustulosis, hyperostosis, osteitis (SAPHO) syndrome (see Chapter 3), and the two diseases may be variants of the same underlying disease. It typically affects children or young adults, is more common in girls, and can have a prolonged, albeit self-limited, course. During clinical exacerbation, the erythrocyte sedimentation rate is elevated, but the C-reactive protein level and white blood count may be normal. Histologically, there is a chronic rather than an acute inflammatory response. It is discussed in this chapter because its imaging appearances are similar to those of pyogenic osteomyelitis.

CRMO affects tubular bones and flat bones, especially the clavicle. In tubular bones the metaphysis is affected, and the lesions appear radiographically as focal trabecular lysis with periosteal reaction. There is variability in the size of the metaphyseal lesions and degree of periosteal response, which sometimes can be the dominant feature, especially in short tubular bones. With healing, the metaphyseal lesions will sclerose, and the periosteal reaction matures as bone-thickening.

The medial and middle portions of the clavicle are affected, are typically enlarged, and acutely can have a lytic destructive appearance with periosteal reaction or a sclerotic appearance. Thickening and hyperostosis are other features of chronic involvement.

Bone scanning with Tc 99m is useful in the workup of patients with suspected CRMO because the multifocality of the disease can be appreciated. Active lesions, even if clinically asymptomatic, will show radiotracer uptake. Disease activity also can be monitored scintigraphically because the quiescent phase shows less intense tracer uptake.

MRI of tubular bones shows marrow edema and periosteal reaction but no adjacent soft tissue edema (unlike pyogenic osteomyelitis). Involvement of the clavicle may have associated soft tissue edema, but this edema is well defined and almost tumoral in appearance compared with the ill-defined edema of true osteomyelitis. Soft tissue abscess is not a feature of CRMO.

SUBACUTE AND CHRONIC BACTERIAL OSTEOMYELITIS

Subacute osteomyelitis can manifest as a Brodie abscess seen radiographically as a geographic area of sclerosis with a lucent center on radiographs and CT. On MRI it usually has low signal intensity on the T_1-weighted sequences and may appear with a heterogeneously high signal intensity on T_2-weighted sequences (Figure 1-8).

Chronic osteomyelitis typically has two appearances. One is the so-called sclerosing osteomyelitis of Garré, in which there is generalized sclerosis of the medullary canal (Figure 1-9). The other appearance is that of markedly thickened periosteal reaction (called an *involucrum*) that wraps around the bone (Figure 1-10). The involucrum is the bone's way of isolating the infection. Typically there is a devitalized bony fragment, called a *sequestrum* (Table 1-2), within the center of the medullary canal of this involved segment of bone. Because the sequestrum does not have a blood supply, antibiotics cannot reach it, and it acts as a safe haven for the offending organism. The sequestrum may not be well seen on radiographs due to the overlying sclerosis of the involucrum. It can, however, be nicely demonstrated on CT (Figure 1-11). An associated feature of such chronic osteomyelitis is a sinus track (called a *cloaca*) through the cortex, which can be quite wide, and which is the body's attempt to expel the sequestrum through a tract in the cortex. A soft tissue sinus track extending to the skin is frequently part of this process.

On MRI, the thickened involucrum is seen as low signal intensity cortical thickening, and the sequestrum may or may not have normal fatty marrow signal intensity. Inactive chronic osteomyelitis can have the normal signal intensity of fatty marrow or the low signal intensity of fibrotic marrow, whereas active chronic osteomyelitis will show edema-like signal intensity. MRI also can demonstrate cortical sinus tracts and soft tissue sinus tracts, typically as linear high signal intensity on T_2-weighted images (Figure 1-12).

Scintigraphic white cell studies are less helpful than they are in acute osteomyelitis because the neutrophil response is diminished in chronic infection. The technetium bone scan can show increased radiotracer uptake, but this merely reflects chronic bony production in response to infection rather than the presence of infection itself. Positron emission tomography (PET) with ^{18}F-fluoro-deoxy-glucose has been reported to have 100% sensitivity and 86% specificity for the evaluation of suspected chronic osteomyelitis, but its cost may be prohibitive for routine use.

INFECTION OF SOFT TISSUE

Soft tissues can be infected independently of the underlying bones. Infection of the skin and subcutaneous tissue is termed *cellulitis* and that of muscle is *infectious myositis*. Radiographically, soft tissue infection is demonstrated as blurring of normal fat planes and swelling. On CT scanning, there is also blurring of fat planes and swelling and increased density of subcutaneous fat due to the inflammatory edema of the infection.

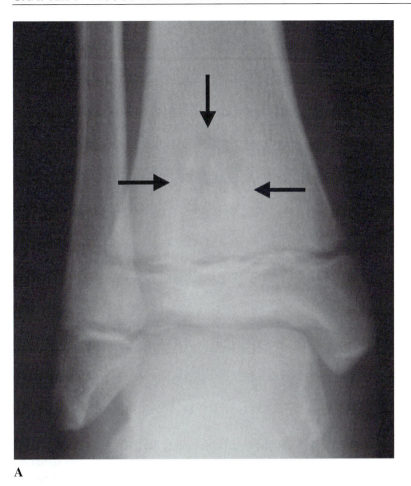

A

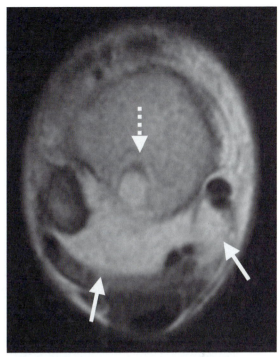

B

FIGURE 1-8. Brodie abscess. *(A)* Anteroposterior radiograph of the distal leg and ankle shows an ill-defined patchy lucency in the distal metaphysis of the tibia (arrows). *(B)* Axial fat-suppressed fast spin-echo T_2-weighted sequence shows the high signal intensity abscess within the bone (dashed arrow) and in the surrounding soft tissue (solid arrows). *(C)* Axial fat-suppressed T_1-weighted sequence after intravenous administration of gadolinium contrast shows the low signal intensity abscess (dashed arrow) and the adjacent soft tissue abscess (solid arrows), both with a surrounding high signal intensity rim.

C

On MRI, cellulitis and myositis are demonstrated by soft tissue swelling and the typical low signal intensity on T_1-weighted and high signal intensity on fat-suppressed T_2-weighted sequences of edema (Figure 1-13). Cellulitis and infectious myositis will enhance with intravenous gadolinium, whereas generalized soft tissue swelling due to benign third spacing of fluid from a non-infectious or non-inflammatory cause typically will not enhance.

The reason for performing advanced imaging in clinically apparent cases of soft tissue infection is to determine the presence of a soft tissue abscess, which might require drainage, and to determine presence of underlying osteomyelitis. CT and MRI can be used for the evaluation of suspected abscess, but intravenous contrast is often required. An abscess appears as a low density mass with an enhancing rim on CT or as a fluid-like mass on MRI that is low signal intensity on T_1-weighted sequences, heterogeneously or uniformly high signal intensity on T_2-weighted sequences, and which has an enhancing rim on T_1-weighted sequences with gadolinium even though the abscess itself does not enhance (Figure 1-14). Sonographically, myositis will appear as a heterogeneous hypoechoic pockmarking of the normal pennate appearance of muscle, and abscess appears as a focal collection that is usually hypoechoic but

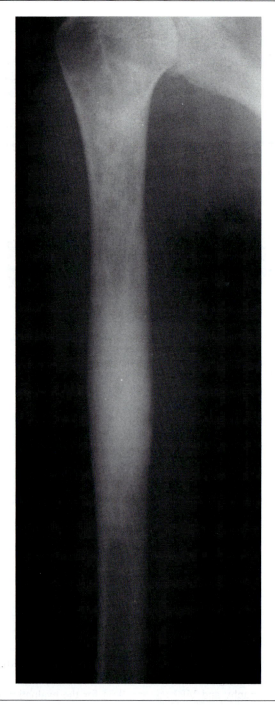

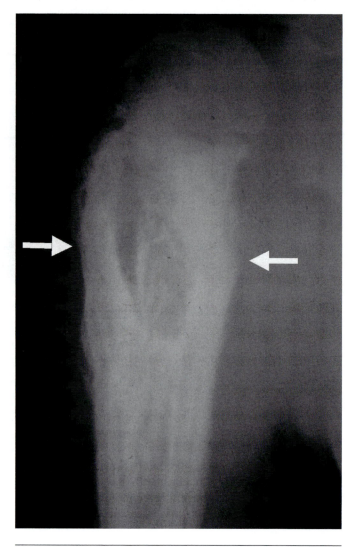

FIGURE 1-10.   Anteroposterior radiograph of the proximal humerus shows marked periosteal thickening (arrows) surrounding a lucent abscess within the bone.

FIGURE 1-9.   Anteroposterior radiograph of the humerus shows chronic sclerosing osteomyelitis with mild fusiform expansion of the shaft.

may have heterogeneous internal echoes due to debris. Power Doppler imaging may not demonstrate hyperemia around the abscess within the first several days of the formation of the abscess.

SEPTIC ARTHRITIS

Infectious organisms can reach the joint through direct inoculation, hematogenous spread, or contiguous spread from an adjacent intraarticular site of osteomyelitis. Radiographically, the earliest signs will be generalized soft tissue swelling and blurring of fat planes about the joint, followed by joint distention due to effusion and synovial thickening. In the septic pediatric hip, the presence of a large joint effusion may actually laterally displace the femoral head, thus showing widening of the medial joint space in comparison with the contralateral normal hip. Periarticular osteopenia also eventually develops, and in pyogenic arthritis there is joint space narrowing early in the disease due to proteolytic enzymes released by the white cell exudate that destroy the articular cartilage; in tuberculous arthritis, the main radiographic features are marked periarticular osteopenia

TABLE 1-2

Entities with a Sequestrum

Chronic osteomyelitis
Fibrosarcoma
Eosinophilic granuloma
Osteoid osteoma (the calcification within the lucent central nidus is not really a sequestrum but it may mimic a small one)

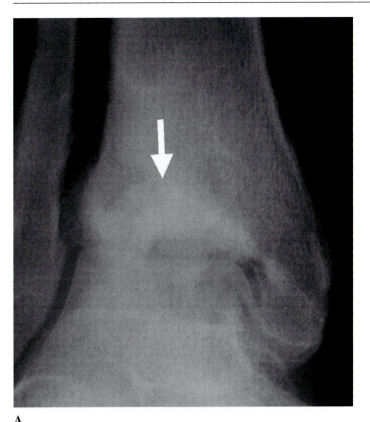

A

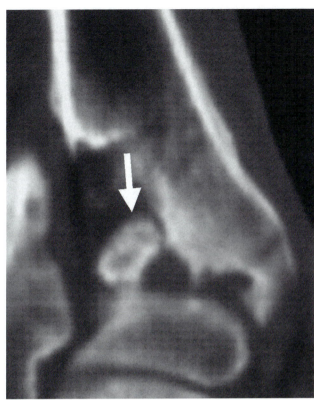

B

FIGURE 1-11.   Sequestrum. *(A)* Oblique radiograph of the ankle shows sclerosis of the distal tibia (arrow) and irregularity of the joint surface. The patient had prior fractures of the distal tibia and distal fibula that resulted in infection. *(B)* Reformatted coronal computed tomographic image shows the dense sequestrum (arrow) within a cavity and the irregularity of the distal articular surface of the tibia.

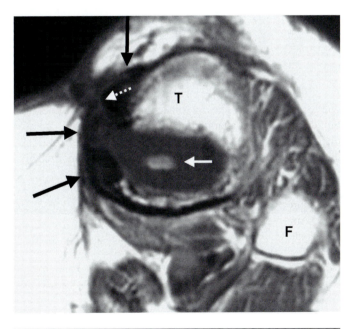

FIGURE 1-12.   Magnetic resonance imaging of chronic osteomyelitis. Axial T_1-weighted image shows a bony sequestrum (solid white arrow) within an area of granulation tissue within the distal tibia (T). Note the thick overlying periosteal reaction (black arrows) and the sinus tract leading to the skin (white dashed arrow). F = fibula.

with relative preservation of the joint space until late in the disease because the chronic inflammatory exudate of tuberculosis lacks the cartilage-destroying proteolytic enzymes (Table 1-3). *Phemister triad* refers to the 3 typical radiographic features of tuberculous arthritis: marked periarticular osteopenia, relative preservation of the joint space, and small periarticular erosions. Erosion of bone also occurs in pyogenic arthritis, concurrently with the cartilage destruction (Figure 1-15).

Sonography and MRI are excellent for the evaluation of a suspected septic joint and will show changes sooner than radiography. However, the presence of a joint effusion per se does not necessarily indicate a septic joint. This is particularly true for pediatric hips, in which a systemic viral infection can cause a transient but painful reactive sterile synovitis. However, the absence of a joint effusion or synovial thickening excludes the presence of a septic joint.

Sonography is particularly useful in children because it can be performed quickly and does not require sedation. Sonography demonstrates a joint effusion as an anechoic or a mildly heterogeneous hypoechoic fluid collection (Figure 1-16). Depending on the acuteness of the process, power Doppler may or may not show hyperemia in the surrounding synovium. A disadvantage of sonography is that it cannot evaluate the underlying bony structures and therefore may miss an early osteomyelitis.

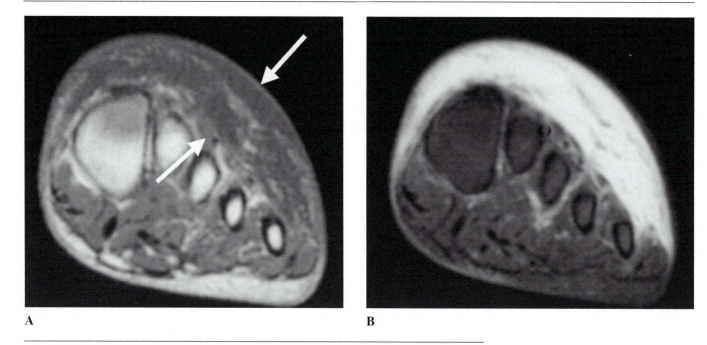

A   **B**

FIGURE 1-13.   Cellulitis. *(A)* Coronal T_1-weighted image of the foot at the level of the metatarsals shows marked swelling and subcutaneous edema of the dorsum of the foot (arrows). *(B)* Corresponding fat-suppressed fast spin-echo T_2-weighted shows the high signal intensity edema. Note that the signal from the underlying bones is normal in both sequences, thus excluding osteomyelitis.

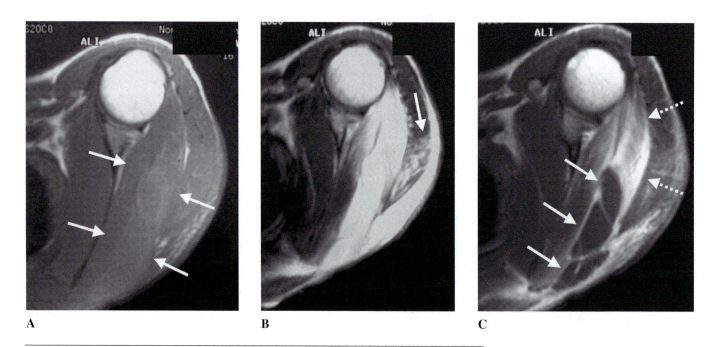

A   **B**   **C**

FIGURE 1-14.   Soft tissue abscess. *(A)* Axial T_1-weighted image of the shoulder shows swelling of the infraspinatus muscle (arrows) with a faint internal high signal intensity outline of the abscess rim. Subcutaneous edema is also present. *(B)* Corresponding T_2-weighted image shows generalized high signal intensity within the muscle and surrounding soft tissue. A distinction between abscess and inflammation cannot be made. Also note the high signal inflammatory edema in the posterior head of the deltoid (arrow). *(C)* Corresponding T_1-weighted image after intravenous administration of gadolinium contrast delineates the septated abscess (arrows) from the adjacent enhancing inflammation (dashed arrows).

TABLE 1-3

Differentiation of Acute Bacterial and Tuberculous Infection

	BACTERIAL	TUBERCULOUS
Bone	Metaphyseal osteolytic lesion with periosteal reaction	1. Metaphyseal osteolytic lesion that can cross the growth plate into the epiphysis 2. Little periosteal reaction in long bones; "spina ventosa" in short tubular bones
Spine	1. Endplate erosions and loss of disc space early in the disease 2. Fusion of the vertebrae without deformity late in the disease 3. Single-level involvement	1. Vertebral body destruction with relative preservation of disc space until late in the disease 2. Subligamentous spread with multilevel involvement 3. Large paravertebral "cold" abscesses 4. Gibbus deformity

Joint	Bone erosions and early loss of joint space	Phemister triad
		  1. Osteopenia
		  2. Bone erosions
		  3. Preservation of the joint space until late in the disease

Abscess	Thick irregular wall with surrounding inflammatory edema	1. Thin smooth wall without surrounding inflammation ("cold") 2. May calcify

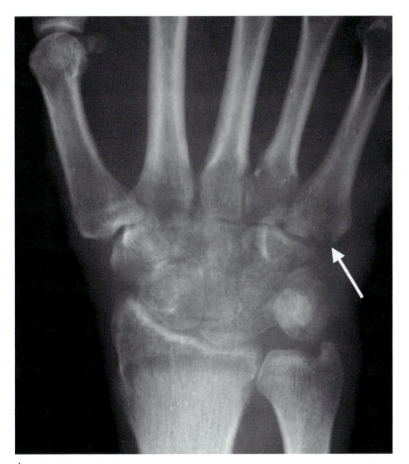 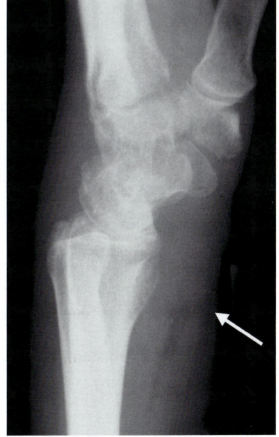

A   **B**

FIGURE 1-15.   Pyogenic septic wrist. *(A)* Anteroposterior radiograph of the wrist shows marked osteopenia of the carpal bones, distal radius and ulnar, and proximal aspects of the metacarpals. Note the radiocarpal and pancarpal narrowing and an erosion in the base of the fifth metacarpal (arrow). *(B)* Lateral radiograph of the same patient shows marked dorsal and volar soft tissue swelling (arrow).

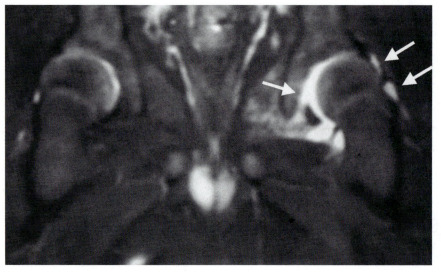

A

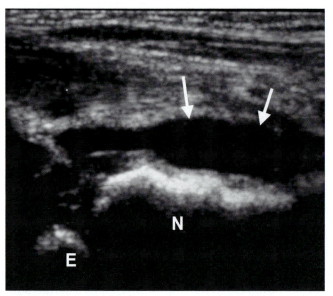

B

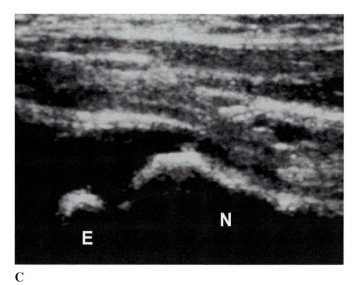

C

FIGURE 1-16. Transient synovitis of the hip in a 2-year-old patient. *(A)* Coronal fat-suppressed fast spin-echo T_2-weighted magnetic resonance image shows high signal intensity joint effusion (arrows) within the left hip. The underlying bony structures are normal. *(B)* Corresponding longitudinal sonogram shows the hypoechoic joint effusion (arrows). Note the early echogenic center of the otherwise cartilaginous hypoechoic capital femoral epiphysis (E) and the echogenic cortex of the femoral neck (N). *(C)* Longitudinal sonogram of the patient's contralateral normal hip shows the hypoechoic cartilage of the capital femoral epiphysis with early ossification (E) but absence of a joint effusion.

MRI is useful for evaluating the joint and the underlying bony structures. Without the use of intravenous contrast, it sometimes can be difficult to distinguish a thickened, infected synovium from joint fluid, because both will have high signal intensity on T_2-weighted sequences. On T_1-weighted images, fluid and synovium have low signal intensity, but sometimes there is subtle difference in the intensity, thereby allowing distinction. The distinction of joint fluid from thickened synovium is optimum with intravenous gadolinium contrast administration, which demonstrates marked enhancement of the inflamed synovium on a T_1-weighted sequence, leaving any joint fluid as low signal intensity (Figure 1-17). Although there is overlap, pyogenic synovitis tends to be thick and irregular, whereas tuberculous synovitis tends to be thin and smooth.

Potential complications of septic arthritis are growth disturbance in children if the physis is involved, osteonecrosis, degenerative arthritis secondary to incongruity of the joint as a result of articular surface destruction or misshaping of the bone, and autofusion of the joint.

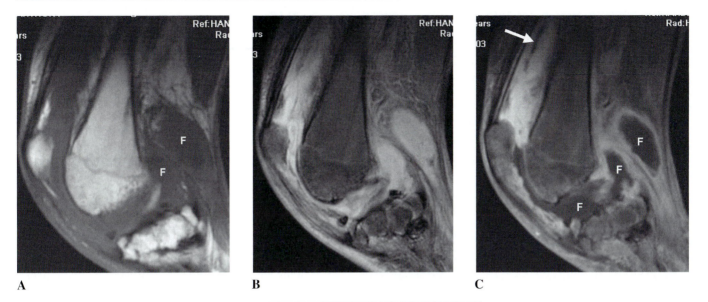

A   B   C

FIGURE 1-17.   Septic knee. *(A)* Sagittal T_1-weighted magnetic resonance image shows marked low signal intensity thickening of the synovium and/or effusion in the knee joint in this patient who had a prior fracture of the proximal tibia. It is difficult to determine how much of this process is fluid or thickened synovium, but notice that, in the posterior aspect of the knee, the center (F) of the process has a lower signal intensity than the rim, suggesting fluid. The posterior collection is an involved Baker cyst. *(B)* Corresponding fat-suppressed fast spin-echo T_2-weighed image shows high signal intensity of fluid and thickened synovium in the joint and in the Baker cyst. *(C)* Fat-suppressed T_1-weighted sequence after intravenous administration of gadolinium contrast shows enhancing thickened synovium in the suprapatellar region with minimal low signal intensity fluid (arrow) and low signal fluid (F) in the joint space and Baker cyst surrounded by high signal intensity enhancing thickened synovium.

INFECTION OF THE SPINE

Vertebral osteomyelitis is usually caused by hematogenous spread to the vertebral body, whereas infection of the intervertebral disc (*infectious discitis*) is due to osteomyelitis of the adjacent vertebral body that secondarily invades the disc or to direct contamination of the disc itself during surgical spine procedures or interventional spine procedures such as discography. Some people prefer the term *spondylodiscitis* because it conveys the intertwined relationship between infection of the vertebrae and intervening disc. In the United States, the most common pyogenic organism to infect the spine is *Staphylococcus aureus*, but tuberculosis is occasionally encountered and may be more common in people from other parts of the world. Immunocompromised people are susceptible to fungal infections and to bacterial and tuberculous diseases.

Radiographically, the hallmarks of pyogenic infection are loss of disc space height and destruction of the vertebral endplates, both of which occur early in the course of the disease, usually within the first few weeks of infection (Figure 1-18). In contrast, tuberculosis of the spine (*Pott disease*) shows marked osteopenia and bone destruction but with relative sparing of the disc space and endplates until late in the course of the disease, typically over several months. A characteristic late sequela of the vertebral and disc destruction of tuberculous involvement of the thoracic spine is the sharply angled kyphotic "gibbus" deformity (Figure 1-19).

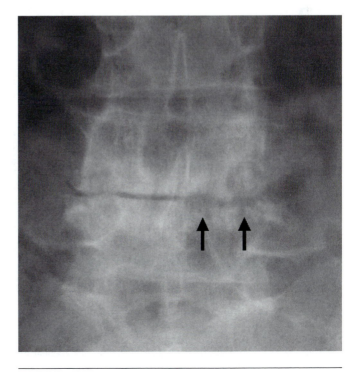

FIGURE 1-18.   Anteroposterior radiograph of pyogenic disc space infection at L4/5 shows disc narrowing and erosion of the endplates (arrows).

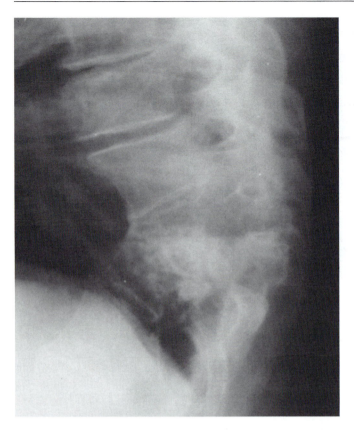

FIGURE 1-19. Lateral radiograph of the thoracal lumbar region shows the kyphotic "gibbus" deformity of old tuberculosis of the thoracic spine.

MRI is more sensitive than radiography and CT for the early detection of vertebral infection by displaying a marrow edema pattern in the adjacent vertebra and endplates. Typically, there is also high signal intensity within the disc on T_2-weighted

imaging and loss of the intranuclear cleft (Figure 1-20). In addition, pyogenic and tuberculous spondylitis can have associated paravertebral and epidural abscesses, but, as previously mentioned, tuberculous abscesses look "cold." The tuberculous infection also can spread into the adjacent psoas muscles, causing large cold abscesses that may track up and down the affected muscle (Figure 1-21). These abscesses may calcify, unlike pyogenic abscesses, and the calcification is best appreciated on radiographs or CT. Tuberculous spondylitis also may demonstrate a subligamentous component involving the anterior longitudinal ligament or the posterior longitudinal ligament, through which the infection can spread to adjacent vertebral levels; the presence of multiple levels of vertebral involvement suggests tuberculosis rather than pyogenic infection, but fungal infection and sarcoidosis of the spine also can have this multilevel appearance. Gadolinium contrast should be administered as part of the MR examination to help distinguish abscess from non-drainable phlegmon. Fungal infections have a predilection for the posterior elements of the spine and may show preservation of normal disc signal intensity and the intranuclear cleft on T_2-weighted imaging even with disc involvement.

A pitfall in the interpretation of disc space infection on MRI is severe degenerative disc disease with disc narrowing, endplate irregularity, and adjacent granulation-type endplate changes. The edema-like pattern in the endplates on either side of the disc can look similar to infection, and the involved regions can show enhancement of the vertebral bodies, endplates, and even portions of the disc with intravenous gadolinium administration. However, if the patient has been complaining of pain for several weeks to months and the MR examination shows no evidence of endplate destruction or paravertebral or epidural abscess, the process is more likely noninfected degeneration rather than a pyogenic process. Moreover, the noninfected patient is afebrile and will not have an elevated white blood cell count,

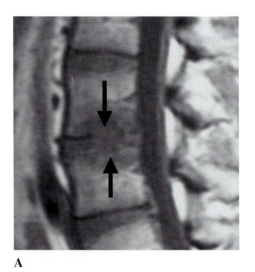

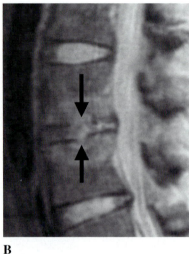

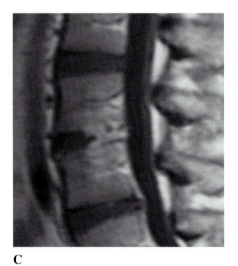

A   B   C

FIGURE 1-20. Pyogenic disc space infection. (*A*) Sagittal T_1-weighted image shows erosion and focal destruction of the cortical black line of the inferior endplate of L3 and superior endplate of L4 (arrows), with surrounding low signal intensity edema. (*B*) Corresponding fat-suppressed T_2-weighted sequence shows the high signal intensity edema in the vertebrae and disc and endplate destruction (arrows). (*C*) Corresponding T_1-weighted sequence after intravenous gadolinium contrast shows enhancement in and around the disc.

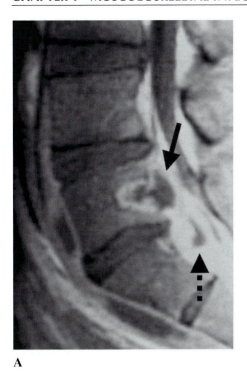

A

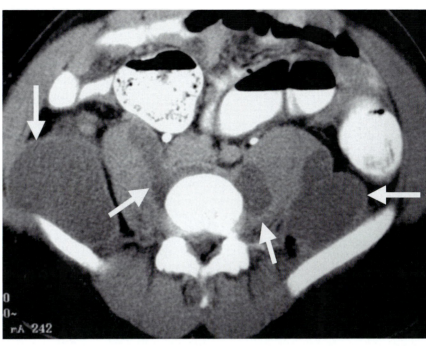

B

FIGURE 1-21. Tuberculous osteomyelitis of the spine. *(A)* Sagittal fat-suppressed T_1-weighted image after intravenous administration of gadolinium contrast shows a low-signal intensity abscess with thick surrounding enhancement in the posterior aspect of the L5 vertebral body (arrow) and in the epidural space (dashed arrow). *(B)* Computed tomographic image of the pelvis of the same patient shows the low density abscesses involving the psoas muscles and iliacus muscles (arrows).

erythrocyte sedimentation rate, or C-reactive protein level. CT can be useful for evaluating endplate irregularities in equivocal cases of infection versus degeneration to determine whether the irregularities are non corticated infectious erosions or corticated degenerative Schmorl nodes. CT also can be helpful for evaluating the degree of frank bone destruction and for guiding percutaneous biopsy. Early investigations with PET scanning suggest that it is more accurate than MRI for distinguishing true infectious spondylodiscitis from severe granulation-type degenerative disc disease (Figure 1-22), but it may not be practical because of its cost. Instead, Ga 67, especially when using single photon emission CT (SPECT) may be a reasonable alternative because it as sensitive and slightly more specific than MRI for viewing spinal infection and surrounding soft tissue involvement (see Fig. 1-22).

A mimicker of disc space infection on radiographs is dialysis spondylo-arthropathy. People on long

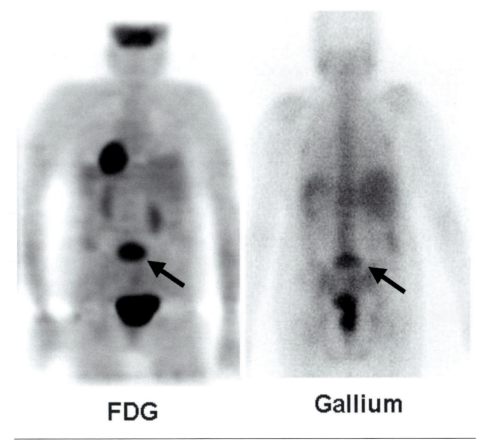

FDG Gallium

FIGURE 1-22. Planar images of the body using positron emission tomography with ^{18}F-fluoro-deoxy-glucose and gallium show increased uptake (arrows) in the L5/S1 region in a patient with infectious spondylitis. *(Courtesy of Dr. Christopher Palestro.)*

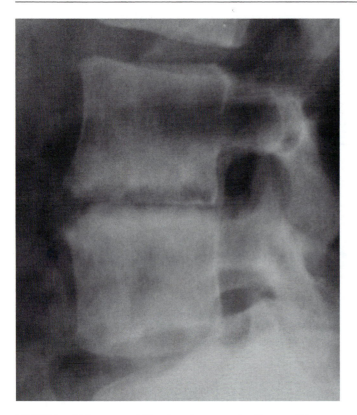

FIGURE 1-23.   Lateral radiograph of a patient with dialysis spondyloarthropathy shows narrowing of the L4/5 disc and disruption of the endplates due to amyloid deposition mimicking acute infection.

term hemodialysis may have accumulation of amyloid in the disc space, with resultant narrowing or loss of the disc space and endplate erosion or destruction (Figure 1-23). The history of hemodialysis and lack of pain with normal C-reactive protein should help to distinguish the two. However, dialysis patients do have a higher than normal risk for developing osteomyelitis.

INFECTION WITH UNDERLYING CONDITIONS

Radiologists are often asked to evaluate the possibility of infection in an area that is complicated by previous surgery or an underlying disease. Common scenarios are the evaluation of an infected prosthesis, suspected infection in the diabetic foot, and suspected infection in a patient with sickle crisis.

Infected Prostheses

Similar to the evaluation of suspected osteomyelitis in uncomplicated areas, the first step in the imaging evaluation of a suspected infected prosthesis is plain radiographs. Because the hip is the most commonly replaced joint, it will be our paradigm. Radiographic findings suggestive of infection include a wide irregular radiolucency around the interface between the cement and the bone (in the case of cemented components) or between the metal and the bone (in the case of non-cemented components) and frank bone destruction (Figure 1-24). However, a distinction

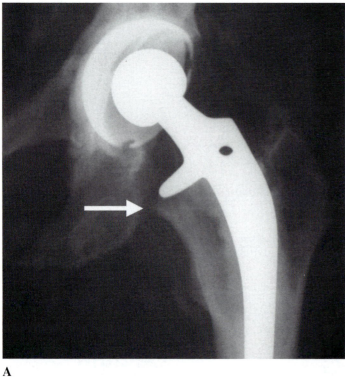

A

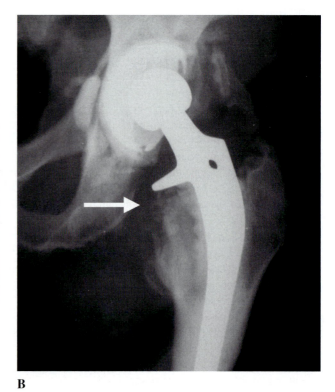

B

FIGURE 1-24.   Infected total hip replacement. *(A)* Initial anteroposterior radiograph shows preservation of bone around the femoral flange (arrow). *(B)* Anteroposterior radiograph 6 months later shows bony destruction around the flange (arrow).

between infectious loosening of a prosthesis and mechanical loosening or loosening due to a non-infectious histiocytic response ("cement disease" or "small particle disease") often cannot be made on a single radiograph. Usually, previous radiographs are necessary for comparison, with mechanical loosening and histiocytic response usually taking a slowly progressive course, whereas an acute infection has a more rapid time course and may look more aggressive. However, even this feature is not reliable because infections can be subclinical and smoldering, leading to slowly progressive loosening in an afebrile patient. The distinction between an infected loose prosthesis and a noninfected loose prosthesis is important because revision arthroplasty in the former case will have to be performed as a 2-stage procedure, with removal of the infected prosthesis, placement of antibiotic-impregnated cement for 6 to 8 weeks, intravenous antibiotic treatment, and placement of the new components, as opposed to a 1-stage revision in the case of a noninfected prosthesis.

The gold standard for the evaluation of the suspected infected joint is aspiration, with gram stain and culture and sensitivity of joint fluid. Although it is considered the definitive diagnostic test, its reported sensitivity is quite variable, ranging from 28 to 92%. Its specificity (the ability to detect true negatives) is more consistent, ranging from 92 to 100%. Some of the reported variability may be due to the patient cohorts, and better results may be obtained if aspiration is reserved for those cases with intermediate or high clinical suspicion of infection.

Various scintigraphic methods are also available for evaluation. Three-phase bone scan can be used but has poor specificity because a cemented femoral component can show increased uptake around the prosthesis for several years after placement, and because a normal non-cemented prosthesis can also show increased radiotracer uptake due to the bony ingrowth that occurs around the prosthesis. Moreover, new areas of radiotracer uptake as compared with areas on prior scans can be caused by infectious and non-infectious loosening. However, because a normal bone scan is reliable for excluding loosening, it might still be used as an initial screening test. Adding a gallium scan to the standard technetium bone scan can improve the diagnostic accuracy for infection: infection is excluded if the gallium scan is normal or has less intense uptake than the corresponding bone scan, and infection is diagnosed when there is uptake of gallium without corresponding technetium uptake or the gallium uptake is more intense than the corresponding technetium uptake.

The combination of labeled white cells and technetium-labeled sulfur colloid has excellent reported results, with sensitivity and specificity as high as 100% and 97%, respectively. The imaging feature of infection is radiotracer spatial mismatch in which there is uptake of the labeled white cells with no uptake of the sulfur colloid (Figure 1-25). PET scanning shows early pro-

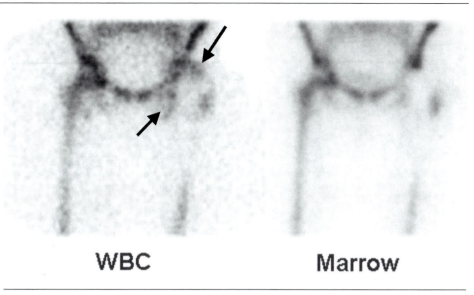

FIGURE 1-25. Planar images of an infected left total hip replacement show areas of abnormal leukocyte activity on the white blood cell study (arrows), without corresponding activity on the sulfur colloid marrow study. *(Courtesy of Dr. Christopher Palestro.)*

mising results, with 90% sensitivity and 89% specificity, but normal persistent post-surgical uptake around the prosthetic head and neck is a potential pitfall in interpretation (Figure 1-26).

Sonography can be used to evaluate the presence of joint effusion associated with an infected prosthesis. It has been suggested that a joint effusion that distends the joint capsule more

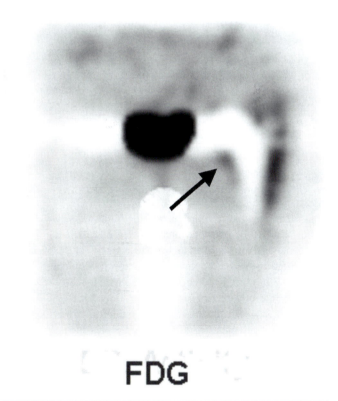

FIGURE 1-26. Positron emission tomographic ¹⁸F-fluoro-deoxy-glucose coronal image of an infected left total hip replacement shows increased activity around the neck area. Although this can be post-surgical in nature, the small focus of increased uptake along the medial aspect of the neck (arrow) is more specific for infection in this patient with an infected total prosthesis. *(Courtesy of Dr. Christopher Palestro.)*

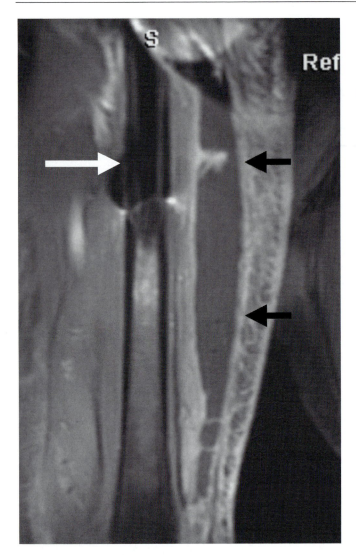

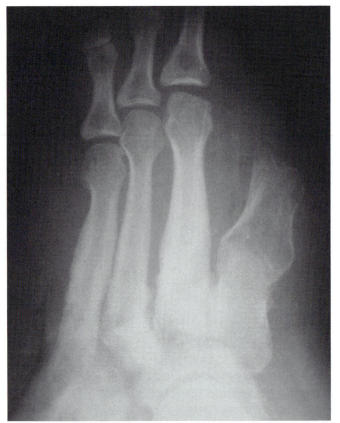

A

FIGURE 1-27. Coronal fat-suppressed T_1-weighted image after intravenous administration of gadolinium contrast in a patient with a total hip replacement shows a long abscess in the vastus lateralis muscle (black arrows). Notice that the dephasing artifact of the femoral stem (white arrow) does not obscure the abscess and that there is no evidence of involvement of the underlying bone.

than 3.2 mm away from the neck of the femur correlates highly with the presence of acute infection. CT and MRI are limited by beam hardening artifact and dephasing artifact, respectively, from the prosthetic components, but newer technical developments such as multidetector CT and MRI metal artifact reduction techniques allow for assessment of the joint space and thus the evaluation of an effusion and of the surrounding soft tissues (Figure 1-27; see Chapter 17). CT also can assess the surrounding bone stock for erosion or lysis.

FIGURE 1-28. Progression of infection in a diabetic foot. *(A)* Anteroposterior radiograph shows sclerosis of the second, third, and fourth metatarsals and neuropathic destruction of the tarso-metatarsal joint. The patient has already undergone amputation of the first toe and the fifth ray. *(B)* Corresponding radiograph 4 months later shows lytic destruction of the third and fourth metatarsals and base of the third toe in this foot infected with pseudomonas. The rest of the third toe had been amputated.

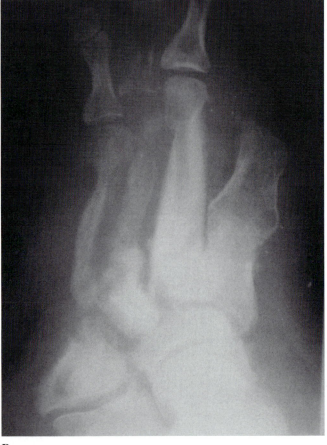

B

The Diabetic Foot

Diabetes unfortunately is common and has many potential medical complications, one of the most common of which is pedal infection. Clinical assessment of the swollen, red, and hot foot for the presence of osteomyelitis is poor, even in the presence of frank ulcer, and the radiologist is therefore often asked to participate in the evaluation.

Radiographs should always be performed first because they may provide the diagnosis by showing trabecular or cortical lysis, and because they give an overview of the anatomy and any underlying complicating structural changes, such as occur in diabetic arthropathy (*Charcot foot*). Previous radiographs are helpful to determine whether any of the abnormalities seen on the current radiographs are acute, suggesting infection (Figure 1-28). In many cases, however, more advanced imaging is needed, and scintigraphic methods or MRI can be performed. A recent meta-analysis of the literature with determination of weighted averages for each modality showed that radiographs have a weighted average with 54% sensitivity and 80% specificity, 3-phase bone scan has 91% sensitivity and 46% specificity,

labeled white cell studies have 88% sensitivity and 82% specificity, and MRI has 92% sensitivity and 84% specificity. Despite the similar sensitivity and specificity between labeled white cell scintigraphy and MRI, MRI has the advantage of providing the anatomic detail and resolution of bones and soft tissues that the surgeon needs to perform debridement or limited resections.

Although the primary sign of marrow edema is the criterion for osteomyelitis, it is usually more difficult to evaluate suspected osteomyelitis in the diabetic foot than in the nondiabetic foot because the diabetic foot is often complicated by underlying neuropathic changes. When evaluating the neuropathic foot, it is helpful to keep in mind that (*a*) normal marrow signal intensity on all pulse sequences excludes osteomyelitis, (*b*) sclerotic marrow usually excludes an acute or active chronic osteomyelitis, and (*c*) marrow edema must be considered to be osteomyelitis until proven otherwise. Thus, MRI is excellent for excluding osteomyelitis if the bone marrow is normal, but it is not as good for diagnosing osteomyelitis because bone marrow edema may be due to infection, may be a result of neuropathic arthropathy as the bones are traumatized, or may represent reactive marrow edema due to adjacent soft tissue inflammation.

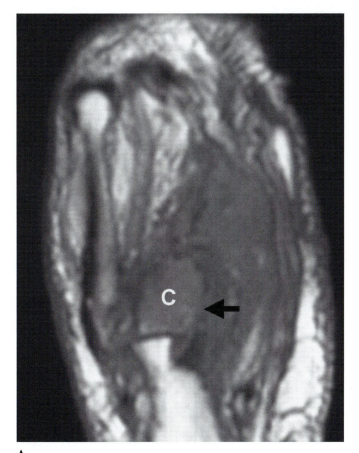
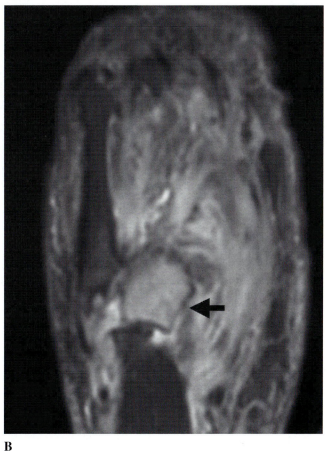

A   **B**

FIGURE 1-29. The "ghost-sign" of osteomyelitis. *(A)* Axial T_1-weighted magnetic resonance image shows low signal intensity within the cuboid (C), with poor definition of the cortex (arrow). Note the marked surrounding soft tissue edema disrupting the fat planes. *(B)* Corresponding fat-suppressed T_1-weighted image after intravenous administration of gadolinium contrast shows uniform enhancement of the cuboid and better outline of the cortical edge (arrow), indicating osteomyelitis.

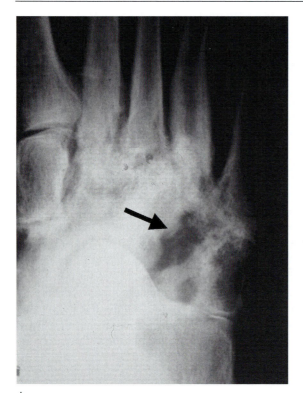

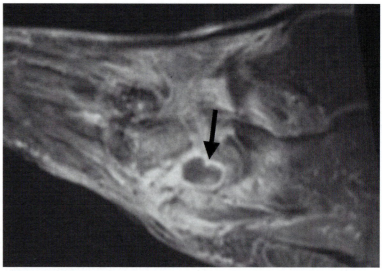

B

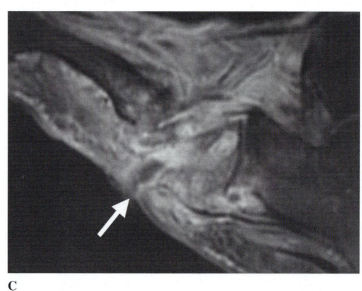

A

FIGURE 1-30. Sinus tract ulcer and abscess in a diabetic patient. *(A)* Anteroposterior radiograph shows destruction of the midfoot and lucency in the cuboid (arrow). *(B)* Sagittal fat-suppressed T_1-weighted image after intravenous administration of gadolinium contrast shows the enhancing abscess (arrow) and *(C)* sinus tract extending from the abscess to the skin surface with a small ulcer (arrow).

C

Secondary signs of osteomyelitis have been described to increase the accuracy of MRI. For example, cortical destruction is a feature of osteomyelitis and not of reactive marrow edema. The "ghost sign" refers to poor definition of the margins of a bone on T_1-weighted images, which become crisp and look normal after contrast administration (Figure 1-29). When the ghost sign is present, osteomyelitis rather than neuropathic arthropathy should be suspected. Other secondary signs include cutaneous ulcer, abscess formation, cellulitis, and sinus tract formation (Figure 1-30), but these processes are, in fact, co-morbid conditions of diabetes that can exist with or without osteomyelitis and that can be causes of reactive marrow edema. Nonetheless, approximately 90% of pedal osteomyelitis cases are due to spread from an adjacent cutaneous ulcer, and ulcers tend to occur at points of pressure on the foot, such as under the first and fifth metatarsal heads, at the tips of the toes and around deformed interphalangeal joints, under the calcaneus, and over the malleoli. The most common locations of osteomyelitis parallel these regions of ulcer location, namely the metatarsal heads,

the phalanges, and the calcaneus. Similarly, more than 90% of abscesses are associated with ulcers, and abscesses also are associated with adjacent osteomyelitis. Abscesses are best evaluated with the use of intravenous gadolinium contrast. Soft tissue infection in the foot does not respect anatomic boundaries and thus can spread from one compartment to another.

Sickle Crisis

The most common organism in sickle osteomyelitis is *Salmonella*, and the dilemma of trying to distinguish infarct from infection as a cause of pain and fever is a common challenge in hospitals that have a large population of patients with sickle cell disease. Unfortunately, both infarction and infection are features of the underlying disease, and radiographs may not be helpful because periosteal reaction and patchy trabecular lysis may be present in both processes. Advanced imaging with scintigraphy, MRI, and sonography can be used to aid in the distinction. Compared with uptake on bone scan, greater uptake of gallium suggests infection, whereas no uptake or less intense uptake of gallium compared with bone scan suggests infarct. A combination of bone scan and sulfur colloid marrow scan suggests infarct if the bone scan shows increased uptake and the marrow study shows decreased uptake, whereas increased uptake on bone scan and normal uptake of sulfur colloid suggests infection. On nonenhanced MRI, infarct and infection have marrow edema, periosteal reaction, and surrounding soft tissue edema; contrast-enhanced MRI suggests infarct if enhancement is thin and linear, whereas patchy and irregular enhancement suggests infection, but such a distinction is often not possible. Sonographically, subperiosteal fluid is present in both conditions, but a thicker collection increases the likelihood of infection. An advantage of sonography is that it can guide a percutaneous diagnostic aspiration of the subperiosteal collection.

SUGGESTED READINGS

Booz MM, Hariharan V, Aradi AJ, Malki AA. The value of ultrasound and aspiration in differentiating vaso-occlusive crisis and osteomyelitis in sickle cell disease patients. *Clin Radiol.* 1999;54:636–639.

Chacko TK, Zhang H, Stevenson K, Moussavian B, Alavi A. The importance of the location of fluorodeoxyglucose uptake in periprosthetic infection in painful hip prostheses. *Nucl Med Commun.* 2002;23:851–855.

Chami M, Daoud A, Maestro M, Lagrange AS, Geoffray A. Ultrasound contribution in the analysis of the newborn and infant normal and clubfoot: a preliminary study. *Pediatr Radiol.* 1996;26:298–302.

Chao HC, Lin SJ, Huang YC, Lin TY. Color Doppler ultrasonographic evaluation of osteomyelitis in children. *J Ultrasound Med.* 1999;18:729–736.

Cheung A, Lachiewicz PF, Renner JB. The role of aspiration and contrast-enhanced arthrography in evaluating the uncemented hip arthroplasty. *AJR.* 1997;168:1305–1309.

Craig JG, Amin MB, Wu K, et al. Osteomyelitis of the diabetic foot: MR imaging–pathologic correlation. *Radiology.* 1997;203:849–855.

Demharter J, Bohndorf K, Michl W, Vogt H. Chronic recurrent osteomyelitis: a radiological and clinical investigation of five cases. *Skeletal Radiol.* 1997;26:579–588.

de Winter F, Van de Wiele C, Vogelaers D, De Smet K, Verdonk R, Dierckx RA. Fluorine-18 fluorodeoxyglucose-positron emission tomography: a highly accurate imaging modality for the diagnosis of chronic musculoskeletal infections. *J Bone Joint Surg Am.* 2001;83:651–660.

Fehring TK, Cohen B. Aspiration as a guide to sepsis in revision total hip arthroplasty. *J Arthroplasty.* 1996;11:543–547.

Fernandez M, Carrol CL, Baker CJ. Discitis and vertebral osteomyelitis in children: an 18-year review [abstract]. *Radiology.* 2002;222:861.

Guhlmann A, Brecht-Krauss D, Gebhard S, et al. Fluorine-18-FDG PET and technetium-99m antigranulocyte antibody scintigraphy in chronic osteomyelitis. *J Nucl Med.* 1998;39:2145–2152.

Guhlmann A, Brecht-Krauss D, Suger G, et al. Chronic osteomyelitis: detection with FDG and PET and correlation with histopathologic findings. *Radiology.* 1998;206:749–754.

Hong SH, Kim SM, Ahn JM, Chung HW, Shin MJ, Kang HS. Tuberculous vs. pyogenic arthritis: MR imaging evaluation. *Radiology.* 2001;218:848–853.

Jurik AG, Egund N. MRI in chronic recurrent multifocal osteomyelitis. *Skeletal Radiol.* 1997;26:230–238.

Kaim A, Ledermann HP, Bongartz G, Messmer P, Muller-Brand J, Steinbrich W. Chronic post-traumatic osteomyelitis of the lower extremity: Comparison of magnetic resonance imaging and combined bone scintigraphy/immunoscintigraphy with radiolabelled monoclonal antigranulocyte antibodies. *Skeletal Radiol.* 2000;29:378–386.

Kraemer WJ, Saplys R, Waddell JP, Morton J. Bone scan, gallium scan, and hip aspiration in the diagnosis of infected total hip arthroplasty. *J Arthroplasty.* 1993;8:611–616.

Lachiewicz, PF, Rogers GD, Thomason, HC. Aspiration of the hip joint before revision total hip arthroplasty. Clinical and laboratory factors influencing attainment of a positive culture. *J Bone Joint Surg Am.* 1996;78:749–754.

Lederman HP, Kaim A, Bongartz G, Steinbrich W. Pitfalls and limitation of magnetic resonance imaging in chronic posttraumatic osteomyelitis. *Eur Radiol.* 2000;10:1815–1823.

Lederman HP, Morrison WB, Schweitzer ME. MR image of analysis of pedal osteomyelitis: Distribution, patterns of spread, and frequency of associated ulceration and septic arthritis. *Radiology.* 2002;223:747–755.

Lederman HP, Morrison WB, Schweitzer ME. Pedal abscesses in patients suspected of having pedal osteomyelitis: analysis with MR imaging. *Radiology.* 2002;224:649–655.

Levistky KB, Hozack WJ, Balderston RA, et al. Evaluation of the painful prosthetic joint. Relative value of bone scan, sedimentation rate, and joint aspiration. *J Arthroplasty.* 1991;6:237–244.

Love C, Patel M, Lonner BS, Tomas MB, Palestro CJ. Diagnosing spinal osteomyelitis: a comparison of bone and Ga-67 scintigraphy and magnetic resonance imaging. *Clin Nucl Med.* 2000;25:963–977.

Love C, Tomas MB, Marwin SE, Pugliese PV, Palestro CJ. Role of nuclear medicine in diagnosis of the infected joint replacement. *Radiographics.* 2001;21:1229–1238.

Miller TT, Randolph DA Jr, Staron RB, Feldman F, Cushin S. Fat-suppressed MRI of musculoskeletal infection: fast T_2 weighted techniques vs. gadolinium-enhanced T_1-weighted images. *Skeletal Radiol.* 1997;26:654–658.

Morrison WB, Ledermann HP, Schweitzer ME. MR Imaging of the diabetic foot. *MRI Clin North Am.* 2001;9:606–613.

Morrison WB, Schweitzer ME, Batte WG, Radack DP, Russel KM. Osteomyelitis of the foot: relative importance of primary and secondary MR imaging signs. *Radiology.* 1998;207:625–632.

Palestro CJ. Radionuclide imaging after skeletal interventional procedures. *Semin Nucl Med.* 1995;25:3–14.

Palestro CJ, Kim CK, Swyer AJ, Capozzi JD, Solomon RW, Goldsmith SJ. Total-hip arthroplasty: periprosthetic indium-111–labeled leukocyte activity and complementary technetium-99m–sulfur colloid imaging in suspected infection. *J Nucl Med.* 1990;31:1950–1955.

Palestro CJ, Kipper SL, Weiland FL, Love C, Tomas MB. Osteomyelitis: diagnosis with (99m) Tc-labeled antigranulocyte antibodies compared with diagnosis with (111) In-labeled leukocytes—initial experience. *Radiology.* 2002;223:758–764.

Palestro CJ, Torres MA. Radionuclide imaging in orthopedic infections. *Semin Nucl Med.* 1997;27:334–345.

Quinn SF, Murray W, Clark RA, Cochran C. MR imaging of chronic osteomyelitis. *J Comput Assist Tomogr.* 1998;12:113–117.

Riebel TW, Nasir R, Nazarenko O. The value of sonography in the detection of osteomyelitis. *Pediatr Radiol.* 1996;26:291–297.

Rosas MH, Leclercq S, Pegoix M, et al. Contribution of laboratory tests, scintigraphy, and histology to the diagnosis of lower limb joint replacement infection. *Rev Rhum Engl Ed.* 1998;65:477–482.

Skaggs DL, Kim SK, Greene NW, Harris D, Miller JH. Differentiation between bone infarction and acute osteomyelitis in children with sickle-cell disease with use of sequential radionuclide bone-marrow and bone scans. *J Bone Joint Surg Am.* 2001;83A:1810–1813.

Soler R, Rodriguez E, Remuinan C, Santos M. MRI of musculoskeletal extraspinal tuberculosis. *J Comput Assist Tomogr.* 2001;25:177–183.

Spangehl MJ, Masri BA, O'Connell, JX, Duncan, CP. Prospective analysis of preoperative and intraoperative investigations for the diagnosis of infection at the site of two hundred and two revision total hip arthroplasties. *J Bone Joint Surg Am.* 1999;81:672–683.

Stumpe KD, Zanetti M, Weishaupt D, Hodler, J, Boos N, Von Schulthess GK. FDG positron emission tomography for differentiation of degenerative and infectious endplate abnormalities in the lumbar spine detected in MR imaging. *AJR.* 2002;179:1151–1157.

Umans H, Haramati N, Flusser G. The diagnostic role of gadolinium enhanced MRI in distinguishing between acute medullary bone infarct and osteomyelitis. *Magn Reson Imaging.* 2000;18:255–262.

Van Holsbeeck MT, Eyler WR, Sherman LS, et al. Detection of infection in loosened hip prostheses: efficacy of sonography. *AJR.* 1994;163:381–384.

William RR, Hussein SS, Jeans WD, Wali YA, Lamki ZA. A prospective study of soft-tissue ultrasonography in sickle cell disease patients with suspected osteomyelitis. *Clin Radiol.* 2000;55:307–310.

Williams RL, Fukui MB, Meltzer CC, Swarnkar A, Johnson DW, Welch W. Fungal spinal osteomyelitis in the immunocompromised patient: MR findings in three cases. *AJNR.* 1999;20:381–385.

Wrobel JS, Connolly JE. Making the diagnosis of osteomyelitis. The role of prevalence. *J Am Podiatr Med Assoc.* 1998;88:337–343.

Yao DC, Sartoris DJ. Musculoskeletal tuberculosis. *Radiol Clin North Am.* 1995;33:679–689.

Zawin JK, Hoffer FA, Rand FF, Littlewood Teele R. Joint effusion in children with an irritable hip: US diagnosis and aspiration. *Radiology.* 1993;187:459–463.

Zhuang H, Chacko TK, Hickson M, et al. Persistent non-specific FDG uptake on PET imaging following hip arthroplasty. *Eur J Nucl Med Mol Imaging.* 2002;29:1328–1333.

Zhuang H, Duarte PS, Pourdehand M, Shnier D, Alavi A. Exclusion of chronic osteomyelitis with F-18 fluorodeoxyglucose positron emission tomographic imaging. *Clin Nucl Med.* 2000;25:281–284.

Zhuang H, Duarte PS, Pourdehand M, et al. The promising role of 18F-FDG PET in detecting infected lower limb prosthesis implants. *J Nucl Med.* 2001;42:44–48.

CHAPTER 2

OSTEONECROSIS

ROBERT SCHNEIDER

Osteonecrosis (ON) is an important cause of bone and joint pain. *Osteonecrosis* means "bone death," and different terms have been used to indicate ON depending on the etiology and location. Because loss of the blood supply to the bone is considered to be the cause of ON, the terms *avascular necrosis* and *ischemic necrosis* are often used, especially when it involves subchondral bone. *Bone infarction* is another synonym for ON and is used when the condition involves the shaft of the bone.

Avascular necrosis itself causes only mild or no pain, but the repair process and revascularization lead to weakening of the bone, which in turn allows subchondral and osteochondral fractures to occur with collapse of the articular surface. The subchondral collapse and subsequent secondary osteoarthritis are responsible for most of the symptoms and disabilities associated with ON. Bone infarcts seldom are the cause of serious symptoms or disability. Although ON can occur in many different bones, the femoral head is the most important site because subchondral collapse and secondary osteoarthritis occur frequently here and have clinical consequences. Diagnostic imaging can diagnose ON during the repair process before segmental collapse and secondary osteoarthritis occurs, but once advanced osteoarthritis is present, it may not be possible (or important) to determine if underlying ON is present.

EPIDEMIOLOGY AND PATHOGENESIS

Etiology

Compromise of the blood supply to bone leading to ON can occur from a number of different mechanisms (Table 2-1): (*a*) direct mechanical disruption of blood vessels that can occur due to trauma; (*b*) occlusion, partial or complete, of arteries that can occur from embolization of fat or gas, from thrombosis due to abnormally shaped cells or thrombophilic conditions, and from angiospasm; (*c*) injury to the arterial wall that can occur from vasculitis or radiation; (*d*) pressure on the arterial wall that can occur from intramedullary deposits such as fat, from intramedullary hemorrhage, or from increased intracapsular pressure due to synovitis, infection, or hemorrhage; (*e*) occlusion of venous outflow that leads to increased intramedullary pressure and resultant decreased arterial inflow; and (*f*) osteoporosis and micro-fractures causing microvascular lesions.

Nontraumatic Osteonecrosis

The actual incidence of ON cannot be determined because asymptomatic ON is often not detected. About 10,000 to 20,000 new cases of ON occur each year in the United States, and ON is the reason for 5 to 18% of total hip replacements. The femoral head is the most frequent site, followed by the humeral head and femoral condyles. Numerous other bones may be involved. The convex surfaces of joints tend to be involved more than the concave. Nontraumatic ON is most frequent between ages 20 and 50 years, with an average age in the mid-30s. Most cases of nontraumatic ON are associated with some underlying cause or risk factor. Corticosteroid therapy and alcoholism are underlying factors in about two thirds of the cases of nontraumatic ON. Other underlying conditions include sickle cell hemoglobinopathy, coagulopathies, hyperlipidemia, Gaucher disease, organ transplantation, dysbarism, high altitude, pancreatitis, gout, pregnancy, and radiation. Other conditions also associated with an increased incidence of ON, such as systemic lupus erythematosus (SLE), Raynaud disease, vasculitis, organ transplantation, and inflammatory bowel disease, are usually treated with corticosteroids, and it is the steroids that are thought to increase the risk for ON. Smoking also increases the risk for ON. About 10 to 20% of cases have no known underlying etiology or risk factors and are classified as "idiopathic." Idiopathic ON tends to occur in older patients. When one hip has ON, there is a 40 to 80% chance that the opposite hip will eventually develop ON.

ON associated with corticosteroid therapy was first described in 1957. The association is greatest with high doses (>30 mg/d of prednisone) of long duration (≥6 months), although many exceptions have occurred. A single dose, even if high, has a lower risk than multiple doses. Chronic low-dose therapy, as often used in asthma, inflammatory arthritis, inflammatory bowel disease, and dermatologic conditions, has a relatively low incidence of ON, especially compared with SLE and organ transplantation. Underlying connective tissue diseases, immune diseases, and vasculitis have a synergistic relationship with corticosteroids in the production of ON. Theories about the cause of corticosteroid-associated ON include fat embolization and intramedullary fat accumulation, hypercoagulability, and vascular damage. Corticosteroid-induced osteoporosis may lead to subchondral insufficiency fractures that may simulate ON. The clinical manifestations of ON usually occur more than 6 months, with an average of 2 to 3 years, after the start of corticosteroid therapy.

TABLE 2-1

Causes of Osteonecrosis

1. Traumatic
    a. Fracture: femoral head, proximal pole of the scaphoid, humeral head, body of the talus
    b. Dislocation
2. Atraumatic
    a. Embolism/thrombosis: sickle cell disease, nitrogen gas bubble ("caisson disease"), fat emboli (pancreatitis, alcoholism), thrombophilic conditions
    b. Vasculitis: lupus, radiation therapy
    c. Compression of arterioles and venous outflow by increased marrow pressure due to fat deposition in the marrow: steroids, alcoholism, Gaucher disease
    d. Compression of feeding arteries by increased intracapsular pressure: synovitis, hemarthrosis, septic arthritis
    e. Osteomyelitis (increased marrow pressure due to inflammatory marrow edema)
    f. Idiopathic
    g. Osteoporosis and microfractures

There is an elevated risk for ON with alcohol intake that increases with increasing consumption both weekly and cumulatively. Weekly consumption of 400 mL/wk (4 drinks daily) increases the risk of ON 10 times. Toxicity to the liver from alcohol causing abnormalities in fat metabolism leading to fat emboli and fat accumulation in the marrow, increased cortisone levels in the blood, and smoking, which is common in alcoholism, may be causative factors.

In sickle hemoglobinopathy, intravascular sickling blocks blood vessels and decreases sinusoidal blood flow, leading to ON including articular surfaces and multiple areas of bone infarction in the metaphyses and diaphyses. In Gaucher disease, sphingolipid-filled macrophages accumulate in the bone marrow due to a genetic abnormality in cerebroside metabolism. This causes compression of blood vessels and increased intramedullary pressure in the bone, reducing blood flow. In dysbarism ("caisson" or decompression disease), nitrogen bubbles are thought to act as gas emboli that block blood vessels.

ON in SLE was first reported in 1960. Thirty to 40% of patients with SLE develop ON. Although most patients with

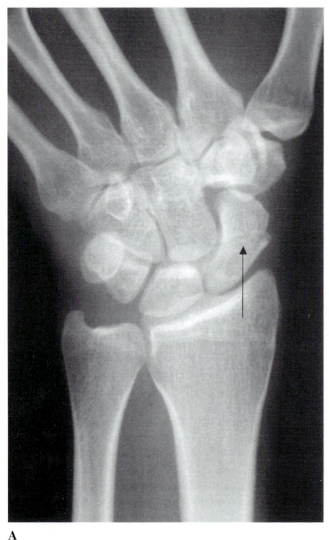

A

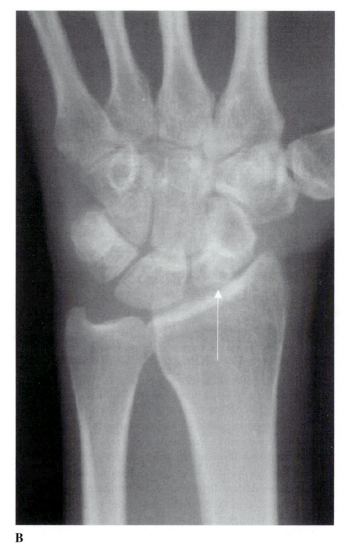

B

FIGURE 2-1.   *(A)* There is a fracture (arrow) of the waist of the scaphoid. *(B)* After the fracture is healed, there is osteonecrosis of the proximal pole of the scaphoid with sclerosis and collapse (arrow).

SLE and ON have received corticosteroids, there are some who have not. Numerous sites are often involved, with correlation with higher mean corticosteroid doses. Antiphospholipid antibodies that are found in SLE predispose to arterial and venous thrombosis and also may be a factor in ON.

The role of intravascular coagulation in the etiology of ON has been emphasized in recent years. Many of the underlying conditions associated with ON also may be associated with increased intravascular coagulation including those conditions discussed above. In addition, hereditary or acquired disorders of coagulation leading to thrombophilia and hypofibrinolysis may be associated with ON. Those causing thrombophilia include resistance to or deficiency of activated protein C, protein S deficiency, and antiphospholipid antibodies. Disorders causing hypofibrinolysis include low tissue plasminogen activator and high plasminogen activator inhibition and high lipoprotein (a). Bacterial and viral infections, autoimmune and hypersensitivity reactions, pregnancy, malignancy, and trauma may lead to venous thrombosis, which causes increased intramedullary pressure and, hence, decreased arterial blood flow and ischemic necrosis of bone.

Posttraumatic Osteonecrosis

ON may occur after fracture or dislocation due to mechanical disruption of the blood supply, particularly in certain bones in which the blood supply is vulnerable or limited (see Chapter 6). The most frequent sites of posttraumatic ON are the femoral head, humeral head, proximal pole of the scaphoid, and the body of the talus. Other sites are possible but less frequent.

Subcapital and transcervical fractures of the femoral neck cross the blood supply to the femoral head and may disrupt it. Intertrochanteric fractures occur distal to the blood supply and rarely cause ON. ON occurs in up to 85% of varus displaced fractures of the femoral neck and in up to 25% of nondisplaced or valgus impacted fractures, and therefore most varus displaced fractures undergo immediate prosthetic replacement of the femoral head. Fractures of the femoral neck in children also have a high incidence of ON, most likely due to the marked trauma necessary for a femoral neck fracture to occur in this age group. Posttraumatic ON of the femoral head also may result from hip dislocation even without fracture; the incidence of ON is extremely high, approaching 100% in patients in whom the hip remains dislocated for longer than 24 hours.

The blood supply to the femoral head is from the medial and lateral femoral circumflex arteries, which usually arise from the profunda femoris artery. There is a ring of arteries around the base of the femoral neck formed posteriorly by the medial circumflex and anteriorly by the lateral circumflex. The ascending cervical branches of the arterial ring give rise to the metaphyseal (inferior) and epiphyseal (superior) retinacular vessels, which can be classified as medial and lateral respectively. Additional blood supply comes from vessels from the ligamentum teres coming through the fovea into the epiphysis. The lateral epiphyseal (superior) retinacular vessels constitute the most important blood supply to the femoral head. In children, the growth plate is a barrier to anastomosis of the epiphyseal and metaphyseal vessels.

With shoulder fractures, posttraumatic ON occurs in about 30% of 3-part and 90% of 4-part fractures. The major blood supply to the humeral head comes from the ascending branch of the anterior humeral circumflex artery, which travels in

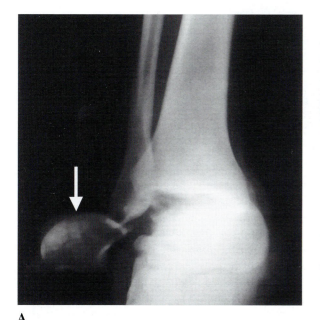

A

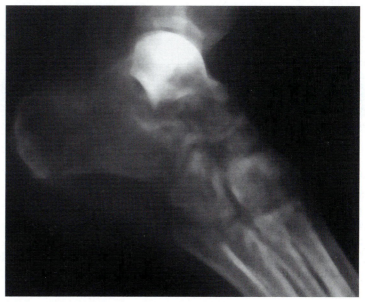

B

FIGURE 2-2.   *(A)* A fracture of the neck of the talus is present with dislocation of the talus (arrow). *(B)* Radiograph 4 months later shows sclerosis in the proximal talus, confirming the diagnosis of osteonecrosis.

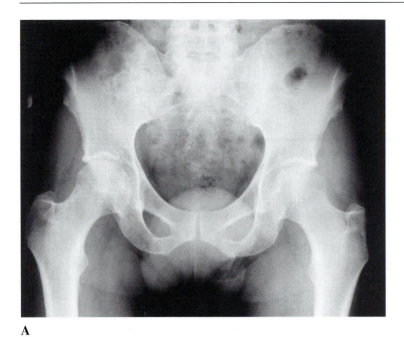

A

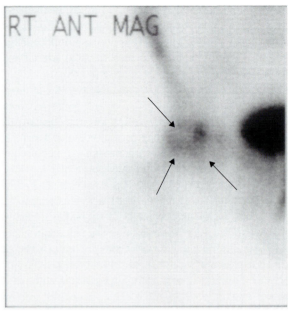

B

C

FIGURE 2-3.   Stage I osteonecrosis of the right femoral head. *(A)* Radiograph shows normal findings or slight bony mottling of the right femoral head. *(B)* Bone scan shows a rim of increased uptake (arrows) surrounding an area of decreased uptake, indicating osteonecrosis. *(C)* Magnetic resonance proton density-weighted coronal (left) and sagittal images (right) show a low signal demarcation line in the right femoral head (arrows).

the bicipital groove. Additional blood supply comes from the posterior humeral circumflex and the arcuate arteries. The collateral circulation is poor, thus making the humeral head vulnerable, especially when the fractures involve the bicipital groove, such as those of the anatomic neck or lesser tuberosity. Symptomatic posttraumatic ON of the humeral head is not seen as frequently as that of the femoral head because collapse of the non–weight-bearing humeral head is less frequent, and because severe fractures often undergo immediate prosthetic replacement of the humeral head.

Posttraumatic necrosis of the proximal pole of the scaphoid occurs in about 15% to 30% of scaphoid fractures. The blood supply to the scaphoid comes from the dorsal and volar scaphoid branches of the radial artery that enter the distal pole of the scaphoid and terminate in the proximal pole. The closer the fracture is to the proximal pole, the higher the incidence of ON. Thus, fractures of the proximal pole of the scaphoid almost always and fractures of the waist of the scaphoid sometimes disrupt the blood supply to the proximal pole, leading to ON. Evidence of ON is seen as increased density in the proximal pole, which may later collapse (Figure 2-1).

Posttraumatic ON of the body of the talus may occur after fractures of the neck of the talus, especially if there is associated dislocation of the tibiotalar or subtalar joints (Figure 2-2). About 60% of the surface of the talus is covered by articular cartilage, and there are relatively few soft tissue attachments to the bone to

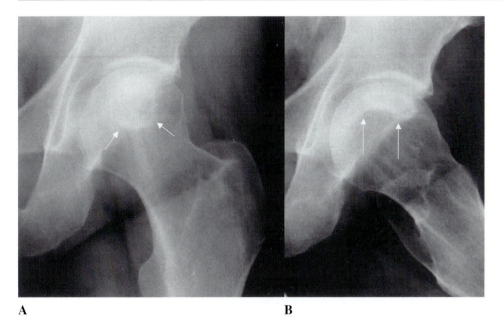

A   B

FIGURE 2-4.   Stage II osteonecrosis. *(A)* Anteroposterior and *(B)* frog lateral radiographs show sclerosis and lucency in the right femoral head without collapse (arrows).

provide extra blood supply. Disruption of the artery of the tarsal canal (the tarsal canal is the posteromedial continuation of the anterolateral sinus tarsi), a branch of the posterior tibial artery, leads to ON of the body or proximal portion of the talus. Radiographically, ON is seen as increased density in the proximal talus. The proximal articular surface may or may not collapse. Lucency within the articular surface of the talar dome (Hawkin sign) represents disuse osteoporosis and indicates that ON is not present.

Classification

There are many classification or staging systems that have been proposed for ON of the femoral head. The first and most widely used is that of Ficat and Arlet, which is based on radiographs:

Stage 0: Normal radiographs and no symptoms (magnetic resonance imaging [MRI] is positive)

Stage I: Normal radiographs or slight mottling of the femoral head and symptomatic (Figure 2-3)

Stage IIA: Mottled sclerosis and lucency within the femoral head with normal contour (Figure 2-4)

Stage IIB: "Crescent sign" (subchondral lucency) without deformity (Figure 2-5)

Stage III: Subchondral collapse and flattening of the head (Figure 2-6)

Stage IV: Secondary osteoarthritis (Figure 2-7)

The Steinberg classification was originally based on radiographs, but information obtained from MRI on the extent of involvement of the femoral head was added (Table 2-2). The Japanese Investigation Committee formulated a classification of

ON based on the location of the necrotic area in relation to the weight-bearing surface of the acetabulum on initial radiographs to determine the prognosis and risk of collapse (Table 2-3).

With the use of MRI, type 2 lesions could be allocated to other types because of visible demarcation lines. Lesions that are lateral at the weight-bearing surface have a worse prognosis. Lesions that are medial rarely progress. The Association Research Circulation Osseous developed a new classification that combines the 4 stages of Ficat and Arlet with the size and location of the lesion (Table 2-4). These classification systems correlate with histopathologic findings, clinical symptoms, and prognosis. Once the crescent sign or collapse of the femoral head

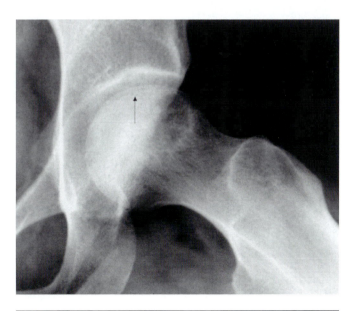

FIGURE 2-5.   Stage IIB osteonecrosis. Frog lateral radiograph shows a subchondral lucency, the "crescent sign" (arrow), in the femoral head without collapse.

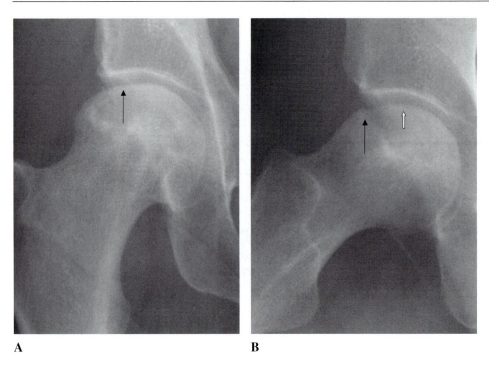

A　　　　　　　　　　　　　　　　　　　**B**

FIGURE 2-6.　Stage III osteonecrosis. *(A)* Anteroposterior radiograph shows sclerosis and lucency in the femoral head with collapse and flattening of the superior aspect of the femoral head (arrow). *(B)* Frog lateral radiograph shows a crescent sign (white arrow) with collapse at the junction of the normal bone and necrotic zone (black arrow).

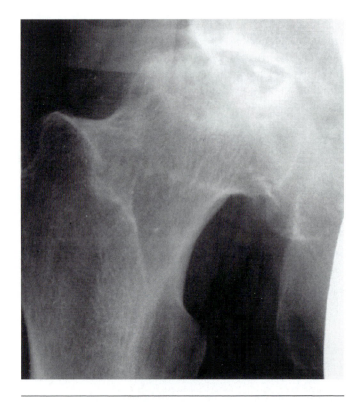

FIGURE 2-7.　Stage IV osteonecrosis. There is secondary osteoarthritis with joint space narrowing and sclerosis.

TABLE 2-2

The Steinberg (Philadelphia) Classification

Stage 0	Normal radiographs, bone scan, and/or MRI
Stage I	Normal radiographs but abnormal bone scan or MRI
A	Mild (<15% of head affected)
B	Moderate (15–30%)
C	Severe (>30%)
Stage II	Lucent and sclerotic changes in the femoral head
A	Mild (<15% of head affected)
B	Moderate (15–30%)
C	Severe (>30%)
Stage III	Subchondral fracture (crescent sign) without flattening
A	Mild (<15% of articular surface)
B	Moderate (15–30%)
C	Severe (>30%)
Stage IV	Flattening of femoral head
A	Mild (<15% of surface and <2 mm depression)
B	Moderate (15–30% or 2–4 mm depression)
C	Severe (>30% or >4 mm depression)
Stage V	Joint narrowing and or acetabular changes
A	Mild
B	Moderate
C	Severe
Stage VI	Advanced degenerative changes

ABBREVIATION: MRI = magnetic resonance imaging.

TABLE 2-3

The Japanese Investigation Committee Classification

Type 1A	Demarcation line appears in the femoral head
Type 1A	Outer end of demarcation line at medial third (non–weight-bearing aspect of the femoral head)
Type 1B	Outer end of demarcation line at middle third
Type 1C	Outer end of demarcation line at lateral third
Type 2	Early flattening but no demarcation line
Type 3	Cystic lesion without demarcation line
Type 3A	Cystic lesion located anteriorly or medially far from the weight-bearing surface
Type 3B	Cystic lesion under the weight-bearing surface

TABLE 2-4

Association Research Circulation Osseous (International) Classification

Stage 0	Normal imaging tests, positive bone biopsy
Stage I	Negative radiographs, positive MRI or bone scan; lesions subdivided into medial, central or lateral, and
A	<15% involvement of the femoral head
B	15–30%
C	>30%
Stage II	Radiographs abnormal with sclerosis, lucency, cyst formation, without collapse of the femoral head on imaging; divided into medial, central or lateral, and
A	<15% involvement of femoral head on MRI
B	15–30%
C	>30%
Stage III	Crescent sign, divided into medial, central or lateral, and
A	<15% crescent sign or <2 mm depression on radiograph
B	15–30% or 2–4 mm depression
C	>30% or >4 mm depression
Stage IV	Secondary osteoarthritis with joint space narrowing, sclerosis, osteophytes, and flattening of the femoral head

ABBREVIATION: MRI = magnetic resonance imaging.

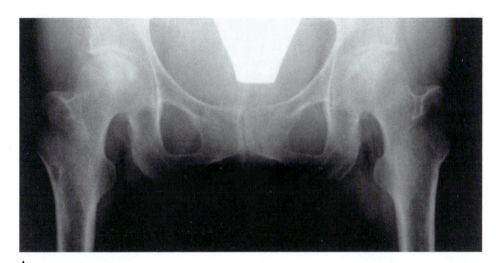

A

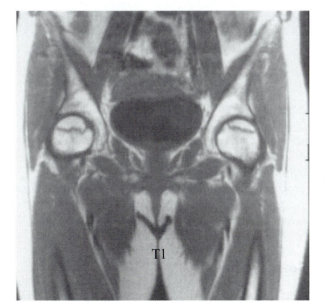

B T1

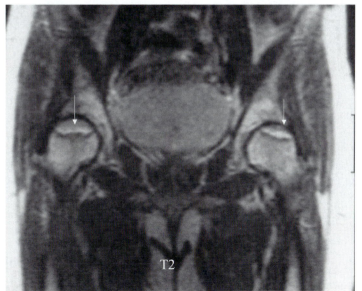

C T2

FIGURE 2-8. Osteonecrosis of the right and left femoral heads. *(A)* Anteroposterior radiograph shows normal findings or slight mottling of the femoral heads. *(B)* Magnetic resonance T_1 image shows a low signal demarcation rim surrounding a necrotic area of normal signal in both femoral heads. *(C)* T_2 image shows a rim of high signal within and parallel to the low signal demarcation rim (arrow). This is the "double-line" sign. The necrotic area within the rim has intermediate signal on T_2- and high signal on T_1-weighted images, indicating fat.

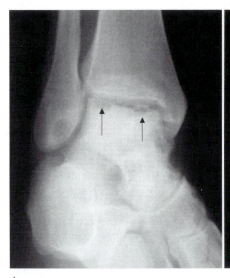
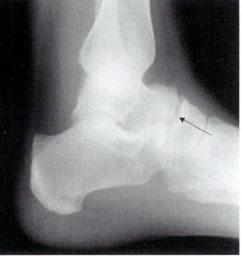

A

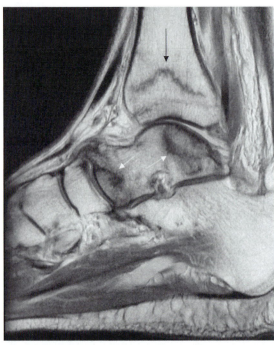

B

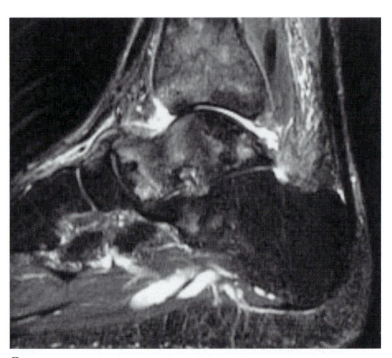

C

FIGURE 2-9. *(A)* Osteonecrosis of the proximal and distal talus (arrows) on anteroposterior (left) and lateral (right) radiographs shows increased density and irregular articular margins. *(B)* Proton density-weighted magnetic resonance image shows low signal areas surrounding normal signal areas in osteonecrosis of the proximal and distal talus (white arrows). There is also an insufficiency fracture of the metaphysis of the distal tibia (black arrow). *(C)* Short tau inversion recovery image shows mixed signal in the necrotic areas, including low, intermediate, and high. The low signal is due to fibrous tissue in the necrotic area.

is present, it is inevitable for secondary osteoarthritis to occur. If the crescent sign or collapse is absent, progression is not inevitable, and the hip may become asymptomatic.

The Mitchell classification is based on the MRI signal characteristics within the necrotic area and does not correlate with the radiographic classification systems:

Type A: Fat signal intensity (high on T_1-weighted imaging [T1WI] and intermediate on T_2-weighted imaging [T2WI])

Type B: Blood signal intensity (high on T1WI and T2WI)

Type C: Fluid signal intensity (low on T1WI and high on T2WI)

Type D: Fibrous signal intensity (low on T1WI and T2WI)

Early in the disease, the ON area may have normal fatty signal intensity (Figure 2-8), but many cases of ON have a mixed signal pattern in the necrotic area (Figure 2-9). Early in ON, the necrotic area may retain the normal fat signal intensity. In the later stages, fibrous tissue may be present and tends to have a worse prognosis. The Mitchell classification has only limited use in determining the prognosis of ON and is basically just a descriptive classification of the MRI appearances.

Pathologic Findings

The histopathologic appearances correlate with the radiographic stages. Initial cell death corresponds to Ficat stage 0, with necrosis of bone and bone marrow. After interruption of the blood supply, the hematopoietic marrow dies within 12 hours; the osteocytes, osteoblasts, and osteoclasts die in 12 to 48 hours; and the marrow fat dies in 2 to 5 days. Cell membranes remain intact for some time. Empty osteocyte lacunae constitute the characteristic histologic feature of ON, but this feature may take weeks to occur. Even with death of the fat cells, the fat within the cells may remain intact and produce the normal fat signal on MRI. The mineral within the bone remains intact, so that radiographs also appear normal. A bone scan may show decreased uptake reflecting decreased vascularity, and dynamic gadolinium-enhanced MRI may show lack of enhancement. This may be more evident in posttraumatic ON because the avascular area tends to be larger than in nontraumatic ON.

Next is the inflammatory response corresponding to Ficat stage I. There is rupture of cell membranes and release of cell contents causing an inflammatory response in the surrounding bone that has been revascularized by ingrowth of new blood vessels. This may cause temporary symptoms resulting from the inflammation. It produces hyperemia in the surrounding normal or revascularized bone, thus mimicking osteoporosis radiographically, whereas the necrotic and avascular area remains unchanged and thus relatively dense radiographically. The inflammatory response may produce a bone marrow edema pattern on MRI with diffuse decreased signal on T1WI and increased signal on T2WI, but whether the bone marrow edema pattern is actually the initial MRI finding in ON is uncertain, and exactly what the histopathology is in the bone marrow edema pattern is not known.

Then there is repair with a reactive interface and bone remodeling corresponding to stages I and II. The repair process begins in the adjacent normal bone, with increased vascularity and granulation tissue at the border with the necrotic zone. New bone is formed at the interface ("creeping substitution" or appositional new bone) and forms a demarcating rim of sclerosis, which is seen on MRI as a rim of decreased signal on T1WI and T2WI (see Fig. 2-8). The granulation tissue and rim of sclerosis form the "double-line sign" on MRI that is characteristic of ON but not always present: on T2WI, the outer rim of sclerosis has low signal intensity, whereas the inner rim of granulation tissue has high signal intensity (see Fig. 2-8). On T1WI, only a single thick rim of low signal is seen. The reactive interface causes bone resorption in the necrotic area, and radiographs may eventually show a region of lucency due to resorption of necrotic bone by invasion of vascular and fibrous tissue, with a surrounding rim of sclerosis from creeping substitution, thus producing a cyst-like appearance on radiographs (see Fig. 2-4). Bone scans in this phase show increased vascularity on the flow and blood pool phases due to the hyperemia and repair process, and the delayed static images usually show an area of increased uptake surrounding an area of decreased uptake (the "cold-in-hot" appearance; see Fig. 2-3, Figure 2-10). This is due to new bone formation around the necrotic area. At this stage of necrosis, there may be complete revascularization of the necrotic area, with resorption of the dead bone and replacement by new bone leading to complete restoration of the bone and recovery. More often, however, there is incomplete recovery, with fibrous tissue preventing complete revascularization and restoration of normal bone.

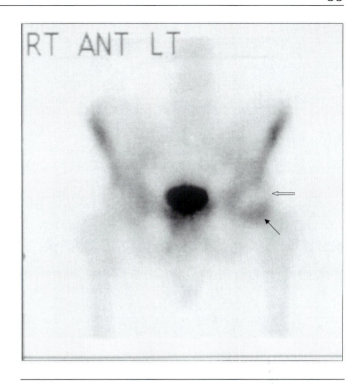

FIGURE 2-10.   "Cold-in-hot sign" of osteonecrosis on a bone scan. There is a rim of increased uptake (black arrow) surrounding an area of decreased uptake (block arrow).

Fracture in the subchondral region (the "crescent sign") may occur (see Fig. 2-5, Figures 2-11 and 2-12) due to (a) fatigue within the necrotic zone, (b) resorption of bone at the reactive interface, or (c) stress at the junction between the thickened trabeculae of the reactive interface and the necrotic bone. On MRI, the bone marrow edema pattern sometimes occurs in the viable bone beneath the necrotic area due to the collapse and fracture. The subchondral fracture eventually leads to collapse, flattening, and deformity of the articular surface. The bone usually collapses at the lateral margin of the fracture in the femoral head.

Collapse of the bone inevitably leads to secondary osteoarthritis corresponding to stage IV. Radiographs show joint space narrowing and osteophyte formation (see Fig. 2-7, Figures 2-13 and 2-14) and may be indistinguishable from primary osteoarthritis, but the gross and microscopic examination nevertheless show evidence of ON. On MRI, the advanced osteoarthritis may mask the underlying demarcation line. The articular cartilage will be thinned or absent over portions of the joint surface.

Increased radiodensity of bone, one of the characteristic radiographic findings of ON, can have 4 causes: (a) relative density due to disuse osteoporosis in the surrounding normal bone. The avascular necrotic bone initially cannot lose mineral because it does not have a blood supply; (b) creeping substitution or appositional new bone, in which new bone is laid down on the dead trabeculae to produce thickened trabeculae at the interface between necrotic and normal bone; (c) saponification of fats, which produces small areas of calcification within the necrotic area; and (d) collapse and impaction of bone causing trabeculae to be closer together. Creeping substitution is probably the most important cause of increased density in nontraumatic ON,

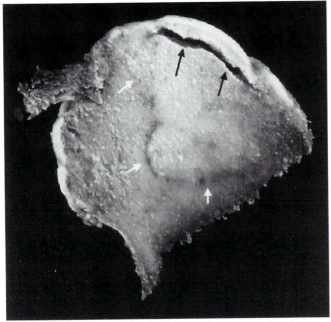

A

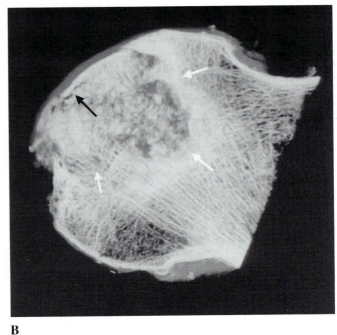

B

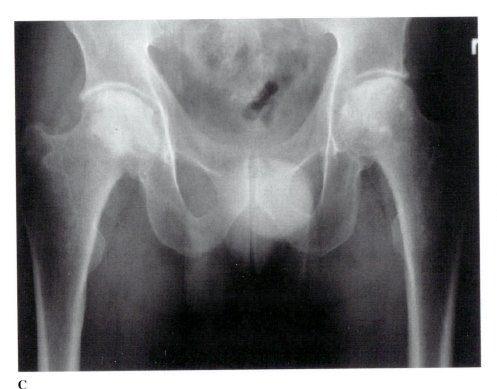

C

FIGURE 2-11. *(A)* Cut specimen and *(B)* cut specimen radiograph of a left femoral head show a wedge-shape area of osteonecrosis in the femoral head. The necrotic area is well demarcated from the normal bone by a reactive interface and rim of sclerosis (white arrows). Bone resorption is present within the necrotic area. A subchondral fracture has occurred in the necrotic area extending to the lateral aspect of the femoral head at the junction of the normal and necrotic bone with collapse of the subchondral cortex (black arrows). *(C)* Anteroposterior radiograph shows sclerosis and lucency in the femoral heads with mild collapse.

whereas relative increased density due to surrounding disuse osteoporosis is prominent mainly in traumatic ON.

Clinical Symptoms

Early nontraumatic ON is usually asymptomatic or only mildly symptomatic. In some cases, there may be initial pain that disappears in 6 to 8 weeks. A noninflammatory synovial effusion may be present. Subsequently, insidious pain may occur with

activity. This usually corresponds with stage III (collapse) or with impending collapse in late stage II, although in some cases pain may be present for many months before radiographs are positive. MRI is positive in about 95% of cases of ON with pain. Pain occurs at rest and eventually even at night in stage IV with secondary osteoarthritis. In traumatic ON, symptomatology is difficult to determine because of the initial pain from the fracture or dislocation itself. Once the pain of the trauma resolves, even patients with secondary ON are usually asymptomatic for months or longer until stage III, when subchondral fracture or

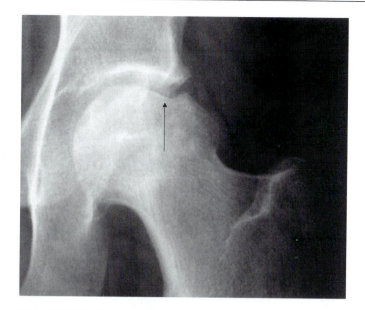

FIGURE 2-12.   Anteroposterior radiograph shows subchondral collapse at the junction of normal and necrotic bone anterolaterally (black arrow).

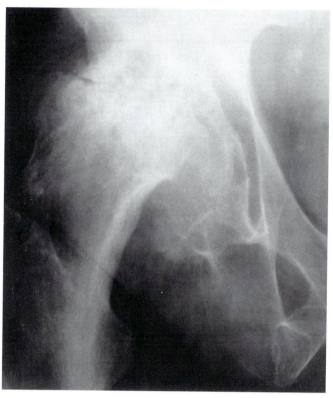

FIGURE 2-14.   Advanced secondary osteoarthritis of the hip due to osteonecrosis.

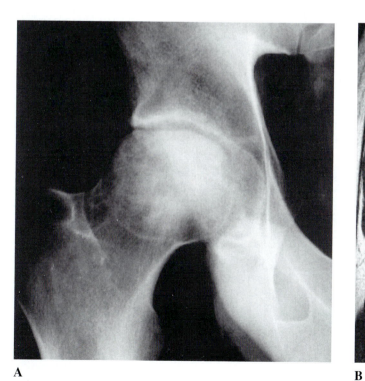

A

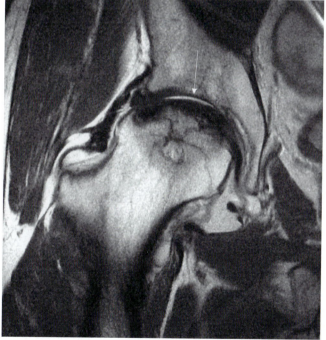

B

FIGURE 2-13.   *(A)* Anteroposterior radiograph depicts osteonecrosis of the right femoral head with sclerosis, lucency, collapse, narrowing of the superolateral aspect of the hip joint, and osteophyte formation at the junction of the femoral head and neck. *(B)* Proton density-weighted coronal magnetic resonance image shows the necrosis with collapse. There is loss of cartilage down to the subchondral bone (arrow). A joint effusion is present.

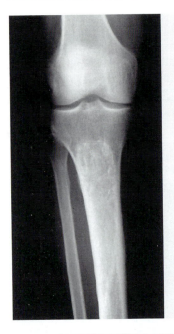
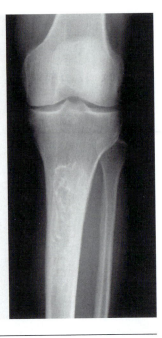

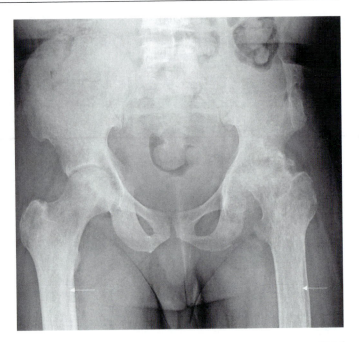

FIGURE 2-15.   Bone infarcts in the right and left tibias with a rim of sclerosis surrounding the area of infarction.

FIGURE 2-16.   Anteroposterior radiograph of a patient with sickle cell anemia, with dense bones due to bone infarction, osteonecrosis of the left femoral head with secondary osteoarthritis, and "bone-within-bone" appearance in the femoral shafts (arrows).

collapse occurs. Sudden severe spontaneous onset of pain with normal radiographs is usually not from ON.

Diagnostic Methods

RADIOGRAPHY.   Radiography is the initial imaging method used to evaluate bone and joint pain and helps determine the presence of arthritis, fracture, neoplastic disease, or other condition that may have clinical symptoms similar to those of ON. The initial radiographs are normal for months after ON occurs because there is no change in the mineral content of the bone. There are three radiographic findings that are characteristic of ON: (*a*) sclerosis, (*b*) lucency, and (*c*) subchondral fracture and collapse. The mottled sclerosis and lucency that are considered to be the earliest radiographic findings in ON are not diagnostic (see Fig. 2-8). Subchondral fracture and collapse were thought to be diagnostic of ON, but subchondral insufficiency and impaction fractures recently have been shown to cause similar findings. A combination of findings including a wedge-shape area of lucency surrounded by a rim of sclerosis plus subchondral fracture is diagnostic (see Fig. 2-11).

Bone infarct of the shaft of the bone has a different appearance. An elongated area of lucency surrounded by a serpiginous rim of sclerosis (the "rising-smoke" appearance) eventually occurs (Figure 2-15). The outer rim of sclerosis helps differentiate a bone infarct from a cartilaginous lesion such as an enchondroma or chondrosarcoma in which there are central calcifications. Periosteal reaction may occur along the shafts of long bones causing a "bone-within-bone" appearance. In patients with sickle cell disease, bone infarcts may cause diffuse bony sclerosis (Figure 2-16). The characteristic H-shape vertebra in sicklers should be differentiated from the biconcave appearance of the vertebral end plates in osteoporosis (Figure 2-17).

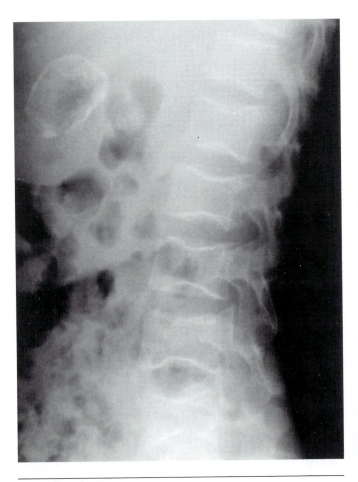

FIGURE 2-17.   Lateral radiograph of the lumbar spine shows "H vertebrae" with depressions in the midportions of the vertebral bodies. There is a large gallstone in the gallbladder.

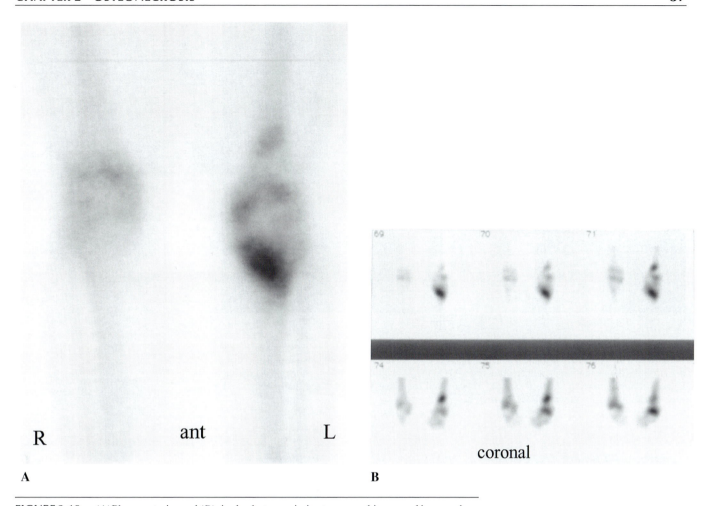

FIGURE 2-18. *(A)* Planar anterior and *(B)* single photon emission tomographic coronal images show areas of increased and decreased uptake in both knees from osteonecrosis. Single photon emission tomography shows the abnormalities better than the planar image in the right knee.

RADIONUCLIDE BONE SCANNING.   Radionuclide bone scanning can diagnose ON when radiographs appear normal and can survey the entire body to identify sites of clinically and radiographically occult ON. With a sensitivity of 75% to 80%, it is more sensitive for ON than radiography but less sensitive than MRI, which has greater than 95% sensitivity. The appearance of the bone scan depends on the stage and the type of ON. Uptake of radionuclide depends on blood flow to the bone and the degree of new bone formation. Absent blood flow produces a cold or photopenic area. Increased blood flow causes increased uptake to a limited degree, but increased bone formation is the main determinant of the degree of uptake of radionuclide. In early ON, when the blood supply is first disrupted, there will be absent vascularity and no uptake. This may be seen in early posttraumatic ON, sickle cell disease, or Legg-Perthes disease, where virtually the entire blood supply to a large portion of bone is disrupted. It is rarely, if ever, seen in nontraumatic necrosis, where only a small area of the bone is affected and the patient is asymptomatic. In nontraumatic ON, the most frequent finding is increased vascularity with increased radionuclide uptake due to the revascularization and hyperemia of the repair process. The characteristic scintigraphic finding is the cold-in-hot appearance with an area of decreased uptake surrounded by a rim of increased uptake (see Fig. 2-10). ON may also show only a focal increased uptake. The increased uptake of ON can be distinguished from degenerative arthritis in which increased uptake occurs on both sides of the joint. Single photon emission tomography increases the sensitivity for the diagnosis of ON because it shows photopenic areas better than routine planar imaging (Figure 2-18). Pinhole collimator scanning also can improve the diagnostic sensitivity by increasing resolution. Bone marrow scanning with technetium Tc 99m sulfur colloid has been used to diagnose traumatic ON in cases in which routine bone scanning with phosphonate complexes was confounded by the high uptake at the fracture site: absent uptake occurs in the necrotic marrow as compared with the opposite side with normal marrow, but variations in the amount of normal marrow can make the diagnosis uncertain in some cases.

MAGNETIC RESONANCE IMAGING.   Dynamic scanning after intravenous injection of gadolinium can depict avascularity by absent enhancement. The MRI findings in ON reflect the repair process, with variable signal intensity as described by the Mitchell classification. The characteristic appearance is the

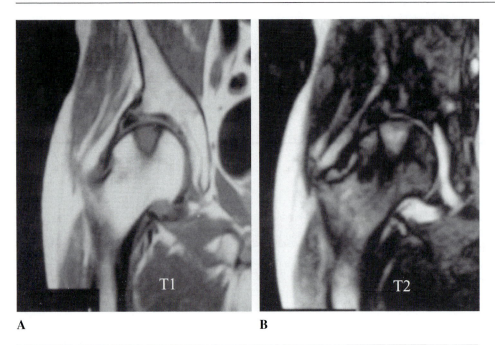

A   B

FIGURE 2-19. Coronal magnetic resonance images of osteonecrosis show a U-shape area of necrosis surrounded by a low signal demarcation rim. (A) On the T_1-weighted sequence, there is decreased signal within the necrotic area. (B) On the T_2-weighted sequence, there is mixed intermediate and high signal. A small synovial effusion is present.

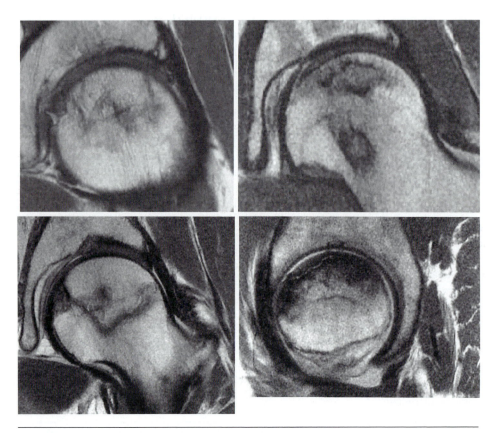

FIGURE 2-20. Proton density-weighted magnetic resonance images in 4 patients with osteonecrosis show different patterns of abnormality within the femoral heads.

U-shape subchondral line demarcating the transition zone between normal and necrotic bone (Figure 2-19). When the demarcating line shows the uniform low signal intensity on T1WI and a "double line" of outer low and inner high signal intensity on T2WI, then the appearance is pathognomonic (see Fig. 2-8C). Other low signal intensity zones of demarcation may take the form of lines, crescents, or round or wedge-shape areas (Figure 2-20). These low signal intensity regions may be due to sclerosis at the interface of the necrotic area or to subchondral fracture in the necrotic area, and it may not be possible to distinguish the two on MRI. T2WI with fat suppression (by frequency-selection technique or short tau inversion recovery technique) is best for showing synovial effusion and the bone marrow edema pattern. It remains controversial as to whether the bone marrow edema pattern is seen as an early finding of ON before focal abnormalities develop. The bone marrow edema pattern that occurs in the femoral neck below the demarcation zone most likely is reaction to collapse or fracture in the necrotic area and not to extension of the area of necrosis. In most cases, the size of the initial necrotic area remains unchanged. The use of surface coils instead of body coils allows higher resolution imaging for identification of demarcation zones and for evaluation of deformity or collapse of the femoral head. High resolution MRI also aids in evaluation of early abnormalities in the articular cartilage before joint space narrowing may be apparent on radiographs.

COMPUTED TOMOGRAPHY. Computed tomography has a limited role in the diagnosis of ON because MRI and bone scanning are more sensitive. On axial images, disruption of the trabecular "asterisk," an area of density in the femoral head caused by intersection of trabeculae, is a sign of ON. The sclerotic rim at the reactive interface may be seen (Figure 2-21). Subchondral fractures and deformity of the articular surface can be evaluated on coronal and sagittal reformatted views and subtle flattening of the head may be better appreciated on such images than on MR images.

Invasive Methods

Intramedullary pressure measurements are done by insertion of a cannula into the intertrochanteric region of the femur. In ON there is elevated pressure in the bone outside the area of necrosis. Intraosseous venography is done by insertion of a needle into the bone of the intertrochanteric region of the femur and injection of contrast material. In ON there is poor flow in the veins with stasis of the contrast in the bone.

Superselective angiography with injection of the medial circumflex artery may show disruption of the superior retinacular vessels in ON of the femoral head. In the future, magnetic resonance angiography may be used to evaluate the vascularity of bone.

Biopsy may be done percutaneously by using a needle, with a core of bone removed for histopathology.

Overall, MRI is the most sensitive and specific method to diagnose ON, but occasionally even MRI may be normal in the very beginning of the process, since it takes time for abnormalities in the marrow fat and bone to develop. Other

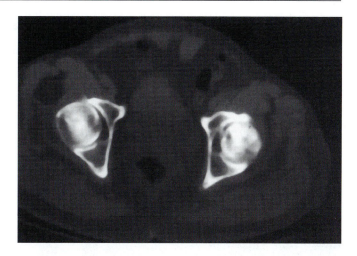

FIGURE 2-21. Computed tomography shows sclerosis in the femoral heads with disruption of the normal trabecular pattern due to osteonecrosis.

techniques such as intramedullary pressure measurements, 3-phase bone scanning, superselective angiography, and biopsy with histopathology may show ON in some cases even when MRI is negative.

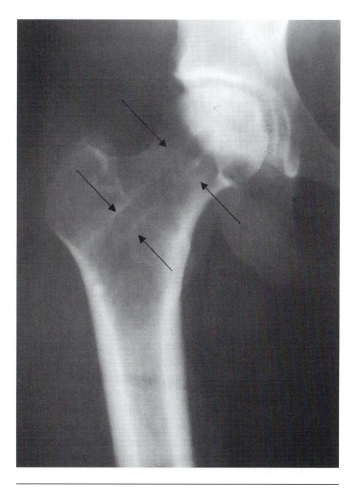

FIGURE 2-22. Core decompression of osteonecrosis of the right femoral head was done with a longitudinal core (arrows) of bone removed from the femoral head and neck.

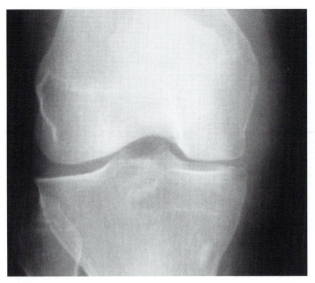

A

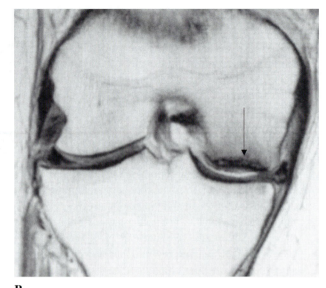

B

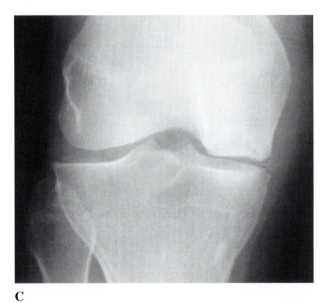

C

FIGURE 2-23.   A 76-year-old woman had sudden onset of severe right knee pain. *(A)* Radiograph is normal except for chondrocalcinosis. Two months later, magnetic resonance imaging shows spontaneous osteonecrosis of the medial femoral condyle. *(B)* Coronal proton density-weighted image shows a demarcation rim (black arrow) surrounding the necrotic area, with a bone marrow edema pattern around it. There is thinning and erosion of the articular cartilage of the medial femoral condyle. The medial and lateral menisci are torn. *(C)* Seven months after the onset of pain, the radiograph depicts sclerosis and lucency, collapse of the medial femoral condyle, and joint space narrowing of the medial compartment.

Treatment of Osteonecrosis

Conservative therapy with the use of crutches and decreased weight bearing is not effective in preventing progression. In patients on corticosteroids, statins may decrease the incidence of ON, most likely by decreasing hyperlipidemia.

Operative management includes core decompression in which a core of bone is taken out of the femoral head and neck (Figure 2-22) or longitudinal holes are drilled in the femoral head and neck, thus relieving intramedullary pressure and bone marrow edema. This procedure is used mainly in stages I and II before collapse has occurred, although it is occasionally used in stage III. Although success with this procedure has been mixed, it can delay or prevent progression in some cases as compared with nonoperative therapy. A potential but uncommon complication is fracture of the femoral neck. Core decompression is used infrequently in sites other than the femoral head.

Bone grafting procedures may be done with vascularized or nonvascularized cortical grafts, usually the fibula, to help support the femoral head. Cancellous grafting also has been used. In the femoral condyles of the knee, osteochondral allografts may be used to replace the necrotic area. In a "trapdoor" procedure, the break in the articular cartilage is opened during surgery, necrotic bone is débrided, and the defect filled with cancellous bone graft.

Rotational or angular osteotomies are used to move the necrotic site away from the weight-bearing area and allow weight bearing on a normal part of the bone. The goal is to preserve the femoral head. These procedures require a long period of non–weight bearing during healing and may make eventual conversion to prosthetic joint replacement more difficult.

The final therapy for most patients with ON of the femoral head is prosthetic joint replacement. Hemiarthroplasty and surface replacement arthroplasty have been used, but total joint arthroplasty is most frequently done for stage III and IV disease. There are reports of higher failure rates in patients who have total joint replacement for ON than for primary osteoarthritis. This may be due to the younger age group for ON, to abnormal bone in ON, or both.

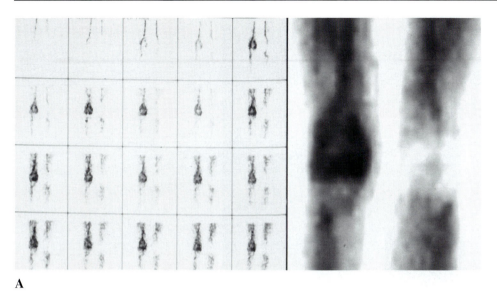

A

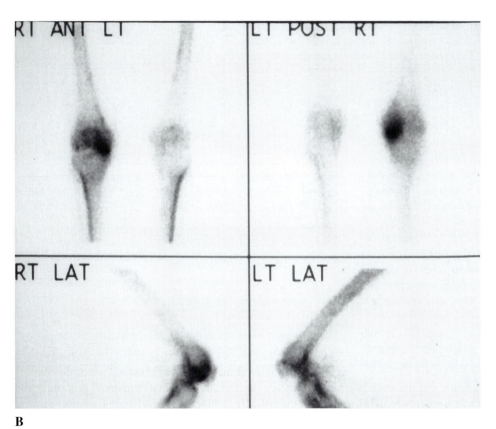

B

FIGURE 2-24.   *(A)* Dynamic flow (left) and blood pool scans (right) show increased vascularity and *(B)* the 3-hour static image shows increased uptake in the right medial femoral condyle from spontaneous osteonecrosis.

Osteonecrosis of the Knee

ON of the knee can be classified as spontaneous or idiopathic ON of the knee and secondary ON associated with corticosteroids or other underlying cause. Spontaneous ON of the knee (SONK) usually occurs in people in their 60s and older, typically elderly women (Figure 2-23). It begins with a sudden onset of pain increasing over a period of weeks. The site is predominantly the weight-bearing aspect of the medial femoral condyle. The lateral femoral condyle is much less common, and the tibial plateau is rare. Initial radiographs may appear normal at the onset of pain or may show an area of flattening, sclerosis, and lucency in the subchondral region. A bony fragment may separate from the articular surface, with an appearance identical to that of osteochondritis dissecans (OCD; see below). There is usually a rapid progression of secondary osteoarthritis leading to total

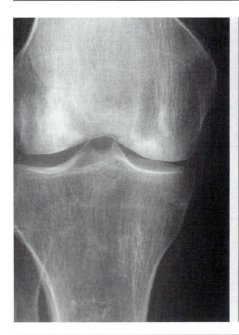
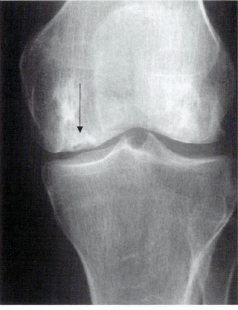

FIGURE 2-25. Secondary osteonecrosis of the knees associated with corticosteroid therapy. AP radiographs of both knees show areas of sclerosis in the medial and lateral femoral condyles bilaterally, and subchondral collapse of the left medial femoral condyle (arrow).

knee replacement in 1 to 2 years. Bone scans show increased vascularity in the early scan phases and a focal area of increased uptake in the femoral condyle in the static phase, even with negative radiographs (Figure 2-24). MRI is also positive at the onset of symptoms, showing subchondral band-like or linear low signal areas surrounded by a bone marrow edema pattern of diffuse low signal on T1WI and high signal on T2WI and short tau inversion recovery STIR images. SONK, rather than being a primary vascular insult, is most likely an insufficiency fracture that progresses to necrosis and thus the term SIFK (subchondral insufficiency fracture of the knee) is probably a more accurate acronym.

Foci of ON in the knee, other than SONK, are usually not painful or have an insidious onset of pain, with relatively slow or even no progression in many cases. They occur in young adults and are secondary to any of the atraumatic causes previously noted. Multiple sites in the knee may be affected, most frequently the lateral femoral condyle and then medial femoral condyle and the tibial plateaus, and may be bilateral (Figure 2-25). Bone infarcts are often present in the femurs and tibias (Figure 2-26).

Septic Necrosis

Infection, either septic arthritis or osteomyelitis, can disrupt the blood supply to bone and cause ON (Figure 2-27). This is most common with septic arthritis or osteomyelitis of the hip in children. Potential resultant complications are growth disturbance of the proximal femur leading to limb length discrepancy and coxa vara deformity. Prompt diagnosis must be made, followed by decompression and debridement, to avoid these complications.

Radiation Necrosis

High dose radiation (30 to 50 Gy) can cause ON. Frequently affected sites include the mandible, skull, sternum, shoulder, and pelvic bones. Radiographic appearances include regions of increased and decreased density, abnormal trabecular pattern, bony collapse, and fracture (Figure 2-28). Irradiated bone is also susceptible to infection and malignant transformation.

Osteochondritis Dissecans

Osteochondritis Dissecans (OCD) is a posttraumatic osteochondral injury. In the clinical setting of acute trauma, the injury is called an *acute osteochondral fracture*; in the setting of remote trauma or chronic overuse from sports or other activities, the abnormality is called *osteochondritis dissecans*. There is a spectrum of injury, ranging from transchondral (affecting only the cartilage), subchondral (affecting only the underlying bone) to osteochondral (affecting the bone and cartilage; Figure 2-29). An initially subchondral injury eventually may lead to disruption of the overlying articular cartilage. Although a similar appearance may be seen in ON and the separated fragment may be partly or completely avascular, the necrosis is secondary to the trauma and not a primary abnormality in the blood supply to the bone.

OCD is most frequent in the knee, with the lateral aspect of the medial femoral condyle affected in 75% of cases, the weight-bearing aspect of the medial femoral condyle in 10%, the lateral femoral condyle in 10%, and the intercondylar region and patella in 5%. The talar dome of the ankle is the second most frequent sight, with the posteromedial aspect slightly more frequent than the anterolateral (Figure 2-30). The capitellum in the

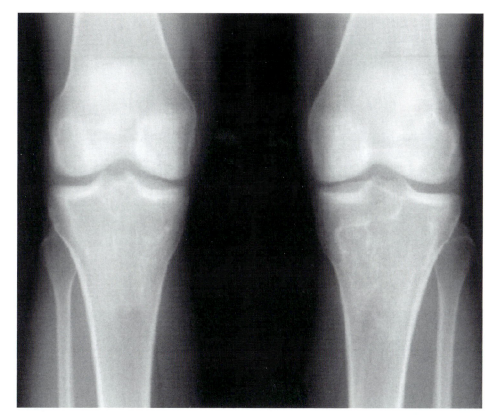

A

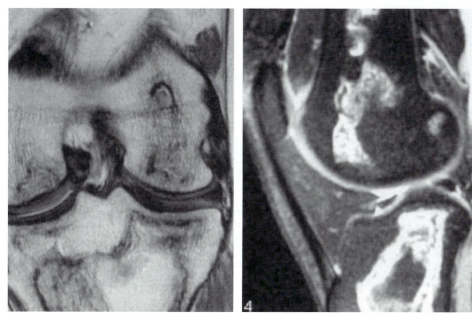

B

FIGURE 2-26. *(A)* Anteroposterior radiograph and *(B)* magnetic resonance imaging (coronal proton density-weighted, left; sagittal STIR, right) show bone infarcts in the distal femurs and proximal tibias bilaterally.

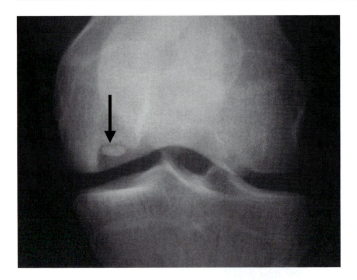

FIGURE 2-29. Osteochondritis dissecans is present in the medial femoral condyle of the knee, with an area of lucency surrounding a bone fragment (arrow).

passing through the articular cartilage and around the osseous fragment, (*c*) the osteochondral defect filled with fluid, and (*d*) a 5-mm or larger fluid-filled cyst in the parent bone adjacent to the lesion. If the stability of the lesion cannot be determined on conventional MR images, direct MR arthrography may be helpful to outline the articular surface or to insinuate between the fragment and parent bone.

Unstable lesions tend to have a poor prognosis for pain and function when treated conservatively. Lesion size is also impor-

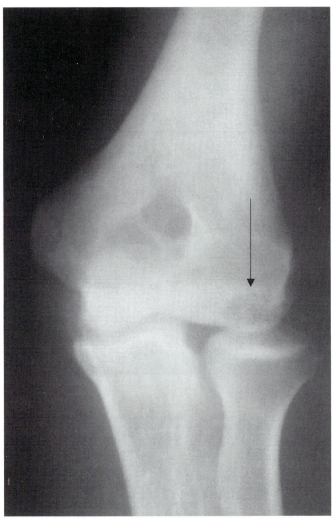

FIGURE 2-31. Osteochondritis dissecans is seen in the elbow, with an area of lucency and sclerosis in the capitellum (arrow).

tant in prognosis, with smaller lesions having a better outcome than larger ones. Thus, the imaging characterization of these lesions has an impact on clinical management.

Transient Bone Marrow Edema Syndrome and Transient Osteoporosis

The *transient bone marrow edema syndrome* is thought to be a transient ischemic attack of the bone that does not progress to frank ON. Patients complain of sudden, spontaneous onset of severe pain. It occurs most often in the femoral head and less commonly in the femoral condyles and the body of the talus. MRI demonstrates diffuse marrow edema without a discrete zone of demarcation to suggest ON or linear abnormality to suggest insufficiency fracture. A joint effusion is usually present. If there is radiographic osteopenia of the affected site, the condition is called *transient osteoporosis* (Figure 2-34).

Transient osteoporosis of the hip was described before the advent of MRI, and the first report was in women in the third

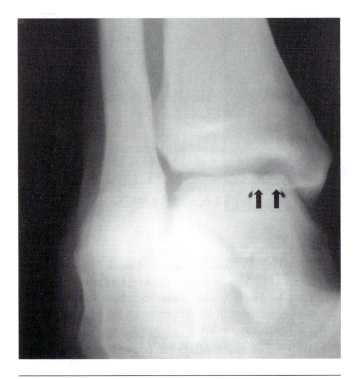

FIGURE 2-30. Osteochondritis dissecans of the ankle, with a focal lucent defect in the medial aspect of the proximal articular surface of the talus (arrows).

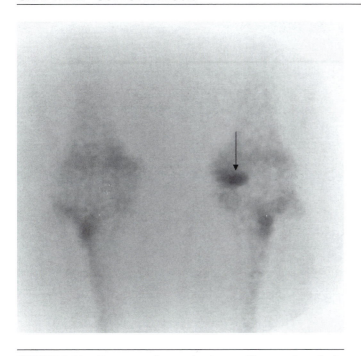

FIGURE 2-32. Bone scan shows a focal area of increased uptake in the left medial femoral condyle (arrow) due to osteochondritis dissecans.

trimester of pregnancy, but more recent and larger series using MRI have shown a mild predominance of middle-age to elderly males. Radiographs may be normal at the initial onset of symptoms and show osteopenia over the ensuing few months. Three-phase bone scan shows marked increased vascularity and uptake in the femoral head extending into the femoral neck to the intertrochanteric region. MRI shows diffuse increased signal intensity on fat-suppressed T2WI and decreased signal on T1WI. There is spontaneous resolution of pain over a period from several months to one year, and the radiographic, scintigraphic, and MRI abnormalities eventually revert to normal.

Although some reports have stated that transient marrow edema syndrome is a precursor or an early stage of ON, very few patients with transient bone marrow edema progress to collapse of the articular surface. It also affects a different group of patients than does ON, with underlying causes such as corticosteroids and alcoholism usually not present. Some cases of transient marrow edema syndrome may be due to subtle insufficiency fractures. The severe pain associated with this condition correlates with the marked bone marrow edema pattern. Core decompression can relieve the symptoms by decreasing the intramedullary pressure, but this treatment is seldom used because the condition is self-limited.

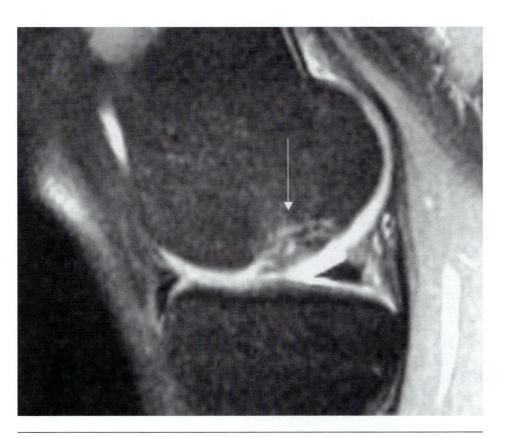

FIGURE 2-33. Fat-suppressed proton density-weighted magnetic resonance image shows linear increased signal in the interface between the bone and the area of osteochondritis dissecans (arrow).

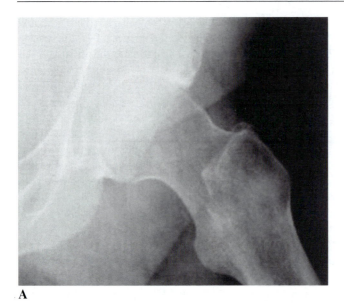

A

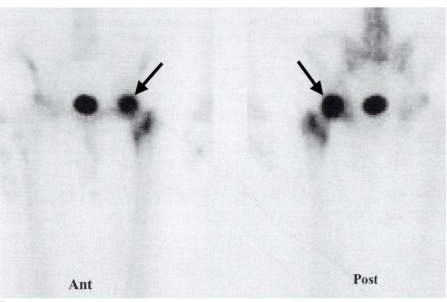

B

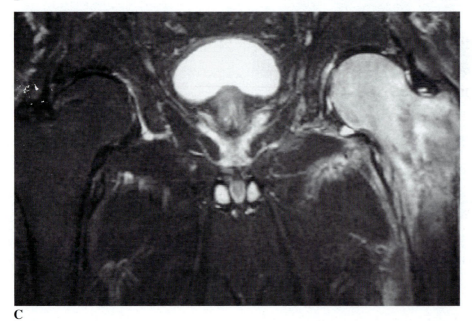

C

FIGURE 2-34.   Transient osteoporosis of the hip. *(A)* Frog lateral view of the left hip shows osteoporosis in the left femoral head. *(B)* Bone scan shows marked uptake in the left femoral head (arrows) extending to the intertrochanteric region. *(C)* Magnetic resonance image shows increased signal intensity on short tau inversion recovery sequence without a demarcation rim in the femoral head.

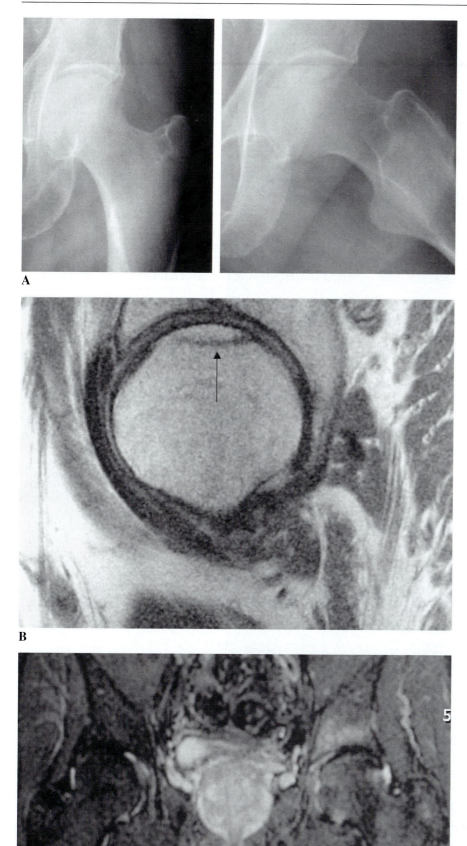

FIGURE 2-35. A 75-year-old female with sudden onset of hip pain. *(A)* Normal radiographs. *(B)* Sagittal proton density-weighted image shows a linear area of decreased signal in the left femoral head (arrow). *(C)* Short tau inversion recovery image shows a bone marrow edema pattern in the left femoral head and neck and in the acetabulum. There was no underlying condition associated with osteonecrosis. The findings are consistent with subchondral insufficiency fracture of the femoral head.

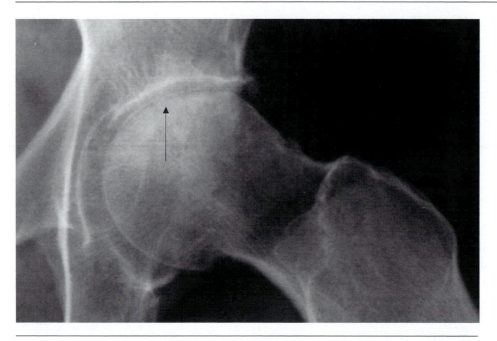

FIGURE 2-36.   Subchondral fracture with a crescent sign (arrow) and hip joint space narrowing. The joint space was normal on radiographs done 3 months before, at the onset of pain.

Subchondral Insufficiency Fractures

Subchondral insufficiency fractures of the femoral head may simulate ON. These fractures tend to occur in elderly females, with sudden onset of severe pain in normal or near normal hips. On MRI, a bone marrow edema pattern is present in the femoral head and neck, and linear, curvilinear, crescentic, or band-like low intensity signal is present in the superior aspect of the femoral head (Figure 2-35). On radionuclide bone scan, there is increased vascularity and uptake in the femoral head extending into the femoral neck. Radiographs may be normal initially or may show a crescent sign similar to that of ON (Figure 2-36). These fractures may heal or may cause collapse of the femoral head and secondary osteoarthritis similar to ON.

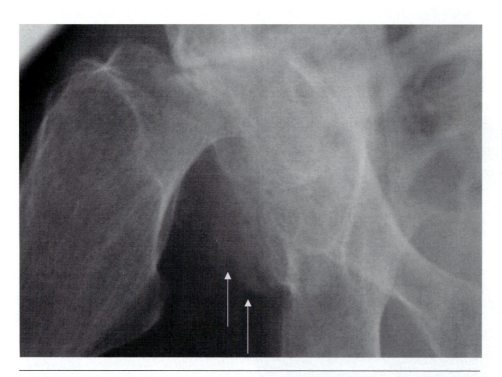

FIGURE 2-37.   Rapidly destructive osteoarthritis of the hip. Radiograph shows marked collapse and fracture of the femoral head with displacement. There is bony debris in the joint (arrows).

In some cases, rapidly destructive osteoarthritis occurs, with marked joint space narrowing developing in less than one year (Figure 2-37) and with severe pain necessitating total joint replacement. Most of these patients are osteoporotic. ON usually has a more insidious onset with a slower progression, with several or more years from onset to joint replacement. In the knee, what used to be called SONK affecting the weight-bearing portion of the medial femoral condyle is now more correctly considered a subchondral insufficiency fracture.

OSTEOCHONDROSES

Osteochondrosis is not a synonym for ON. The osteochondroses are a group of conditions affecting mainly children and teenagers and characterized by fragmentation, irregularity, sclerosis, and small size of epiphyses and apophyses (secondary growth centers). Although originally thought to be due to ON, it is now recognized that the osteochondroses are a heterogeneous group of conditions of various etiologies such as ON, growth disturbances, normal variants of growth, and posttraumatic abnormalities.

Legg-Perthes Disease

Legg-Perthes disease is true ON of the ossification center of the femoral capital epiphysis in the hip in children ages 3 to 12 years, with is peak at ages 4 to 8 years. Boys are involved 5 to 6 times more frequently than girls. Bilateral involvement occurs in 10% to 20% but not usually at the same time. Delayed bone age is often present in these patients. Clinical findings are limp, pain in the hip, thigh, or knee, and limited motion of the hip. Absent or decreased blood flow to the femoral head occurs. Some

hypotheses for this finding include thrombophilia with arterial thrombosis, increased venous pressure due to synovial effusion causing increased pressure in the joint capsule, and trauma. The blood supply to the femoral head is more vulnerable in children than in adults due to the barrier of the growth plate preventing flow from the metaphysis to the epiphysis. The ossification center of the femoral capital epiphysis becomes necrotic with loss of the blood supply, whereas the cartilaginous femoral head remains viable because it is nourished by synovial fluid. Revascularization always occurs with bone resorption leading to fragmentation and collapse of the ossification center of the femoral capital epiphysis. Radiographs early in the disease may show only widening of the distance from the pelvic "teardrop" to the medial aspect of the femoral head. Later radiographic findings include the crescent sign of subchondral fracture, collapse of the head, and fragmentation and decreased size of the ossification center of the femoral head (Figure 2-38). Re-ossification of the head may lead to a normal appearance or to residual deformity, with flattening and broadening of the femoral head and neck, known as *coxa plana* or *coxa magna*, respectively. Symptoms may precede radiographic findings, but bone scans and MRI usually will be positive. Bone scans show decreased or absent vascularity manifest as decreased uptake in the entire femoral head in the early stages of the condition (Figure 2-39) and increased vascularity and uptake in the metaphysis followed by the femoral head in the later stages. MRI in the early stage shows decreased signal intensity in the ossification center of the femoral head on T1WI and increased or normal signal intensity on T2WI. Moreover, the shape of the cartilaginous femoral head can be assessed on MRI.

The younger the patient is at onset, the better the prognosis is for restoration of the normal contour of the femoral head. Abnormal cartilaginous and osseous growth may lead to lateral displacement of the ossification center of the femoral head.

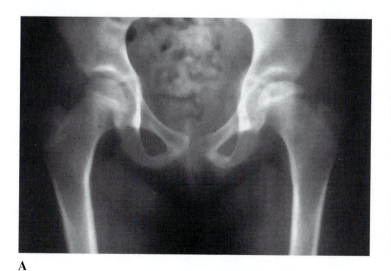

A

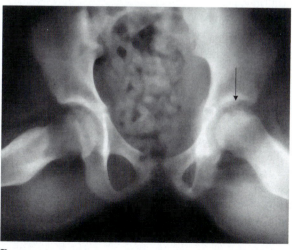

B

FIGURE 2-38. Legg-Perthes disease of the left hip. *(A)* Anteroposterior and *(B)* frog lateral radiographs show decreased size and increased density of the ossification center of the left femoral capital epiphysis. Collapse of the anterolateral aspect of the left femoral head is seen on the frog lateral image (arrow).

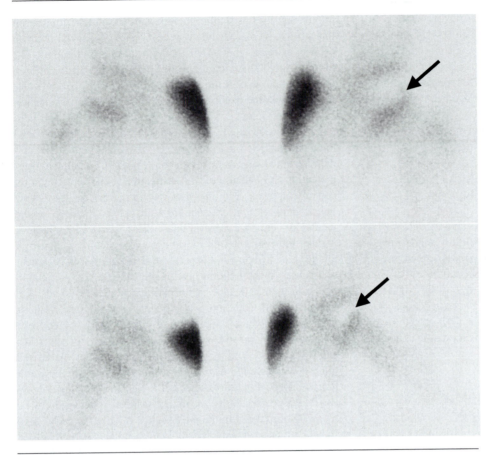

FIGURE 2-39.   There is absent uptake of radionuclide in the entire left femoral head on anterior and frog lateral pinhole collimator views of the bone scan (arrows).

Radiolucent areas due to uncalcified cartilage occur in the femoral neck. The most frequent differential diagnosis for hip pain in this age group when radiographs are normal is transient synovitis of the hip. Bilateral symmetrical fragmentation of the femoral heads may represent multiple epiphyseal dysplasia rather than Perthes disease. Meyer dysplasia, a normal variant of ossification that starts with a fragmented femoral head ossification center in very young children that goes on to become normal, also can mimic Perthes disease.

Köhler Disease

Köhler disease involves the tarsal navicular bone. Initially, a normal navicular becomes flattened and sclerotic, most likely due to a decrease in the blood supply leading to ON (Figure 2-40). It is most frequent between ages 5 to 10 years and is more common in boys than in girls. There is usually a sudden onset of pain and limp, with tenderness over the navicular and often soft tissue swelling. Re-ossification and restoration of the normal shape of the navicular always occurs, suggesting that this condition may be a variation of growth and not a real abnormality. However, the progression from a normal navicular to collapse in addition to symptoms should differentiate Köhler disease from a normal growth variation.

Kienböck Disease

In Kienböck disease, there is collapse and fragmentation of the lunate of the wrist (see Chapter 11; Figure 2-41). It occurs most commonly between ages 20 and 30 years, more often in males than in females, and more in those engaged in heavy labor. Most likely it is a condition of repetitive trauma leading to ON. Most cases are associated with negative ulnar variance, but most patients with negative ulnar variance do not develop Kienböck disease. Radiographs may be normal at the outset of symptoms. Sclerosis subsequently occurs, with a normal shape of the lunate followed by collapse and fragmentation of the lunate and by secondary osteoarthritis. Most symptomatic patients present at the stages of sclerosis or collapse. The Lichtman classification divides the disease into stages based on the radiographic appearance and is useful for determining therapy:

Stage I: Normal radiographs or a linear fracture

Stage II: Increased density of the lunate

Stage IIIA: Sclerosis and fragmentation of the lunate, without changes in carpal alignment

Stage IIIB: Carpal collapse, with fixed volar flexion of the scaphoid

Stage IV: Pancarpal osteoarthritis

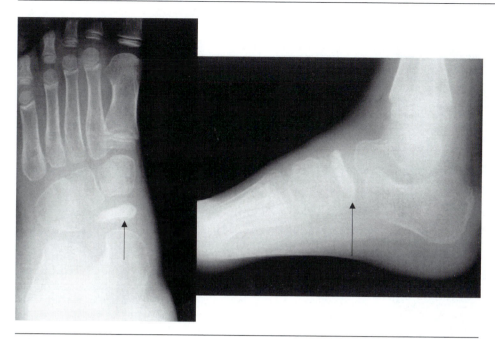

FIGURE 2-40. Köhler disease with sclerosis and collapse of the tarsal navicular bone (arrows).

The diagnosis can be made in patients with normal radiographs using MRI or radionuclide bone scanning. On MRI, there is decreased signal intensity on T1WI and usually increased signal intensity on T2WI or short tau inversion recovery images. This signal may involve the radial portion or entire lunate. On bone scanning, there is increased uptake localized to the lunate due to the repair process.

Freiberg Infraction

Freiberg infraction is collapse of the articular surface of the metatarsal head, most frequently the second, then the third, and very uncommonly the first and fifth (Figure 2-42). It can occur in any age, but adolescence is most common. It affects females more commonly than males, with a ratio of about 5 to 1. It is most likely due to repetitive trauma leading to ON. It is often associated with a long second metatarsal as compared with the first, which may place excessive stress on the second metatarsal head. Early radiographic findings may include only subtle increased density in the metatarsal head, fissuring of the epiphysis, and widening of the joint. Flattening of the metatarsal head then occurs with depression of the articular surface. The cortex becomes thickened. An osteochondral fragment may be present. The final stage is secondary osteoarthritis. In the early stage, when radiographs are normal or equivocal, MRI and radionuclide bone scanning will be positive showing marrow edema and increased uptake, respectively.

Osgood-Schlatter Disease

Osgood-Schlatter disease is the clinical triad of anterior knee pain, swelling, and heterotopic ossification around the insertion of the patellar tendon on the tibial tubercle (see Chapter 13; Figure 2-43). It occurs between ages 11 and 15 years, more often in boys. It is a microavulsion injury of the patellar tendon due to repetitive contraction of the extensor mechanism. It is not an avulsion fracture through the growth plate of the anterior tibial tubercle, nor is it ON. Initially, only soft tissue swelling, thickening of the patellar tendon, and edema in the anterior infrapatellar fat pad may be the only radiographic findings, but eventually heterotopic ossification develops, which may cause a bump on the anterior aspect of the knee near the tibial tubercle. This condition should not be confused with bony fragments, which may normally be present around the anterior tibial tubercle from multiple ossification centers or incomplete fusion, but which are asymptomatic and not associated with soft tissue swelling.

Blount Disease (Tibia Vara)

Blount disease is a growth disturbance of the medial aspect of the proximal tibial metaphysis that leads to a varus deformity of the tibia. ON is not present in this condition. The infantile form begins before age 3 years, and the adolescent type occurs between ages 10 and 14 years. The infantile form tends to occur in patients who are early walkers and in obese African American children who have physiologic bowing of the tibias. It is bilateral in more than 50% of cases and more commonly affects boys. It is most likely related to axial overload, with excessive compression of the medial growth plate leading to decreased growth with disordered enchondral ossification of the epiphysis, physis, and metaphysis. The radiologic appearance occurs after age 2 years, when the medial tibial growth

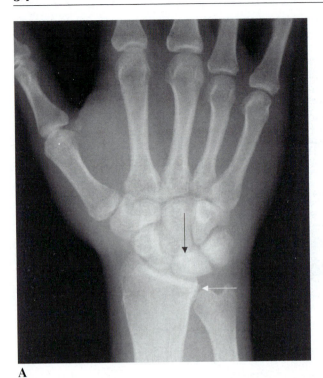

A

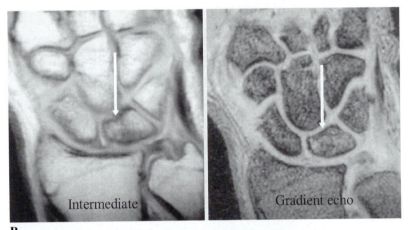

Intermediate   Gradient echo

B

FIGURE 2-41. Kienböck disease with mild sclerosis of the lunate. *(A)* Radiograph shows negative ulnar variance, with the ulna shorter than the radius (white arrow). The lunate (black arrow) is normal but *(B)* Magnetic resonance images display decreased signal in the lunate on the proton density-weighted image (left), and increased signal on the gradient-echo image (right). *(C)* Another patient with marked collapse of the lunate (arrow) and negative ulnar variance.

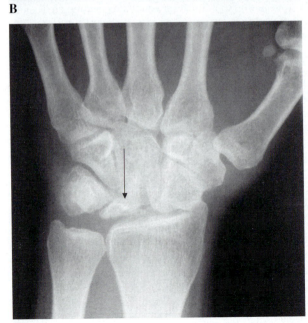

C

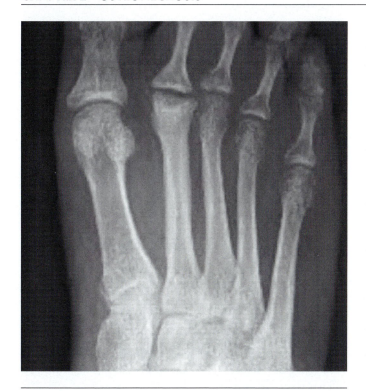

FIGURE 2-42. Freiberg infraction with collapse and flattening of the second metatarsal head. There is cortical thickening of the shaft of the second metatarsal.

disturbance can be differentiated from normal physiologic bowing. The Langenskiöld classification of this condition has 6 stages, beginning with irregularity of the medial metaphysis with beaking, progressing to various degrees of depression of the medial metaphysis and deformity of the medial epiphysis, and then to premature fusion of the medial tibial growth plate (Figure 2-44). Adolescent Blount disease is less frequent than infantile, is usually unilateral, and causes less severe varus deformity. It is thought to be related to premature fusion of a portion of the growth plate.

Scheuermann Disease

Scheuermann disease is a growth disturbance of the spine. Although Scheuermann hypothesized that it was due to ON of the ring apophyses of the vertebrae, it now is recognized as a growth disturbance caused by herniation of disk material through the endplates, most likely from trauma or compression stress, and is not related to the ring apophysis or ON. The radiologic criteria for Scheuermann disease are a kyphotic angle greater than 40°, anterior wedging of 5° or more of 3 or more consecutive vertebrae, Schmorl nodes with irregularity of endplates, and disk space narrowing (Figure 2-45). It most commonly involves the thoracic spine and may involve the upper lumbar spine. Scoliosis is often present. The anterior portion of the vertebra is affected because the posterior portion is supported by the posterior elements. Scheuermann disease has to be differentiated from "round back" (abnormal kyphosis without endplate abnormalities).

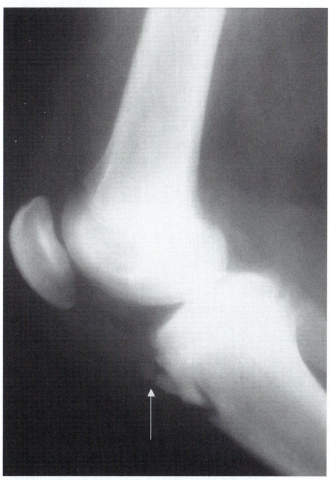

FIGURE 2-43. Osgood-Schlatter disease. There is fragmentation of the ossification center of the apophysis of the anterior tibial tubercle (arrow), swelling of the patellar tendon, and increased density in the Hoffa fat pad.

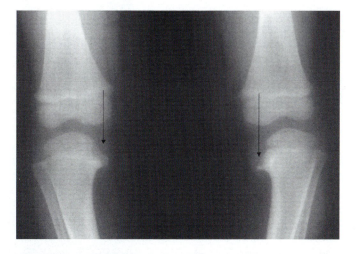

FIGURE 2-44. Blount disease. At age 4 years, there is a growth disturbance of the medial metaphyses and epiphyses that is more severe in the left knee (arrows), with depression of the medial metaphyses and resultant tibia vara.

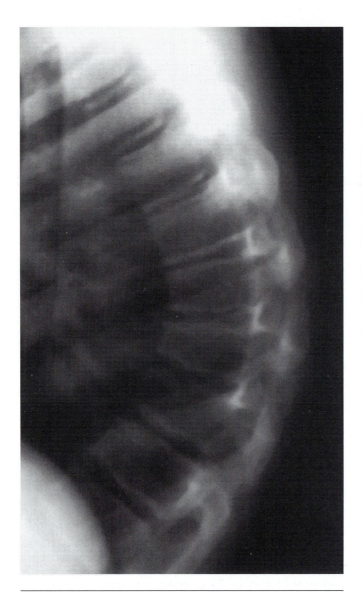

FIGURE 2-45. Scheuermann disease with accentuation of the thoracic kyphosis, anterior wedging of vertebrae with irregularity of the endplates, Schmorl nodes, and disk space narrowing.

FIGURE 2-46. Panner disease of the elbow in a child with sclerosis and subchondral lucency in the capitellum of the humerus (arrow).

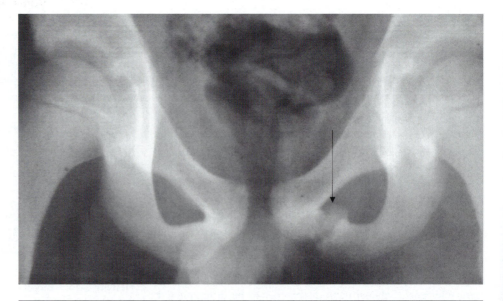

FIGURE 2-47. Asymmetry in the ischiopubic synchondrosis, with the right fused and the left incompletely fused (arrow).

Sever Disease

Sever disease is the term used for the clinical finding of a painful calcaneal apophysis consisting of inflammation of the calcaneal apophysis with posterior heel pain and swelling. It is most frequent in boys ages 10 to 12 years and is made worse by running or jumping. The diagnosis cannot be made radiographically. The radiographic findings of increased density, fragmentation, and irregularity of the calcaneal apophysis are in fact the normal appearance of the apophysis.

Panner Disease

Panner disease affects the capitellum of the elbow, with fragmentation and sometimes subchondral lucency, but without collapse (Figure 2-46). There is localized pain and tenderness, and it occurs mainly in boys ages 5 to 10 years. It is self-limited, with restitution of the normal appearance with no residual abnormality. It is due most likely to ON, but the exact etiology is unknown. It is analogous to Legg-Perthes disease of the hip and should be differentiated from OCD of the capitellum, which occurs in adolescent athletes with a fully ossified capitellar apophysis due to repetitive microtrauma and often leads to residual deformity and arthritic disease.

Van Neck Disease

Van Neck disease was described as an irregular bubbly appearance of the ischiopubic synchondrosis but is actually a normal variant in ossification that occurs before fusion of the synchondrosis. The age of fusion of the synchondrosis varies and one side may fuse before the opposite (Figure 2-47). The synchondrosis may even fuse and reopen. It is not associated with clinical symptoms.

Other Osteochondroses

Sinding-Larsen-Johansson disease describes fragmentation and pain at the secondary ossification center of the inferior pole of the patella (Figure 2-48). It is most likely an avulsion injury of the proximal aspect of the patellar tendon. It occurs in adolescents. Patients with cerebral palsy may have this condition due to spastic paralysis of the quadriceps muscle.

Friedrich disease affects the medial aspect of the clavicle at the sternoclavicular joint. It occurs mainly in young and middle-age women and most likely is due to chronic trauma.

Calve disease is vertebra plana (Figure 2-49). The most common cause is Langerhans cell histiocytosis (eosinophilic granuloma) and occurs mainly in children.

Kümmel disease is ON of the vertebral body after trauma. The vertebral body is collapsed and has intraosseous vacuum phenomenon (Figure 2-50).

Preiser disease is sclerosis and collapse of the carpal scaphoid without a history of prior fracture or underlying condition or corticosteroid use. It is most likely due to ON.

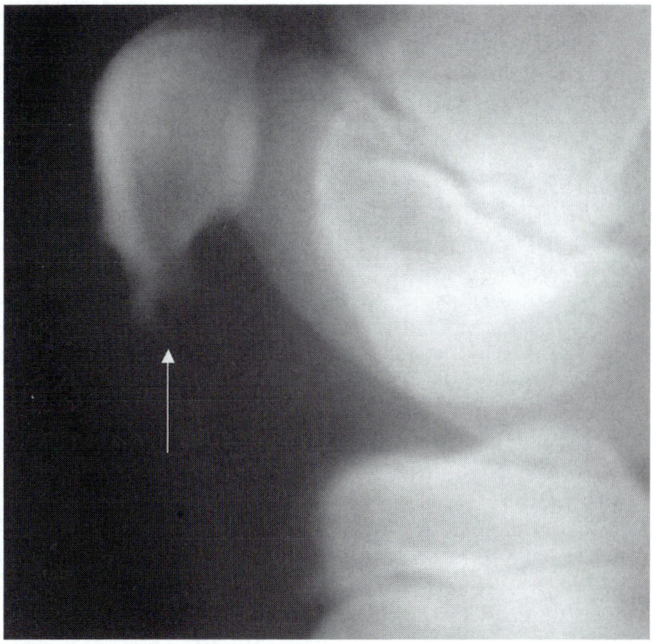

FIGURE 2-48. There is deformity of the inferior aspect of the patella at the insertion of the patella tendon (arrow), representing Sinding-Larsen-Johansson disease.

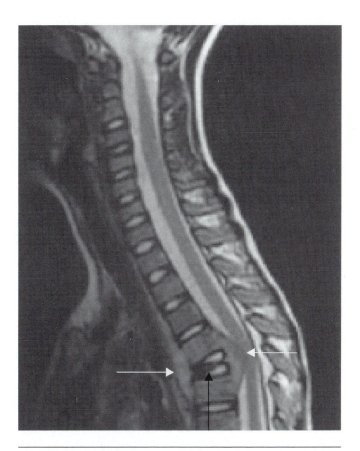

FIGURE 2-49. Vertebra plana of T5 due to Langerhans cell histiocytosis. Sagittal T_2-weighted magnetic resonance image shows a flattened T5 vertebral body (black arrow), with a para spinal soft tissue mass (white arrows) compressing the thecal sac and spinal cord.

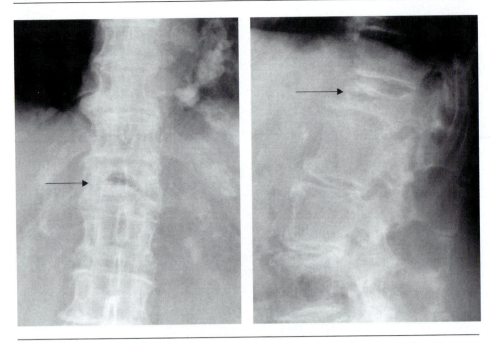

FIGURE 2-50. Kümmel disease. Radiographs show a compression fracture of L1, with gas or "vacuum phenomenon" in the vertebral body (arrows).

Thiemann disease affects the epiphyses of the middle phalanges, most frequently in the third finger, but may also involve other fingers symmetrically. It is most likely due to ON.

SUGGESTED READINGS

Arlet J. Nontraumatic avascular necrosis of the femoral head. Past, present, and future. *Clin Orthop.* 1992;277:12–21.

Beltran J, Knight CT, Zuelzer WA, et al. Core decompression for avascular necrosis of the femoral head: correlation between long-term results and preoperative MR staging. *Radiology.* 1990;175:533–536.

Borges JL, Guille JT, Bowen JR. Kohler's bone disease of the tarsal navicular. *J Pediatr Orthop.* 1995;15:596–598.

Brower AC. The osteochondroses. *Orthop Clin North Am.* 1983;14:99–117.

Chang CC, Greenspan A, Gershwin ME. Osteonecrosis: current perspectives on pathogenesis and treatment. *Semin Arthritis Rheum.* 1993;23:47–69.

Davids JR, Blackhurst DW, Allen BL Jr. Radiographic evaluation of bowed legs in children. *J Pediatr Orthop.* 2001;21:257–263.

De Smet AA, Ilahi OA, Graf BK. Untreated osteochondritis dissecans of the femoral condyles: prediction of patient outcome using radiographic and MR findings. *Skeletal Radiol.* 1997;26:463–467.

Dihlmann W. CT analysis of the upper end of the femur: the asterisk sign and ischaemic bone necrosis of the femoral head. *Skeletal Radiol.* 1982;8:251–258.

Douglas G, Rang M. The role of trauma in the pathogenesis of the osteochondroses. *Clin Orthop.* 1981;158:28–32.

Duda SH, Laniado M, Schick F, Claussen CD. The double-line sign of osteonecrosis: evaluation on chemical shift MR images. *Eur J Radiol.* 1993;16:233–238.

Forst J, Forst R, Heller KD, Adam G. Spontaneous osteonecrosis of the femoral condyle: causal treatment by early core decompression. *Arch Orthop Trauma Surg.* 1998;117:18–22.

Froberg PK, Braunstein EM, Buckwalter KA. Osteonecrosis, transient osteoporosis, and transient bone marrow edema: current concepts. *Radiol Clin North Am.* 1996;34:273–291.

Goffin E, vande Berg B, Pirson Y, Malghem J, Maldague B, van Ypersele de Strihou C. Epiphyseal impaction as a cause of severe osteoarticular pain of lower limbs after renal transplantation. *Kidney Int.* 1993;44:98–106.

Goldfarb CA, Hsu J, Gelberman RH, Boyer MI. The Lichtman classification for Kienbock's disease: an assessment of reliability. *J Hand Surg [Am].* 2003;28:74–80.

Guerra JJ, Steinberg ME. Distinguishing transient osteoporosis from avascular necrosis of the hip. *J Bone Joint Surg Am.* 1995;77:616–624.

Hayes CW, Conway WF, Daniel WW. MR imaging of bone marrow edema pattern: transient osteoporosis, transient bone marrow edema syndrome, or osteonecrosis. *Radiographics.* 1993;13: 1001–1012.

Hernigou P, Lambotte JC. Volumetric analysis of osteonecrosis of the femur. Anatomical correlation using MRI. *J Bone Joint Surg [Br].* 2001;83:672–675.

Holman AJ, Gardner GC, Richardson ML, Simkin PA. Quantitative magnetic resonance imaging predicts clinical outcome of core decompression for osteonecrosis of the femoral head. *J Rheumatol.* 1995;22:1929–1933.

Kawasaki M, Hasegawa Y, Sakano S, et al. Prediction of osteonecrosis by magnetic resonance imaging after femoral neck fractures. *Clin Orthop.* 2001;385:157–164.

Kim YM, Ahn JH, Kang HS, Kim HJ. Estimation of the extent of osteonecrosis of the femoral head using MRI. *J Bone Joint Surg [Br].* 1998;80:954–958.

Kim YM, Oh HC, Kim HJ. The pattern of bone marrow oedema on MRI in osteonecrosis of the femoral head. *J Bone Joint Surg [Br].* 2000;82:837–841.

Koo KH, Kim R. Quantifying the extent of osteonecrosis of the femoral head. A new method using MRI. *J Bone Joint Surg [Br].* 1995;77:875–880.

Koo KH, Ahn IO, Kim R, et al. Bone marrow edema and associated pain in early stage osteonecrosis of the femoral head: prospective study with serial MR images. *Radiology.* 1999;213:715–722.

Lavernia CJ, Sierra RJ, Grieco FR. Osteonecrosis of the femoral head. *J Am Acad Orthop Surg.* 1999;7:250–261.

Lecouvet FE, van de Berg BC, Maldague BE, et al. Early irreversible osteonecrosis versus transient lesions of the femoral condyles: prognostic value of subchondral bone and marrow changes on MR imaging. *AJR.* 1998;170:71–77.

Magid D, Fishman EK, Scott WW Jr, et al. Femoral head avascular necrosis: CT assessment with multiplanar reconstruction. *Radiology.* 1985;157:751–756.

Mitchell DG, Steinberg ME, Dalinka MK, Rao VM, Fallon M, Kressel HY. Magnetic resonance imaging of the ischemic hip. Alterations within the osteonecrotic, viable, and reactive zones. *Clin Orthop.* 1989;244:60–77.

Mont MA, Hungerford DS. Non-traumatic avascular necrosis of the femoral head. *J Bone Joint Surg [Am].* 1995;77:459–474.

Murray PM, Weinstein SL, Spratt KF. The natural history and long-term follow-up of Scheuermann kyphosis. *J Bone Joint Surg [Am].* 1993;75:236–248.

Ohzono K, Saito M, Sugano N, Takaoka K, Ono K. The fate of non-traumatic avascular necrosis of the femoral head. A radiologic classification to formulate prognosis. *Clin Orthop.* 1992;277:73–78.

Patel DV, Breazeale NM, Behr CT, Warren RF, Wickiewicz TL, O'Brien SJ. Osteonecrosis of the knee: current clinical concepts. *Knee Surg Sports Traumatol Arthrosc.* 1998;6:2–11.

Plakseychuk AY, Shah M, Varitimidis SE, Rubash HE, Sotereanos D. Classification of osteonecrosis of the femoral head. Reliability, reproducibility, and prognostic value. *Clin Orthop.* 2001;386:34–41.

Plancher KD, Razi A. Management of osteonecrosis of the femoral head. *Orthop Clin North Am.* 1997;28:461–477.

Plenk H Jr, Gstettner M, Grossschmidt K, Breitenseher M, Urban M, Hofmann S. Magnetic resonance imaging and histology of repair in femoral head osteonecrosis. *Clin Orthop.* 2001;386:42–53.

Resnick D. Osteochondroses. In: Resnick D, ed. *Diagnosis of Bone and Joint Disorders.* Philadelphia: WB Saunders, 2002:3686–3741.

Resnick D, Sweet D, Madewell J. Osteonecrosis: pathogenesis, diagnostic techniques, specific situations, and complications. In: Resnick D, ed. *Diagnosis of Bone and Joint Disorders.* Philadelphia: WB Saunders, 2002:3599–3685.

Ryu JS, Kim JS, Moon DH, et al. Bone SPECT is more sensitive than MRI in the detection of early osteonecrosis of the femoral head after renal transplantation. *J Nucl Med.* 2002;43:1006–1011.

Shimizu K, Moriya H, Akita T, Sakamoto M, Suguro T. Prediction of collapse with magnetic resonance imaging of avascular necrosis of the femoral head. *J Bone Joint Surg [Am].* 1994;76:215–223.

Steinberg ME, Hayken GD, Steinberg DR. A quantitative system for staging avascular necrosis. *J Bone Joint Surg [Br].* 1995; 77:34–41.

Sugano N, Takaoka K, Ohzono K, Matsui M, Masuhara K, Ono K. Prognostication of nontraumatic avascular necrosis of the femoral head. Significance of location and size of the necrotic lesion. *Clin Orthop.* 1994;303:155–164.

Theodorou DJ, Malizos KN, Beris AE, Theodorou SJ, Soucacos PN. Multimodal imaging quantitation of the lesion size in osteonecrosis of the femoral head. *Clin Orthop.* 2001;386:54–63.

Urbaniak J, Jones J, eds. *Osteonecrosis—Etiology, Diagnosis, and Treatment.* Chicago: American Academy of Orthopaedic Surgeons, 1997.

Vande Berg BC, Malghem J, Goffin EJ, Duprez TP, Maldague BE. Transient epiphyseal lesions in renal transplant recipients: presumed insufficiency stress fractures. *Radiology.* 1994;191:403–407.

Vande Berg BC, Malghem J, Lecouvet FE, Maldague B. Magnetic resonance imaging and differential diagnosis of epiphyseal osteonecrosis. *Semin Musculoskelet Radiol.* 2001;5:57–67.

Williams JS Jr, Bush-Joseph CA, Bach BR Jr. Osteochondritis dissecans of the knee. *Am J Knee Surg.* 1998;11:221–232.

Yamamoto T, Bullough PG. Spontaneous osteonecrosis of the knee: the result of subchondral insufficiency fracture. *J Bone Joint Surg [Am].* 2000;82:858–866.

Yamamoto T, Kubo T, Hirasawa Y, Noguchi Y, Iwamoto Y, Sueishi K. A clinicopathologic study of transient osteoporosis of the hip. *Skeletal Radiol.* 1999;28:621–627.

Zizic TM. Osteonecrosis. *Curr Opin Rheumatol.* 1991;3:481–489.

CHAPTER 3

ARTHRITIS

WILLIAM MORRISON / JOHN CARRINO

Descriptions of joint maladies date back to the days of Hippocrates, and manifestations of arthritis have been detected in skeletons of prehistoric humans. However, historical descriptions of arthritis and theories of their cause were often fanciful, lacking scientific substance. For example, as late as the 1500s it was thought that "rheumatic phlegm" was responsible for causing joint disease when it flowed from the brain to the extremities. Maladies of the joints were commonly referred to under the nonspecific blanket term "rheumatism" or were attributed to "the gout." This confounds efforts to track separate diseases through history. Attempts to more accurately classify arthritides were not made until the 17th and 18th centuries, as clinical diagnosis improved. In the 20th century, the advent of radiography had a major impact on diagnosis and characterization of the arthritides.

Arthritis is a broad topic; diseases of many categories have articular manifestations. Articular findings on radiographs may represent the early presentation of a clinically silent process, may aid the characterization of a clinically suspected process, or may represent an articular manifestation of a known disease process.

Despite the development of more advanced imaging modalities, radiologic analysis of arthritis remains based primarily on radiographic findings, in association with a thorough history and physical examination, coupled with serologic evaluation and occasionally joint fluid analysis. A thorough knowledge of arthritides and arthropathies is essential for the general radiologist and sub-specialist alike, as questions about arthritis are literally a daily occurrence in clinical practice.

ARTICULAR ANATOMY

The three basic types of anatomic joints are fibrous, cartilaginous, and synovial. Nonanatomic joints include pseudarthroses and coalitions.

In a fibrous articulation, the bones are joined by fibrous tissue. Some examples are the cranial sutures and the tibiofibular syndesmosis. In cartilaginous articulations, cartilage connects the bones. The cartilage can be hyaline, fibrocartilage, or a combination of both. The pubic symphysis and intervertebral discs are cartilaginous joints. A synchondrosis has intervening hyaline cartilage; an example is the physeal growth plate.

A pseudarthrosis is an anomalous joint occurring where there should be a more fixed articulation or no articulation at all. This is most commonly associated with a fracture that does not heal with osseous bridging, with continued motion at the junction. The other form of pseudarthrosis occurs at an anatomic syndesmosis, such as the os trigonum and bipartite, or multipartite, variations of bones, such as occur at the patella. These junctions are normally composed of fibrous tissue; chronic or acute stress can break the fibrous connection and form a mobile articulation that can undergo osteoarthritic change.

Coalitions are abnormal connections between bones; there may be solid osseous fusion between the bones or there may be intervening fibrous or cartilaginous tissue. Common areas involved include calcaneonavicular and subtalar coalitions in the ankle, lunate-triquetrum coalition in the wrist, and vertebral body fusion, especially in the cervical spine.

Joints also can be subdivided in terms of the degree of motion allowed by the articulation. The three groups are (*a*) synarthroses, in which there is no motion normally (eg, the cranial sutures); (*b*) amphiarthroses, which have flexible fibrous or cartilaginous intervening tissue serving a "cushioning" function (eg, intervertebral discs and pubic symphysis); and (*c*) diarthrodial joints, which allow a wide range of motion. Diarthrodial joints are also called *synovial joints*; they are the main focus of this chapter and are reviewed in detail.

Diarthrodial joints exist in a wide variety of types suited to their function. Sliding-type joints, such as spinal facets, allow smooth flexion, extension, and rotation of the spine. Hinge-type joints (historically referred to as a *ginglymus*) allow the majority of motion in one plane; limited motion in other directions enhances stability of these joints (eg, the ankle joint). Ball-cup–type joints allow for a large range of motion in multiple directions, as in the hip and glenohumeral joints. Other joints are combinations of these basic structures, in particular the elbow joint, which acts as a hinge joint at the ulnar-trochlear articulation but allows for a great degree of rotation of the hand because of the ball-cup configuration of the radiocapitellar articulation. At the knee there is also a complex articulation that includes a sliding-type articulation at the patellofemoral articulation and a flattened hinge-type articulation at the tibiofemoral joint that allows slight rotation. The sacroiliac joint is an interesting articulation because it functions as an amphiarthrosis with only mild flexibility allowed, yet has a synovial portion at its anteroinferior aspect. It is a combination joint with fibrous connections at its posterosuperior aspect (Figure 3-1).

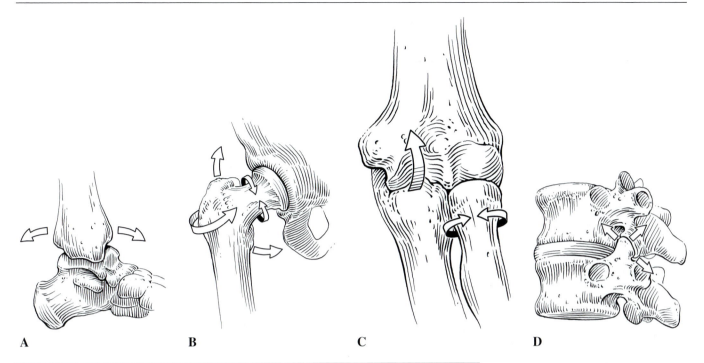

FIGURE 3-1. Different diarthrodial joint configurations. *(A)* Ankle: a hinge-type joint. *(B)* Hip: a ball/cup-type joint. *(C)* Elbow: a combination hinge and ball-cup. *(D)* Facet (zygapophyseal): a sliding-type joint.

STRUCTURE OF SYNOVIAL JOINTS

Synovial joints are composed of a capsule lined by a thin synovial membrane surrounding the articular surfaces that are covered with hyaline cartilage (Figure 3-2).

The capsule is composed of fibrous tissue that joins tightly with the periosteum of bone at the joint margin. The capsule restricts some of the range of motion of the joint, thus providing stability; joint capsules often contain focal bands of relative thickening that further stabilize the joint. For example, the glenohumeral ligaments of the shoulder are *condensations*, or linear strips of thickening of the joint capsule.

The capsule is lined with a thin membrane called the *synovium*. The synovium has an inner layer of specialized cells (normally just a few cells thick) surrounded by a sub-intima composed of loose areolar tissue, lymphatic channels, and a rich capillary plexus. The synovium projects into the joint as microscopic villi that greatly increase the surface area of the lining. These villi and the synovium in general become thickened and enlarged in chronic inflammation or injury.

The synovium performs a variety of important functions. The articular cartilage is avascular and derives its nutrients from the synovial fluid, which is in part a dialysate of plasma secreted from the subintimal capillary network within the synovial lining. The synovium also secretes a mucinous material into the joint, which, in conjunction with a physiologic amount of fluid, acts as a lubricant to allow a relatively frictionless gliding motion between articular surfaces. The synovium also serves a phagocytic function by clearing debris and dead cells from the synovial fluid.

The synovium attaches to the margins of the joint adjacent to the edge of the articular cartilage, called the *bare area* because

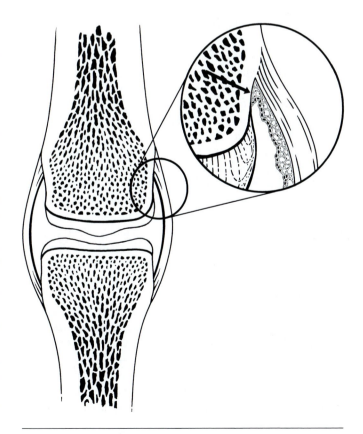

FIGURE 3-2. Structure of a synovial joint. Blow-up shows the "bare area," between the capsule and articular cartilage (arrow).

the cortical bone in this location is devoid of overlying protective articular cartilage and periosteum. This area is important because it is the site of early "marginal" erosions resulting from synovial proliferation related to inflammatory arthropathies.

Cartilage exists in two forms, hyaline cartilage and fibrocartilage. Hyaline cartilage coats the articular surfaces of synovial joints, thereby providing a smooth surface for efficient articular motion. It also provides a shock-absorbing quality for the joint against axial loading and shearing forces. This quality is a result of the complex structure of hyaline cartilage; collagen microfibrils within the cartilage are arranged in a curved lattice pattern, vertically oriented at the junction with subchondral bone, curving to become parallel to the cartilage surface. These microfibrils are surrounded by a background of chondrocytes and mucopolysaccharides, in particular chondroitin sulfate. Hyaline cartilage is highly hydrated, composed of 60 to 80% water; however, water content decreases later in life, which predisposes to injury and degeneration due to loss of the shock-absorbing function.

Hyaline cartilage is avascular; it derives nutrients from the synovial fluid, the transport of which are facilitated by pumping action during use of the joint. In fact, patients with paralysis may experience cartilage loss in the affected extremities due in part to diminished cartilage nutrition. Cartilage thickness varies depending on the joint; the thickest cartilage in the body is in the patellofemoral joint, where the cartilage is normally up to 5 or even 7 mm thick.

The other type of cartilage is fibrocartilage. In some joints, including the temporomandibular joint and the triangular fibrocartilage of the wrist, the sternoclavicular joint, and the acromioclavicular joint, the fibrocartilage exists as a disc within the joint. These discs primarily provide shock absorption and force distribution, but in some joints the disc may also facilitate motion. This is particularly seen in the temporomandibular joint, in which the disc translates forward as the jaw is opened, and, to a lesser extent, the menisci of the knee. The intervertebral discs are also composed partly of fibrocartilage surrounded by dense collagen fibers, together known as the *anulus fibrosis*, with a central core of gelatinous material called the *nucleus pulposus*.

Fibrocartilage appears in other joints as a wedge-shape structure attached to the margin of the joint, as in the menisci of the knee and the labrum of the shoulder and acetabulum. These structures provide not only shock absorption and distribution of forces (especially in the knee) but also stability. Stability is an important function of the glenoid labrum in particular, because the glenohumeral joint is inherently unstable. The fibrocartilaginous labrum lines the rim of the osseous glenoid like an O-ring, which increases the surface area of the articulation. This may also provide a small suction effect, thus keeping the humeral head in place. The dense collagenous structure and low water content of these structures result in the magnetic resonance imaging (MRI) appearance of low signal intensity on T_1-weighted (T1W) and T_2-weighted (T2W) images. These fibrocartilaginous discs, menisci, and labra are avascular and, when torn, generally there is no healing potential except at the periphery, where some vascularity is present.

Other structures in or adjacent to joints are fat pads, ligaments, tendons, sesamoid bones, and bursae. Fat pads help cushion

joints; they may be intracapsular or extracapsular. Radiographically, they are important because their displacement away from the joint can be helpful in diagnosis of joint effusion or synovial proliferation.

Ligaments are strong and relatively inelastic and are composed of collagen fibers that help stabilize joints. They can be inside the joint (such as the anterior and posterior cruciate ligaments of the knee), part of the capsule itself (as in the glenohumeral ligaments of the shoulder, which are bands of capsular thickening), or outside the capsule (eg, the collateral ligaments of the knee). Some tendons are also incorporated into the capsule; this allows fluid from the joint to extend into the tendon sheath. The best example is the long head of the biceps tendon, which originates from the superior glenoid labrum and extends through the shoulder joint adjacent to the humeral head before it turns 90° to enter the bicipital groove between the greater and lesser tuberosities. Other tendons, such as the popliteus tendon of the posterolateral knee and the flexor hallucis longus tendon of the ankle, pass by joints and their sheathes may communicate with the associated joints.

Sesamoid bones are often incorporated into the capsule, as are the tibial and fibular sesamoids of the first metatarsophalangeal joint; when associated with joints, sesamoid bones are covered on the articular side with hyaline cartilage and undergo similar arthritic changes as the rest of the joint.

Bursae mainly function as "pads" that cushion areas undergoing chronic stress from friction, although some are merely potential spaces in which fluid can collect in trauma or inflammation. The majority are anatomic structures that are normally present, usually in areas of expected stress (eg, the olecranon bursa of the elbow); others, called *adventitial* bursae, are not normally present but form in response to unusual stresses (eg, bursae occurring over an exostosis or a large accessory navicular).

ORIGIN OF RADIOGRAPHIC FINDINGS OBSERVED IN VARIOUS ARTHRITIC PROCESSES AND RADIOGRAPHIC APPROACH

When reviewing radiographs of patients with suspected arthritis, it is useful to go through a checklist of findings before verbalizing a differential diagnosis (Tables 3-1 and 3-2). This serves a number of functions: it aids identification of all pertinent findings; it organizes and standardizes thought patterns, which aids formulation of a differential diagnosis; and it communicates to

TABLE 3-1

Basic Radiographic Approach to Arthritis

Soft tissues
Mineralization
Joint space/subchondral bone
Erosions
Proliferation
Deformity
Distribution

TABLE 3-2

Arthritis and Gender

Arthritides more common in
    Males
        Gout
        Ankylosing spondylitis
        Reiter disease
    Females
        Rheumatoid arthritis
        Connective tissue disease
    Same
        Osteoarthritis
        Psoriasis

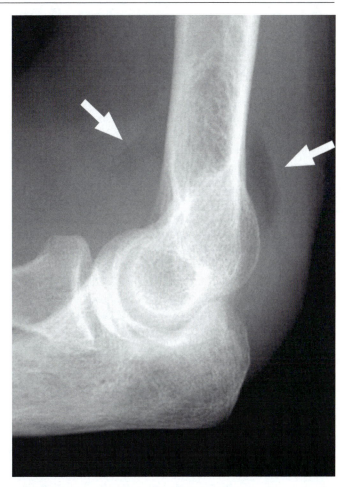

FIGURE 3-3. Joint effusion. Lateral radiograph of the elbow of a patient with a large effusion shows displacement of the anterior and posterior fat pads (arrows).

the clinician or reviewer that a differential has been arrived at by using logic rather than luck or instinct. A standard approach such as that popularized by Brower, Resnick, and others involves evaluation of the soft tissues, bone mineralization, the joint and subchondral bone, erosions, proliferation, deformity, and distribution of disease. These categories are discussed separately with regard to abnormalities seen in different disease processes and the etiology of these findings.

Soft Tissues

EFFUSION/SYNOVIAL PROLIFERATION. Effusion is a common finding in many of the arthritides, not only in the inflammatory arthropathies but also commonly in joints with osteoarthritis. Effusions in some joints are detectable radiographically by displacement of periarticular fat planes or by asymmetric widening of the joint. Some examples are the elbow joint, in which displacement of the anterior fat pad (the "sail sign") or visualization of the posterior fat pad (normally "hidden" from view within the olecranon fossa) on the lateral view indicates a joint effusion (Figure 3-3); the hip joint, in which an effusion may be seen as asymmetric widening of the medial joint (a finding less useful in the adult population, in whom there may be asymmetric joint narrowing from cartilage loss simulating an effusion on the other side) or asymmetric bowing of the extracapsular fat planes (an unreliable sign in the hip); and the knee joint, in which soft tissue density in the region of the suprapatellar recess with separation of the suprapatellar fat from the pre-femoral fat indicates presence of an effusion.

Effusions in the joints of the digits present as fusiform, or band-like, swelling around the proximal interphalangeal joint (PIP) or distal interphalangeal joint (DIP) joints, a common finding in many of the inflammatory arthropathies and in septic arthritis. At the metacarpophalangeal joint (MCP) or metatarsophalangeal joint (MTP) joints, effusion may be seen radiographically as increased opacity over the joint on the anteroposterior view or dorsal soft tissue swelling on the lateral view. Effusion within the radiocarpal and midcarpal joints of the wrist is best seen on the lateral view as diffuse dorsal soft tissue swelling over the carpus.

One caveat in the radiographic diagnosis of a joint effusion is that synovitis or synovial thickening, such as in rheumatoid

arthritis or pigmented villonodular synovitis, may look similar.

Classically, psoriatic arthritis and Reiter disease have diffuse swelling of one or more digits ("sausage digit") that generally represents a combination of tenosynovitis, joint effusion, and subcutaneous edema.

BURSITIS. Bursitis can be mechanical or inflammatory. Mechanical bursitis is seen in areas of chronic friction or pressure; the classic example is olecranon bursitis, which can result from excessive leaning on the elbows. The eponym for mechanical olecranon bursitis is "student's elbow" or "plumber's elbow." Mechanical bursitis is also common in the foot due to poorly fitting footwear or foot deformities.

Because bursae are synovial-lined structures similar to joints, inflammatory bursitis occurs in a number of synovial-based disorders. In rheumatoid arthritis and seronegative spondyloarthropathy, bursae can become enlarged, filled with fluid, and proliferative inflammatory synovial tissue. This process can cause erosion of the adjacent bone. Inflammatory bursitis also may be associated with crystalline disorders, classically gout and calcific bursitis (also called *hydroxyapatite deposition disease,* or HADD). These inflammatory processes also have a predilection for areas of friction, especially the olecranon bursa and the foot, in particular the retrocalcaneal bursa, although bursae anywhere may become involved. Calcific bursitis has a different distribution, most commonly affecting the subacromial/subdeltoid bursa of the shoulder, a result of rupture of hydroxyapatite (HA) crystal deposits within the rotator cuff tendons into the adjacent bursa, with subsequent acute inflammation of the bursa. Inflammatory and mechanical forms of bursitis are susceptible to superimposed infection.

SOFT TISSUE CALCIFICATION.   Certain patterns of soft tissue calcification are associated with arthropathies. HA deposition can occur in bursae and within tendons and around joint capsules. HADD rarely appears within joints, but can cause an acute, destructive arthropathy resembling neuropathic disease or an aggressive infection. Vascular calcifications are commonly seen in extremities of diabetic patients in whom neuropathic osteoarthropathy may occur. In chronic renal failure, periarticular deposition of calcium salts, called *tumoral calcinosis*, may be present in addition to vascular calcification. Dense, coarse deposits of HA are seen in the soft tissues of the distal extremities in lupus (associated with joint subluxation) and in scleroderma (which can be associated with a rheumatoid-like pattern of disease in the hands and wrists). In scleroderma, the soft tissues of the distal digits often become thinned and superimposed on acroosteolysis, which is referred to as a "whittled" or "pencilled" appearance of the digit. Longitudinally oriented linear calcification of peripheral nerves has been described in leprosy, which causes a mutilating neuropathic disorder in the affected extremity.

SOFT TISSUE MASSES.   Soft tissue masses of various etiologies can be seen in association with different arthritides; in rheumatoid arthritis, rheumatoid nodules (inflammatory granulomatous subcutaneous lesions) can be seen, especially in the hands and other areas exposed to increased friction, such as the elbows and feet. Gouty tophi also form in the hands and feet in patients with chronic gout, predominantly in those who do not seek medical care until late in the disease, as these tophi take years to form. Tophi and rheumatoid nodules do not commonly calcify, although they may be of relatively high radiographic density. Sarcoidosis also can present with focal soft tissue masses in the digits and are commonly associated with the classic radiographic appearance of a "lacy" trabecular pattern in the middle and distal phalanges of the affected digits, often with cortical destruction or erosion. Focal soft tissue prominence associated with arthritis also may be caused by ganglia or synovial cysts, which can extend from joints or tendon sheaths in osteoarthritis or chronic inflammatory arthropathies.

Mineralization

Demineralization, or osteopenia, is viewed on radiographs as decreased density of bone that begins as loss of trabeculae followed by cortical thinning. Periarticular osteopenia is a classic

characteristic of rheumatoid arthritis, in which synovial hyperemia and decreased use of the affected joints causes bone resorption; this can be an early finding in the disease process. However, the appearance of periarticular osteopenia is nonspecific; it can be seen in other conditions resulting in temporary immobilization of the extremity and in reflex sympathetic dystrophy and can be simulated by suboptimal radiographic technique.

Diffuse osteopenia is seen in elderly patients with osteoporosis, which may be superimposed on various arthropathies seen in this population. Paralysis also results in osteopenia, and cartilage loss can occur in affected joints due to cartilage malnutrition. Various medications also can cause diffuse osteopenia, including steroids that are often included in treatment regimens for inflammatory arthropathies.

Increased bone density or preservation of density is one characteristic seen in joints affected by osteoarthritis and neuropathic osteoarthropathy. Preservation of bone density with destructive arthropathy is not specific to neuropathic disease and may be seen in psoriatic arthritis, Reiter disease, gout, and a variant of rheumatoid arthritis called *robust rheumatoid arthritis* (Table 3-3).

The Joint Space and Subchondral Bone

JOINT NARROWING.   Joint narrowing is due to cartilage thinning. Because the mechanism of cartilage loss is different in different types of arthritis, the pattern of joint narrowing can be

TABLE 3-3

Mineralization

Osteopenia
    Diffuse
        Osteoporosis
        Metabolic disease (osteomalacia, hyperparathyroidism)
        Medications (eg, steroids)
        Immobilization
    Periarticular
        Rheumatoid arthritis
        Juvenile chronic arthritis
        Septic arthritis
        Reflex sympathetic dystrophy
        Immobilization
        Reiter disease (early)
        Psoriatic arthritis (early)
Preservation of bone density with arthritis
    Nonerosive
        Osteoarthritis
        Calcium pyrophosphate dihydrate arthropathy
        Synovial osteochondromatosis (may cause scalloping)
    Erosive
        Erosive osteoarthritis
        "Robust" rheumatoid arthritis
        Neuropathic arthropathy
        Gout
        Reiter disease
        Psoriatic arthritis
        Pigmented villonodular synovitis (erosive in small capacity joints)
        Amyloid

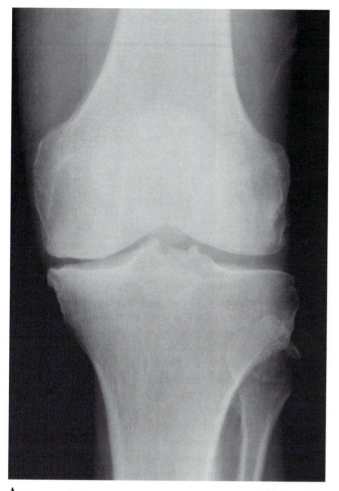 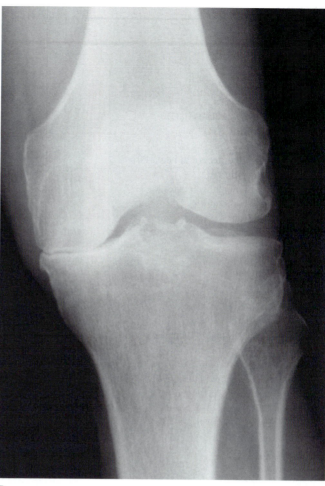

A   B

FIGURE 3-4.   Joint narrowing: importance of the weight-bearing view. Anteroposterior radiographs of the knee of the same patient obtained in supine position *(A)* and with weight bearing *(B)* show that loss of cartilage (seen here in the medial compartment) may be more apparent on the weight-bearing view.

very important in consideration of a differential diagnosis, especially when evaluating weight-bearing joints. In inflammatory arthropathies and septic arthritis, the joint narrowing is typically uniform, or "concentric." The classic appearance of joint narrowing in osteoarthritis is asymmetric, eg, at the superior aspect of the hips and the medial compartment of the knees. In the knees, chronic meniscal tears may contribute to asymmetric tibiofemoral joint narrowing. Joint narrowing of the knees may not be radiographically apparent without weight-bearing views (Figure 3-4 and Table 3-4).

CHONDROCALCINOSIS.   Chondrocalcinosis is radiographically visible mineralization of hyaline cartilage or fibrocartilage due to deposition of calcium pyrophosphate crystals; the knee is most commonly affected, and in the knee the fibrocartilaginous menisci are most commonly involved. Chondrocalcinosis is often observed on radiographs and has been reported with many conditions, but only osteoarthritis, gout, primary hyperparathyroidism, and hemochromatosis have firm associations. Crystalline arthritis related to intraarticular calcium pyrophos-

phate in the absence of these other conditions is called *pseudogout* or *calcium pyrophosphate dihydrate (CPPD) arthropathy*. Osteoarthritis in unusual locations (eg, glenohumeral, elbow, wrist, or isolated patellofemoral involvement of the knee) suggests CPPD arthropathy and a search for chondrocalcinosis in the affected joint and in other locations such as the symphysis pubis, hip, shoulder, and wrist should be made (Table 3-5).

THE SUBCHONDRAL WHITE LINE.   Subchondral bone is generally visualized radiographically as a thin white line. In various inflammatory arthritides, this white line can appear indistinct or even absent due to subtle erosive change, typically beginning at the bare area of bone adjacent to the margin of the articular cartilage. Another classic location for loss of this thin white line is at the sacroiliac joint. Early inflammatory arthropathies appear as loss of the distinctness of the normal thin subchondral line. Further involvement may lead to cartilage loss and erosions at the anteroinferior, synovial portion of the sacroiliac joint, causing a paradoxical appearance of joint widening. As

TABLE 3-6

Sacroiliac Joint Disease

Bilateral symmetric
  Ankylosing spondylitis
  Inflammatory bowel disease
  Osteitis condensans ilii (iliac side only)
Bilateral asymmetric
  Psoriatic arthritis
  Reiter disease
  Rheumatoid arthritis
  Osteoarthritis
Unilateral
  Infection
  Psoriatic arthritis
  Reiter disease
  Postoperative (from iliac bone graft donor site)
Pseudo-sacroiliitis
  Hyperparathyroidism (due to subarticular bone resorption)
  Adolescence (subchondral white line not well defined)
  Osteoarthritis (due to anterior bridging osteophytes)

intraarticular bodies are also seen in synovial osteochondromatosis, a condition in which metaplastic synovium forms cartilage that may mineralize. If the intraarticular bodies are of similar size and more numerous than expected for the degree of osteoarthritis in the joint, synovial osteochondromatosis should be considered, especially in a young adult with a monoarticular process. Degenerative bodies tend to be varied in size and shape. Multiple small fibrous bodies called *rice bodies* (because they resemble grains of rice) also can be seen in various inflammatory arthropathies, in particular rheumatoid arthritis.

These bodies have various appearances on MR images because they can be composed of many different substances: meniscal fragments are generally dark on T1W and T2W sequences; hyaline cartilage signal is partly dependent on its degree of hydration and sequence parameters but is generally intermediate on T1W and T2W images; calcifications within bodies can result in areas of low signal on T1W and T2W images, but, if ossified, the central signal follows that of fatty marrow, which is bright on T1W and dark to intermediate on T2W images (depending on fat suppression). The variable and often heterogeneous signal characteristics can make bodies difficult to detect on MR images. Presence of intraarticular fluid or gadolinium contrast surrounding the fragments optimizes detection. Computed tomography (CT) is also useful for evaluation of quantity, size, and location of calcified bodies; intraarticular administration of air or dilute iodinated contrast aids evaluation.

ANKYLOSIS. Ankylosis, or fusion of a joint, is the end stage of various, but usually inflammatory, processes; fusion is most commonly associated with juvenile chronic arthritis, ankylosing spondylitis (affecting the spine and sacroiliac joints), and psoriatic arthritis. It also can occur at the interphalangeal joints in erosive osteoarthritis and at the wrist in rheumatoid arthritis. Other causes include trauma, infection, frostbite, and thermal or electrical burns. Functional ankylosis due to osseous bridging around joints without actual obliteration of the joint space

itself also can occur about the hip in paralyzed people, after arthroplasty, and in fibrodysplasia ossificans progressiva, a heritable condition in which ligaments, tendons, and fascia ossify (Table 3-8).

Erosions

Erosions are associated with numerous processes, but location of erosions in the joint, distribution (which joints are affected), and margination of the erosions are useful features to differentiate various etiologies. Erosions can be central (articular surface), marginal (at the bare area next to the attachment of the synovial membrane), or periarticular (Figure 3-10, Tables 3-9, and 3-10).

CENTRAL EROSIONS. These erosions occur in the central aspect of the joint, in places typically covered by articular cartilage. Articular cartilage is usually protective against erosive processes, so central erosions are generally associated with severe overlying cartilage loss. The classic disorder associated with central erosive changes is erosive osteoarthritis, which typically involves the distal interphalangeal joints of the hands; however, central erosions also can be seen after severe cartilage loss in inflammatory and crystalline arthropathies. The classic radiographic appearance is marked joint narrowing associated with a central depression in the articular surface, an appearance that has been likened to the shape of a seagull in flight (Figures 3-11 and 3-12).

MARGINAL EROSIONS. Marginal erosions occur at the bare area, a rim of articular bone devoid of cartilage adjacent to the capsular insertion of the synovium (Figures 3-13 and 3-14). In inflammatory arthropathies, the proliferative synovium erodes the adjacent unprotected bone; early in the erosive process, the cortex at the marginal zone becomes indistinct. Later a more discrete erosion forms, which initially may have ill-defined margins. As the disease becomes quiescent or goes into remission, these erosions may develop a thin, sclerotic margin. If the disease progresses, more severe erosion of the articular surface can result in an "arthritis mutilans" pattern in which the articular surface becomes "pencilled" and "telescoped," or shortened, with the distal bone advancing into the proximal bone. Marginal erosions in seronegative spondyloarthropathy may have a proliferative quality, with a "fluffy" or "whiskered" appearance and adjacent periostitis (Figures 3-15 and 3-16).

Although septic arthritis is covered in Chapter 1, it is essential at this point to briefly discuss this topic, because it should be in the differential diagnosis of an erosive arthropathy. Early on, radiographs will show only a joint effusion or fusiform soft tissue swelling around the joint. The articular cartilage is a relative barrier to infection of the underlying bone, so osseous involvement will begin as marginal erosions at the bare area. As cells in the joint fluid release chondrolytic factors, the cartilage erodes and more uniform joint narrowing occurs (cartilage destruction is generally more rapid in bacterial infections than in tuberculous or fungal infections, which may preserve the articular cartilage until late in the disease course). Periarticular osteopenia may

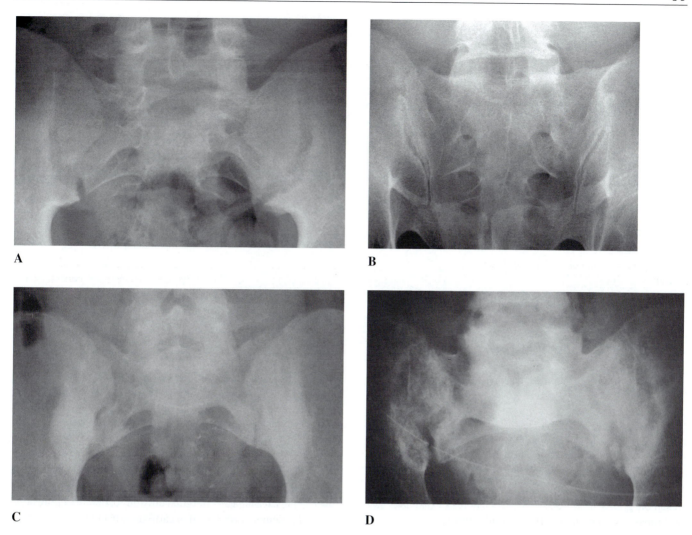

A

B

C

D

FIGURE 3-6. Sacroiliac joint pitfalls. *(A)* Radiograph of an adolescent showing normal absence of the subchondral line and false widening of the sacroiliac joint, which can be seen during development. *(B)* Radiograph of an elderly individual with osteoarthritis of the sacroiliac joints and bridging anterior osteophytes. Osteophytes and subchondral sclerosis blur the subchondral line and simulate joint fusion on the radiograph. *(C)* Radiograph of a female with osteitis condensans ilii, showing sclerosis on the iliac side of the joint. *(D)* Radiograph of a patient with chronic renal failure and secondary hyperparathyroidism, showing subchondral bone resorption at the sacroiliac joints.

occur at the affected joint due to hyperemia. When a monarticular joint effusion or fusiform periarticular swelling presents acutely in a nontraumatic setting, or erosive change is seen in a single joint, septic arthritis should be considered.

PERIARTICULAR EROSIONS. Periarticular erosions result from gouty tophi or other soft tissue masses outside the joint; they are often described as resembling a "rat bite," ie, a defect with a thin sclerotic rim and overhanging edges. However, this classic radiographic pattern of tophaceous gout is not as commonly seen as periodic acute gouty attacks due to intraarticular urate crystal formation. This more typical clinical presentation can lead to inflammatory marginal erosions and eventually to osteoarthritis in chronically affected joints (Figures 3-17 and 3-18).

Erosions also can occur in locations other than joints, such as at attachments (entheses) of tendons, ligaments and fascia, or adjacent to bursae. This may occur in patients with inflammatory

arthropathies such as psoriatic arthritis and Reiter disease. These disorders can cause an inflammatory enthesopathy or bursitis, both of which can erode the underlying bone. Characteristically, these erosions are proliferative in appearance, with ill-defined or fluffy margins (see Figure 3-18). Rheumatoid arthritis and gout less commonly affect the entheses but commonly cause an inflammatory bursitis, which can cause erosion of the underlying bone.

PITFALLS. Normal bone contours can simulate the appearance of erosions depending on patient positioning. A classic example of pseudoerosion is the normal notch at the base of the proximal phalanges of the hands; these notches are attachment sites for intrinsic muscles but often are interpreted as erosions. True erosions at the metacarpophalangeal joints are usually associated with some alteration of the joint space or surrounding soft tissue. Normal contours of the metacarpal and metatarsal

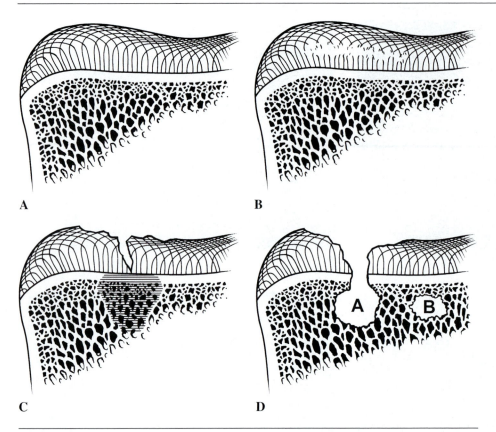

FIGURE 3-7. Articular cartilage degeneration. *(A)* Normal hyaline cartilage with network of microfibrils. These fibrils originate at right angles to the subchondral bone and curve to a horizontal orientation at the cartilage surface; they provide structural integrity and shock absorption. *(B)* Breakage of the microfibril network occurs early in the process of cartilage degeneration. *(C)* As cartilage degenerates, the surface becomes irregular, and fissures and defects develop. Joint fluid may enter the subchondral bone. *(D)* Cysts may form in the subchondral bone, which often communicate with the joint through fissures in cartilage (A). Cavitations may also occur in the subchondral bone, forming cysts which do not communicate with the joint (B).

Proliferation

OSTEOPHYTES AND ENTHESOPHYTES. Both osteophytes and enthesophytes (collectively called *spurs*) are osseous projections from the bones; osteophytes form at the margins of joints, whereas enthesophytes form at the entheses (attachment sites of tendons, ligaments, or fascia). Osteophytes follow hyaline cartilage loss or other internal joint derangement, such as ligament or fibrocartilage damage. These injuries alter the mechanics of the joint, causing clinical or subclinical instability that adds stress to the joint periphery; the underlying bone responds by forming osseous projections at the joint margins. This serves to increase the surface area of the articulation and buttress the margins, which may help improve stability for a time. A similar process can result in "cortical buttressing," which occurs as the joint degenerates and additional stresses are placed on the margins. The terminus of the periosteum responds by laying down new bone at the junction of the epiphysis and metaphysis, thus thickening the cortex; this process is observed most commonly at the hips and knees.

With continued abnormal stress, osteophytes slowly enlarge and

heads and of the carpal bones also can appear as areas of rarefaction simulating early erosions when viewed at certain obliquities.

In addition, scalloping of the cortex can occur from chronic mass effect from the soft tissues or adjacent periosteum; this can appear as a periarticular erosion. Some entities that can cause cortical scalloping are ganglion cyst, giant cell tumor of the tendon sheath (especially in the digits of the hands or feet), nerve sheath tumor, vascular malformation, and periosteal chondroma. Sarcoidosis also can result in periarticular cortical scalloping or frank cortical destruction, especially in the digits of the hand (middle and distal phalanges in particular), which may be associated with diffuse or focal soft tissue prominence; in general, when there is cortical scalloping or destruction, there is also underlying trabecular alteration with a lacy pattern that is characteristic of sarcoidosis.

Resorption of bone at the entheses, capsular attachments, and beneath the periosteum due to hyperparathyroid conditions also can simulate erosions. This resorption can be differentiated from inflammatory erosions by relative preservation of the joint space and other stigmata such as acroosteolysis, radial side subperiosteal location of bone resorption at the middle phalanges of the fingers, tumoral calcinosis, and vascular calcifications.

eventually may restrict range of joint motion, as in the elbow and ankle. They also may impinge on adjacent nerves, as at the neural foramina of the spine, where spurs from the facet joints, uncovertebral joints, or posterior endplates impinge the exiting nerve root or the spinal cord itself. A similar situation occurs in the elbow in throwing athletes who can form marginal osteophytes that can impinge on the ulnar nerve as it passes through the cubital tunnel.

Less commonly, osteophytes can form on the articular surface itself due to overlying hyaline cartilage injury; this can be seen as a flat, button-like projection of bone from the articular surface, or merely as irregularity of the articular surface. This form of osteophyte formation is especially common in the knee from cartilage loss in osteoarthritis or as a sequela of remote osteochondral impaction injury (eg, at the lateral femoral condyle with anterior cruciate ligament tear).

Enthesophytes result from chronic pull at sites of tendon, ligament, or fascial attachment and are usually asymptomatic. Some common examples are the calcaneal spurs at the insertion of the Achilles tendon and origin of the plantar fascia (the latter is often linked to clinical plantar fasciitis, yet most people with a spur in this location are asymptomatic). Enthesopathy (a nonspecific term for an abnormality of these sites of attachment) can result

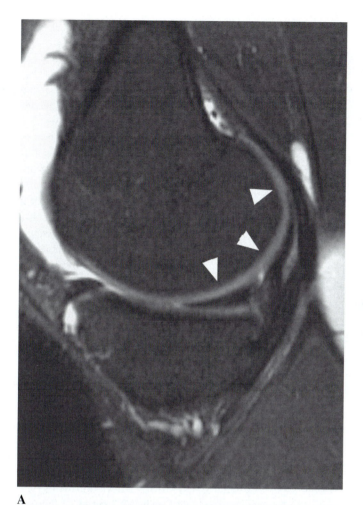

A

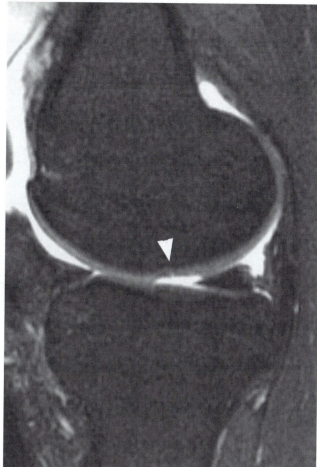

B

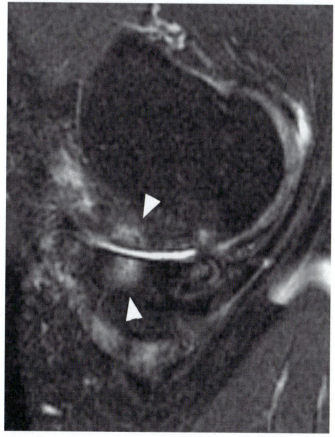

C

FIGURE 3-8. Cartilage degeneration. Sagittal T_2-weighted fat-suppressed fast spin echo images of the knee. Note low signal wedge-shape fibrocartilaginous menisci. *(A)* Normal hyaline cartilage (arrowheads). *(B)* Small partial-thickness cartilage defect with fissure (arrowhead). *(C)* Cartilage defect with formation of discrete subchondral cyst (arrowheads).

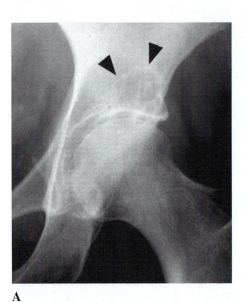

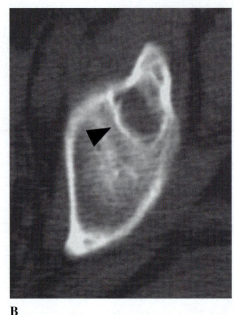

A   B

FIGURE 3-9. Subchondral cystic change: the supraacetabular cyst. *(A)* Anteroposterior radiograph shows osteoarthritis with superior hip joint narrowing and an acetabular cyst with a thin, sclerotic margin (arrowheads). *(B)* Computed tomography of the hip show a well-defined lucency at the superior acetabular margin with the sclerotic rim (arrowhead).

either from overuse, in entities such as lateral epicondylitis (also called "tennis elbow"), or from inflammation in seronegative spondyloarthropathy. Juxtaarticular periostitis also can be seen in proliferative inflammatory arthropathies, including psoriatic arthritis and Reiter disease.

PERIOSTITIS.   Periosteal thickening or "whiskering" of the periosteal margin adjacent to joints also can occur in seronegative spondyloarthropathy, especially in the digits in psoriatic arthritis and Reiter disease.

TABLE 3-7

Prominent Subchondral Cysts or Lucencies

Joint narrowed
  Nonuniform
    Primary osteoarthritis
    Secondary osteoarthritis (trauma)
    Calcium pyrophosphate dihydrate arthropathy
    Gout (late)
  Uniform
    Rheumatoid arthritis
    Secondary osteoarthritis (inflammatory arthropathy)
    Hemophilic arthropathy
Joint preserved
  Amyloidosis
  Tuberculous arthritis (early)
  Gout (early)
  Pigmented villonodular synovitis
  Synovial osteochondromatosis

Deformity

Various arthritides are associated with joint deformities, which include subluxation and dislocation, angulation (flexion and hyperextension or varus and valgus), instability, telescoping, and frank joint destruction. For example, joint subluxations that are easily reducible (in the absence of erosions), especially in the hands, is a classic characteristic of systemic lupus erythematosus (SLE) and Jaccoud arthropathy, a rare condition occurring in association with rheumatic fever. Subluxation and destructive changes describe a neuropathic joint, or arthritis mutilans, from severe involvement by inflammatory arthropathies, especially psoriatic arthritis. Subluxations, especially of the hands and feet, are also common in rheumatoid arthritis with more severe or chronic involvement.

Angular deformities at various joints are common in rheumatoid arthritis, especially in the digits, with ulnar deviation at the MCP joints and Boutonniere and swan neck deformities of the digits, which is discussed in more detail later. Varus or valgus angulation is also common in other arthropathies, in particular osteoarthritis, where asymmetric cartilage loss may occur (especially in the knee). Angular deformity of the interphalangeal joints is also common in osteoarthritis, but is most prominent in the inflammatory subgroup of the disease, erosive osteoarthritis (Table 3-11).

Distribution

A description of the distribution of affected joints is one of the most useful factors in generation of a differential diagnosis because many arthritides have a characteristic pattern of joint

TABLE 3-8

Joint Ankylosis

Juvenile chronic arthritis
Ankylosing spondylitis
Psoriatic arthritis
Reiter disease
Rheumatoid arthritis
Erosive osteoarthritis
Surgical fusion
Developmental coalition
Paralysis

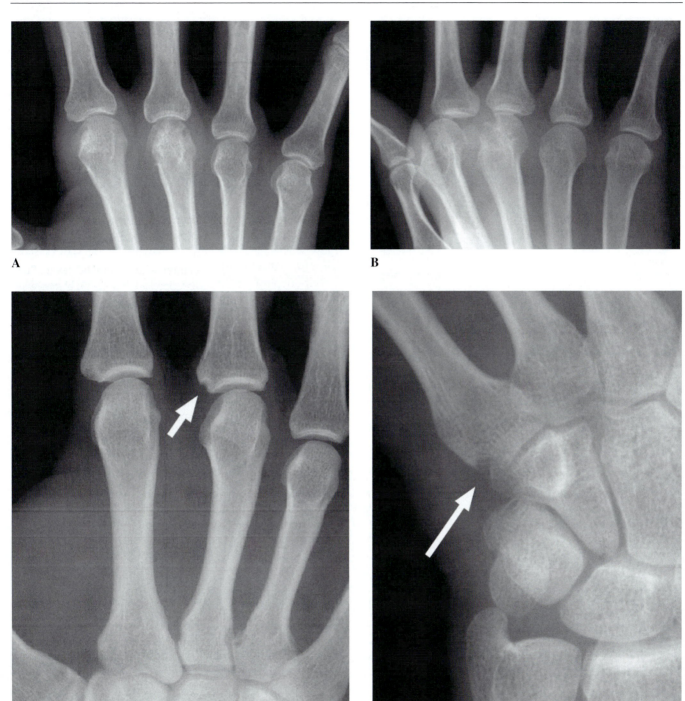

A

B

C

D

FIGURE 3-10.   Detection of erosions in the hand: the Norgaard view and pitfalls. *(A)* Anteroposterior and *(B)* Norgaard (reverse oblique) views of the metacarpophalangeal joints demonstrate improved visualization of erosions at the metacarpal heads on the Norgaard view. Also note soft tissue swelling and joint narrowing at the second and third metacarpophalangeal joints, with mild subluxation at the second metacarpophalangeal joint. *(C)* Anteroposterior view of the hand shows a classic "pseudoerosion" at the base of the proximal phalanx, an appearance caused by insertion of intrinsic muscles. Note the well-defined margin and absence of other manifestations of inflammatory arthropathy, as seen in A and B. *(D)* Anteroposterior view of the wrist shows another common site for a pseudoerosion, at the base of the fifth metacarpal.

TABLE 3-9

Arthritis with Erosions

Central
    Erosive osteoarthritis
    Thermal injury
    Psoriatic arthritis (late)
    Reiter disease (late)
Marginal
    Rheumatoid arthritis
    Psoriatic arthritis ("fuzzy")
    Reiter disease ("fuzzy")
    Gout
    Mixed connective tissue disease
    Multicentric reticulohistiocytosis
Periarticular
    Gout

TABLE 3-10

Arthritis without Erosions

Primary osteoarthritis
Secondary osteoarthritis not caused by inflammatory arthropathy
    (eg, trauma)
Calcium pyrophosphate dihydrate arthropathy
Acromegaly
Hemochromatosis
Jaccoud arthropathy
Systemic lupus erythematosus

in joints predisposed to minor trauma, such as the digits, elbows, and weight-bearing joints, especially the knees and ankles, and may be asymmetric. A monarticular arthropathy raises a separate differential that includes posttraumatic osteoarthritis, septic arthritis or postinfectious osteoarthritis, pigmented villonodular synovitis, and synovial osteochondromatosis (Tables 3-12 and 3-13).

APPROACH TO DISCUSSION OF AN ARTHRITIS CASE

As unknowns, in a clinical setting or in a case conference, arthritis cases can be a daunting experience because findings may be

involvement. Osteoarthritis of the hands, for example, characteristically involves the base of the thumb and the interphalangeal joints. Rheumatoid arthritis classically involves the carpus and MCPs in a bilaterally symmetric pattern. Reiter disease rarely involves the hands but does favor the foot. Psoriatic arthritis favors the digits of the hand. Hemochromatosis classically affects the second and third MCPs. Hemophilia is seen predominantly

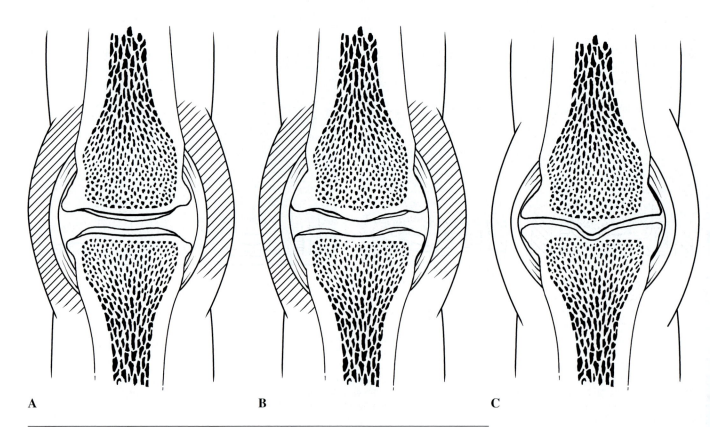

A   B   C

FIGURE 3-11.   Development of central erosions. *(A)* Early. Cartilage thinning is present, related to underlying osteoarthritis. Superimposed inflammation causes a joint effusion and results in fusiform soft tissue swelling around the joint. *(B)* A central depression begins to form in the articular surface. *(C)* Late. The central depression deepens, which along with marginal osteophytes, deform the articular surfaces into a "seagull" configuration. This pattern is typical of erosive osteoarthritis.

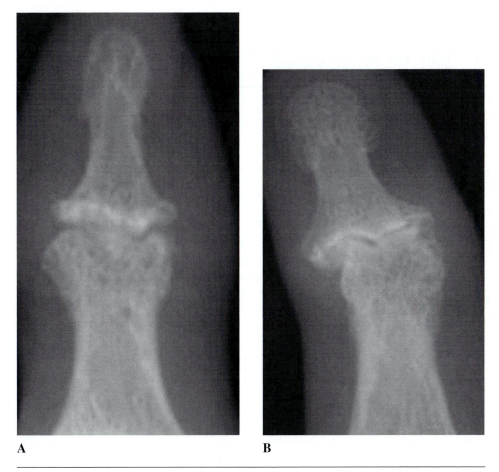

A   B

FIGURE 3-12. Progression of erosive disease: central erosions in erosive osteoarthritis, distal inter-phalangeal (DIP) joints. *(A)* Early central erosion with slight depression of the articular surface. Note joint narrowing and osteophytes. *(B)* Late erosion with advancing deformity of the articular surface and more severe joint narrowing. Note the seagull shape of the joint.

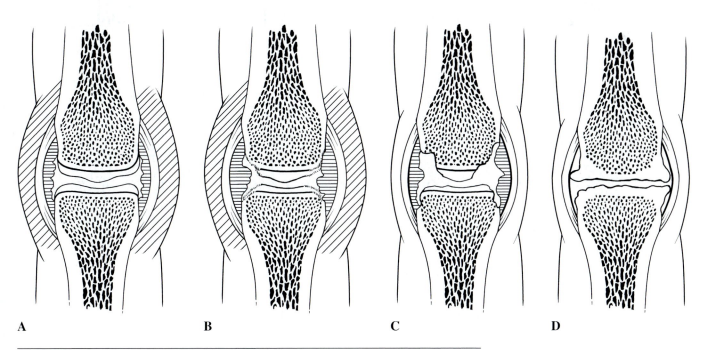

A   B   C   D

FIGURE 3-13. Development of marginal erosions. *(A)* Synovial proliferation with joint effusion and fusiform soft tissue swelling around the joint. *(B)* Early marginal erosion related to synovial proliferation and inflammation (pannus) at the "bare area." Note ill-defined borders of the early erosions. *(C)* As erosions become more chronic, they may persist and undergo healing response, with development of sclerotic borders. *(D)* Chronic synovial inflammation can result in diffuse cartilage loss with uniform joint narrowing and secondary osteoarthritis.

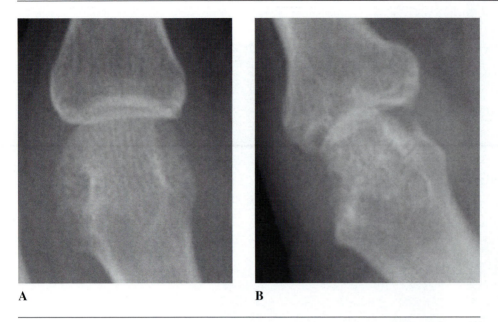

FIGURE 3-14.   Progression of erosive disease: marginal erosions in rheumatoid arthritis, metacarpophalangeal joints. *(A)* Early marginal erosion with lucency and loss of the cortical line at the bare area. There is also joint narrowing and soft tissue swelling, representing a joint effusion. *(B)* Late erosion.

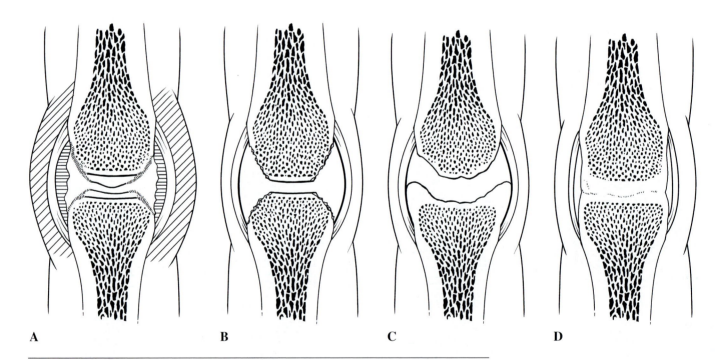

FIGURE 3-15.   Development of proliferative erosions. *(A)* Erosions associated with psoriatic arthritis and Reiter's disease characteristically have a "fluffy" or "whiskered" appearance. *(B)* If the underlying disease goes into remission, the erosions may heal with residual irregularity of the articular margins. *(C)* Severe involvement can cause extensive destruction of the articular surfaces, called "arthritis mutilans." This appearance can also be seen with severe forms of nonproliferative arthropathies, including rheumatoid arthritis, mixed connective tissue disease, and multicentric reticulohistiocytosis. *(D)* Chronic involvement by psoriatic arthritis or Reiter's disease can cause joint fusion, predominantly in the digits. Peripheral ankylosis can also be observed in patients with rheumatoid arthritis, especially juvenile rheumatoid arthritis.

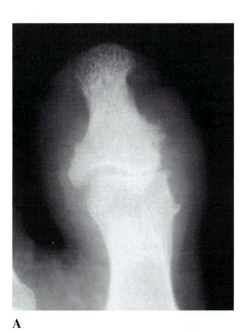

A

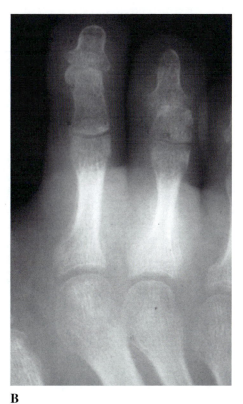

B

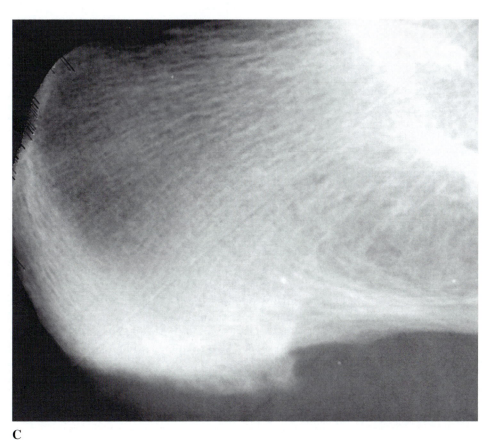

C

subtle or may be so severe as to overwhelm attempts at description; either possibility can lead to long periods of silence that are not looked on favorably by the clinician or the examiner. Also, as is the problem in many areas of radiology, "the patients don't read the textbooks"; the classic patterns presented in textbooks are not always seen. Arthritides can appear in mixed patterns, further confusing the matter; for example, osteoarthritis may occur in addition to other arthropathies or may occur secondary to cartilage loss in these disorders, and characteristics of both can be present in the same joints. One should remember that atypical manifestations of common disorders are more common than typical manifestations of uncommon disorders.

1. Always use a standard checklist of findings, especially in evaluation of hand and wrist radiographs; the approach (soft tissues, mineralization, joint narrowing, erosions, proliferation, deformity, and distribution) outlined in each disease subsection of this chapter is useful, but any checklist should cover all the pertinent findings. Verbalize all steps on the checklist, even if negative ("I don't see any erosions"), to avoid periods of silence and to organize thoughts.

2. If there is a mixed pattern of erosive arthropathy and osteoarthritis, consider the possibility of superimposed secondary osteoarthritis and evaluate the distribution and pattern of the erosions to arrive at a differential.

3. If there is an atypical pattern, consider evaluation of other joints; a more characteristic pattern may emerge. For example, if the pattern is atypical in the hands, consider obtaining radiographs of the feet.

FIGURE 3-16.   Proliferation in seronegative spondyloarthropathy (figures are of patients with Reiter disease). *(A)* Proliferative erosions at the interphalangeal joint of the great toe. *(B)* Periostitis in a phalanx of the toe. *(C)* Proliferative enthesophyte of the calcaneus.

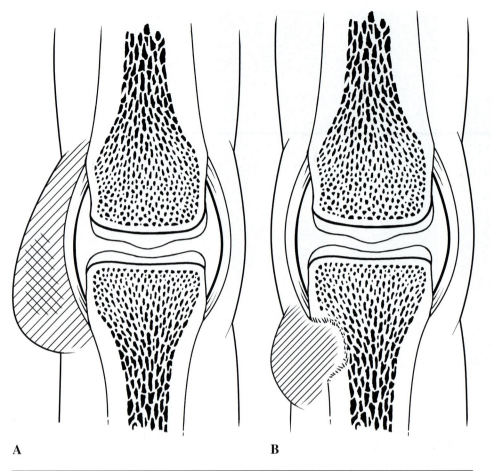

A   B

FIGURE 3-17.   Development of periarticular erosions. *(A)* Radiodense but non-calcified periarticular mass representing a gouty tophus. *(B)* The tophus erodes the underlying bone in a juxta-articular location.

4. To differentiate an articular disease from periarticular disorders, look for involvement of both articular surfaces.

5. Become well-versed in the wide range of human anatomic variations and pitfalls, both real and artifactual, that can simulate the findings associated with arthropathies.

IMAGING OF ARTHRITIS

Radiography

Radiography remains the primary radiologic modality for evaluation of arthritis. In the early stages of arthritis, abnormalities may be very subtle. Identification of these subtle findings is dependent on high quality radiographic technique. Quality control is very important to ensure that patient positioning and radiographic technique are adequate to allow visualization of the findings listed in the prior section. Multiple views of the affected joint are essential for detection of all relevant findings. In some areas of the body, "special" radiographic views in addition to or instead of the routine views are helpful for identification of these findings, such as the Norgaard view ("ball-catcher's view") of the hands, which helps identify early marginal erosions.

Computed Tomography

CT has limited utility in diagnosis and management of arthritis but can be used to more accurately evaluate complicating factors associated with arthritides, such as location and quantity of intraarticular bodies before surgical intervention (especially in conjunction with arthrography using air and a small amount of iodinated contrast) and identification of osteophytes impinging on adjacent nerves. It can help verify the presence of lesions of the articular surface, such as osteochondral defects or coalitions across joints, when radiographs are indeterminate. CT can also be useful for preoperative quantification of the degree of osteoarthritis, especially in smaller joints with complex surfaces. CT can be useful in early detection of sacroiliitis if radiographs are negative or indeterminate.

Ultrasound

Ultrasound is much more sensitive to the presence of joint effusion and erosions than radiographs. Addition of power Doppler offers potential for the evaluation of synovial vascularity that may be related to disease activity in inflammatory arthropathies and therefore may be used to assess effectiveness of antiinflammatory therapy.

Magnetic Resonance Imaging

MRI can be useful for identification of tenosynovitis, joint effusions, synovial proliferation, cysts, ganglia, erosions, and cartilage loss. A great deal of research activity over the past few years has been devoted to imaging of cartilage, partly in response to several clinical advances that hold promise for the treatment of cartilage damage. As these therapies become more commonly used, it is likely that MRI will play a major role in evaluation of early cartilage damage.

MRI is especially useful in evaluation of synovial disease. Degree of synovial proliferation is easily assessed; because the synovial tissue is highly vascular, thickened or inflamed synovial tissue enhances brightly after intravenous administration of gadolinium on T1W fat-suppressed images. In normal joints, the synovial membrane is very thin, only a few cells thick, and there is minimal to no perceptible enhancement. The finding of synovial thickening and enhancement on MRI, however, is

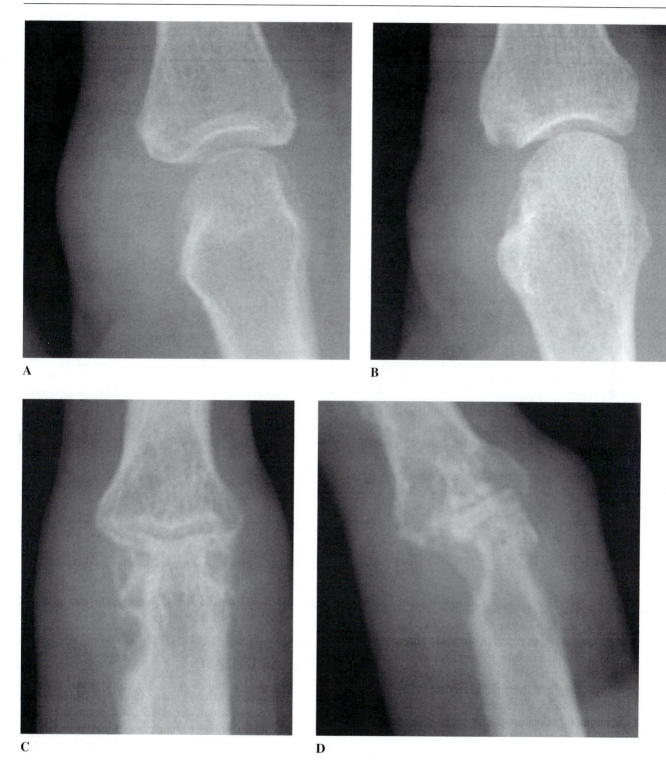

FIGURE 3-18.   Progression of erosive disease: periarticular erosions in gout. *(A)* Asymmetric periarticular soft tissue mass from gouty tophus. Slight loss of definition of adjacent cortical margin indicates site of developing erosion. *(B)* Small erosions developing on the adjacent phalanx and metacarpal. Note absence of involvement of the opposite side of the joint, unlike erosions formed from a primary synovial process. *(C)* Early periarticular erosion with asymmetric involvement of the joint from the adjacent soft tissue mass. Note the sharp margins of the erosion and the "overhanging edge," or "rat bite," appearance. *(D)* Late erosive disease from gout. Severe joint narrowing and central erosions are also present.

TABLE 3-11

Joint Malalignment

With erosions
    Rheumatoid arthritis
    Psoriatic arthritis
    Reiter disease
    Multicentric reticulohistiocytosis
Without erosions
    Systemic lupus erythematosus
    Jaccoud arthropathy
    Severe osteoarthritis
    Trauma, internal derangement
    Neuropathic arthropathy
    Pseudosubluxation (positioning, effusion)

nonspecific and can be seen in many inflammatory and noninflammatory arthropathies.

Detection of synovial proliferation can be useful in a variety of situations. For example, it has been used for confirmation of sacroiliitis when disease is clinically suspected but radiographs are negative or indeterminate. Also, MRI can be helpful for identification of synovial proliferation around the dens of the upper cervical spine in patients with rheumatoid arthritis.

MRI also may be useful for detection of complications of arthritis and its treatment, especially in early diagnosis of avascular necrosis in patients on chronic steroid therapy. Tendon tears, seen with increased frequency in patients on steroid therapy and patients with rheumatoid arthritis and gout, are optimally evaluated with MRI. MRI can be used as a sensitive tomographic technique for early detection of joint erosions.

Scintigraphy

Scintigraphy has a limited role in evaluation of arthritis. Three-phase bone scan using technetium 99m MDP can detect synovial hyperemia on the vascular and blood pool phases and periarticular uptake on the delayed phase in joints affected by inflammatory arthritis, but uptake is nonspecific and generally is not used for narrowing the differential diagnosis in cases of suspected arthropathy. However, bone scan can be useful in identifying the number and distribution of joints involved and can help distinguish an articular from a nonarticular process based on location of uptake at the joint versus the juxtaarticular bone. Because uptake of radiotracer is nonspecific, skeletal

TABLE 3-12

Monarticular Arthropathy—Differential Diagnosis

Secondary osteoarthritis (eg, posttraumatic or instability)
Septic arthritis
Gout
Synovial osteochondromatosis
Pigmented villonodular synovitis

TABLE 3-13

Common Distribution of Various Arthropathies

Primary osteoarthritis
    Base of thumb, digits, weight-bearing joints, spine
    Bilateral asymmetric (upper extremity asymmetry depends on
        side dominance)
Rheumatoid arthritis
    Wrist, MCPs, MTPs (especially the fifth), shoulders, C spine,
        knees, hips
    Bilateral symmetric (refers to distribution; severity may vary)
Psoriatic arthritis
    IPs, MCPs, MTPs, sacroiliacs
    Bilateral asymmetric
Reiter disease
    IPs (feet), MTPs, sacroiliacs
    Bilateral asymmetric
Ankylosing spondylitis
    L > T > C spine, sacroiliacs, hips
    Bilateral symmetric
Gout
    First IP (foot), first MTP, Lisfranc, scattered hand/wrist joints
    Bilateral asymmetric
Neuropathic arthropathy (related to diabetes; other causes less
        common)
    Lisfranc, hindfoot
    Unilateral or bilateral asymmetric
Hemophilia
    Weight-bearing joints: ankles, knees
    Bilateral symmetric
    Upper extremities: elbows, digits, shoulders
    Bilateral asymmetric or scattered
Juvenile chronic arthritis
    Knees, hips, ankles
    Bilateral symmetric

ABBREVIATIONS: C = cervical, IP = interphalangeal, L = lumbar, MCP = metacarpophalangeal, MTP = metatarsophalangeal, T = thoracic.

scintigraphy should be evaluated in conjunction with radiographs of areas with abnormal uptake.

ARTICULAR DISEASES

Articular diseases can be categorized loosely as degenerative, synovial, collagen vascular, deposition, and neuropathic diseases. Degenerative diseases include primary and secondary osteoarthritis. The synovial category is divided into inflammatory (included are autoimmune diseases such as rheumatoid arthritis and nonautoimmune diseases such as small particle disease) and noninflammatory proliferative (such as pigmented villonodular synovitis and synovial osteochondromatosis) disorders. Examples of collagen vascular disease associated with arthritis are scleroderma and mixed connective tissue disease. Deposition diseases include gout, calcium pyrophosphate deposition disease, hemochromatosis, amyloid, and others. Infectious entities are discussed in Chapter 1. There is overlap between the diseases in these categories, and some disorders do not fit well into one category. However, this categorization serves to organize thought processes when reviewing cases.

DEGENERATIVE DISORDERS

Osteoarthritis

Osteoarthritis, commonly called *degenerative joint disease*, is by far the most common articular disease and may present in primary or secondary forms. Osteoarthritis results from cartilage loss; this loss can be from primary cartilage damage related to chronic joint wear or injury or from secondary cartilage erosion related to various underlying disorders such as inflammatory or crystalline arthropathy, septic arthritis, or recurrent intraarticular hemorrhage. Radiographic hallmarks of osteoarthritis are non-uniform joint narrowing, osteophytes, subchondral sclerosis, and subchondral cysts.

PRIMARY OSTEOARTHRITIS.   In primary osteoarthritis, the degenerative process is due to an abnormality of the articular cartilage initiated by cartilage dehydration, loss of proteoglycans, and disruption of the collagen framework. It generally occurs in older individuals and in weight-bearing joints, such as the hips, knees, and spine, and joints that have undergone chronic stress or overuse, such as the joints of the hand or the shoulder and elbow joints of throwing athletes. In acromegaly, the articular cartilage is abnormally thick, and nutrients from the synovial fluid may not penetrate to the deeper portions, resulting in early cartilage degeneration. Other entities can predispose to cartilage loss: lack of transport of nutrients from the synovial fluid into the avascular articular cartilage related to decreased "pumping action" of articular motion in paralyzed joints can predispose to primary cartilage degeneration, and individuals with epiphyseal dysplasias may have abnormal overlying cartilage that is more susceptible to injury and wear.

SECONDARY OSTEOARTHRITIS.   In secondary osteoarthritis, factors extrinsic to the articular cartilage result in eventual cartilage loss and degeneration of the joint. A common cause is chondrolytic enzymes within the synovial fluid. These enzymes may originate from inflammatory synovial tissue, as in rheumatoid arthritis, or from release of lysosomal enzymes from dead cells in the synovial fluid, as seen in septic arthritis, crystalline disorders including gout and CPPD arthropathy, and chronic hemarthroses. Other primary synovial processes that can result in secondary osteoarthritis are synovial osteochondromatosis, pigmented villonodular synovitis, and multicentric reticulohistiocytosis. Appearance and distribution of these arthropathies are presented in separate sections devoted to each disorder.

Joint instability and articular incongruity are common causes of secondary osteoarthritis; etiologies of joint instability include ligament and fibrocartilage tears (such as anterior cruciate ligament [ACL] and meniscal tears in the knee) and tears of certain tendons, the muscles of which are secondary joint stabilizers (particularly the rotator cuff tendons). Examples of articular incongruity include deformity of the articular surfaces related to intraarticular fracture, avascular necrosis with articular collapse, developmental deformity, Paget disease (with expansion of the end of the bone), and other deforming processes. Osteoarthritis from these processes is considered secondary because the degenerative process does not originate as an intrinsic abnormality

TABLE 3-14

Primary versus Secondary Osteoarthritis

Primary osteoarthritis (primarily cartilage problem)
    Overuse
    Age
    Obesity (weight-bearing joints)
    Acromegaly (cartilage malnutrition)
    Epiphyseal dysplasia (abnormal cartilage)
Secondary osteoarthritis (problem originates outside the cartilage)
    Trauma/instability
    Septic arthritis
    Rheumatoid arthritis/juvenile chronic arthritis, other inflammatory
      arthropathies
    Hemophilia, recurrent hemarthrosis
    Crystalline arthropathies, hemochromatosis
    Joint incongruity (eg, Paget, developmental deformity)
    Synovial osteochondromatosis
    Pigmented villonodular synovitis
    Avascular necrosis

---

of the hyaline cartilage. Direct impaction injury of the hyaline cartilage can also result in acute chondrolysis and accelerated primary osteoarthritis (Table 3-14).

GENERAL IMAGING FINDINGS.   In large joints, especially the knees and hips, joint effusions are common, although the amount is usually small. Asymmetric soft tissue prominence can be seen in the digits, mainly due to large underlying osteophytes.

Erosions are absent unless the osteoarthritis is secondary to diffuse cartilage loss from an underlying inflammatory arthropathy or other etiology outlined at the beginning of this section. Erosive or inflammatory osteoarthritis is a related entity, which is discussed at the end of this section.

Bony proliferation, especially in the form of osteophytes, is a basic finding characterizing osteoarthritis. Unaffected joints almost always have rounded margins; early osteophyte formation is seen as "sharpening" of the edges of the joint (notable exceptions are the uncovertebral joints and facet joints, which start off sharp and become rounded and blunted as osteophyte formation progresses).

Joint deformity is a feature of severe osteoarthritis. Large osteophytes at the margins of the interphalangeal joints cause hard, focal prominences at the interphalangeal joints. There also may be angular deformities at the interphalangeal joints. Cartilage loss at one side of the affected joint can cause a varus or valgus deformity, most commonly observed in the knees. With more severe cartilage loss and joint instability, subluxation can occur; this can cause an angular appearance of the interphalangeal joints and proximal migration of the first metacarpal at the cariometacarpal (CMC) joint. Subluxation of the tibia also can be seen at the knee. Subluxation of degenerated spinal facet joints in association with disc degeneration results in spondylolisthesis of the vertebral bodies.

The distribution of osteoarthritis corresponds to patterns of chronic use or overuse. Weight-bearing joints are typically affected, especially the knees. In most people, the brunt of weight bearing at the knees is across the medial tibiofemoral

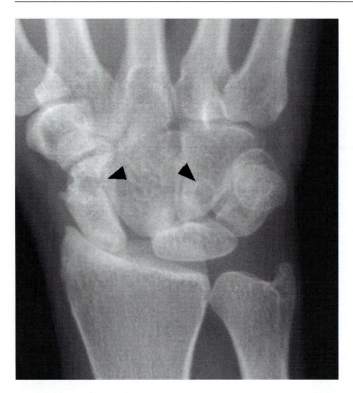

FIGURE 3-20. Carpal instability with scapholunate widening and scapholunate advanced collapse. Secondary osteoarthritis is evident by radioscaphoid and intercarpal joint narrowing, subchondral sclerosis, and carpal cysts in the hamate and scaphoid (arrowheads).

Knees. Osteoarthritis of the knees is very common; the primary form is typically seen in obese or older individuals, is bilateral and usually symmetric, and is most severe in the medial compartment, with joint narrowing, marginal osteophytes, and subchondral cysts (Figure 3-23). With medial involvement a varus deformity can result, which further shifts weight bearing through the medial compartment; thus creating a cascade accelerating the degenerative process. In this subset of patients, a high tibial osteotomy is often performed to shift weight bearing more to the center of the joint.

Knee injuries are very common in contact sports, skiing, and other activities, and osteoarthritis due to meniscal or cruciate ligament injury is commonly seen in a younger population as a result; the distribution in this case is asymmetric, limited to the injured side, and more severely affects the compartment in which the meniscus was torn. Meniscectomy is performed to reduce pain and locking, but it does not prevent (and actually may hasten) development of osteoarthritis; meniscal transplantation does not appear to prevent the degenerative process. Osteoarthritis is also accelerated after cruciate ligament injury. Cruciate ligament reconstruction is performed mainly to restore joint stability; whether it helps prevent progression of osteoarthritis is controversial.

Although it is not a weight-bearing joint, patellofemoral joint osteoarthritis is commonly seen in older individuals in conjunction with involvement of the medial and lateral compartments (*tricompartmental osteoarthritis*). However, cartilage degeneration and subsequent osteoarthritis can occur in younger individuals who have tracking abnormalities of the patella or instability of the extensor mechanism. This process has a number of potential etiologies. One source of tracking abnormalities is an abnormal *Q angle*, the angle between the origin of the rectus femoris (at the anterior inferior iliac spine), the patella, and the insertion of the patellar tendon at the anterior tibial tuberosity. This angle is increased in some individuals, especially females, and action of the quadriceps muscle tends to sublux the patella laterally. A developmentally shallow patellar sulcus and "high-riding" patella (patella alta) contribute to tracking abnormalities and patellofemoral instability. Prior traumatic patellar dislocation with tearing of the medial retinaculum and, perhaps more importantly, the medial patellofemoral ligament, which anchor the patella medially, can also cause chronic instability; other people have excessive tightening of the lateral retinaculum, which can tilt the patella laterally. This latter condition is called *excessive lateral pressure syndrome* when it results in cartilage degeneration in the lateral aspect of the patellofemoral joint. An atypical pattern of osteoarthritis also can be observed in CPPD arthropathy; when chondrocalcinosis is seen and there is predominant patellofemoral osteoarthritis, this entity can be suggested.

Ankles and Feet. In the ankle, mild changes of osteoarthritis are common in the elderly, with small osteophytes at the margins of the medial and lateral malleoli and the anterior margins of the joint. More severe osteoarthritis is usually secondary to joint incongruity from intraarticular fracture or to instability related to ligamentous damage (Figure 3-24), especially the syndesmosis, which presents radiographically as widening of the tibiofibular interval with asymmetry of the joint medially versus laterally. In these settings, a severe, debilitating osteoarthritis can result, which may require joint fusion; it is important to detect syndesmotic injury early and treat with fixation.

Some individuals exhibit large spurs at the anterior margin of the ankle joint, which most likely represent chronic avulsive stress from the anterior capsular attachments. These spurs can cause deep peroneal nerve impingement and limitation of dorsiflexion, a condition called *anterior impingement*. Chronic osseous abutment of these matching spurs from the tibia and talus can lead to formation of intraarticular bodies and early osteoarthritis. A similar process can occur at the posterior ankle, called *posterior impingement*. Individuals with a large os trigonum (normally attached to the talus by a fibrous syndesmosis), especially those who perform activities requiring extreme plantarflexion (such as ballet dancers and gymnasts), can form a painful pseudarthrosis through the junction. The subtalar joint also undergoes osteoarthritic degeneration predominantly secondary to prior trauma, typically calcaneal fracture with resultant incongruity of the joint or instability due to ligamentous injury. The Lisfranc (tarsometatarsal) joint also can undergo degeneration from instability. This is usually initiated by a twisting injury of the midfoot, with tearing or avulsion of the Lisfranc ligament extending from the medial cuneiform to the second metatarsal base. Initial radiographs may be interpreted as normal due to missed subtle subluxation or the small avulsion fragment; accelerated osteoarthritis can result from the instability.

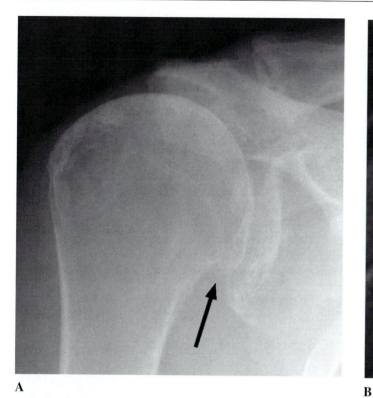

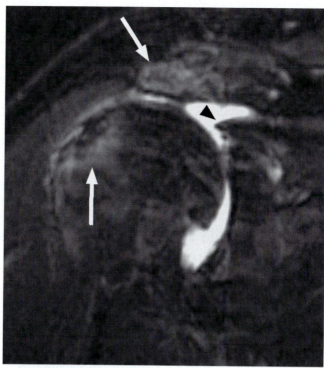

A   B

FIGURE 3-21.   Rotator cuff arthropathy. *(A)* Anteroposterior view of the shoulder shows high-riding humeral head with abutment on the acromion consistent with rotator cuff tear; note remodeling of the acromion and humeral subchondral sclerosis from the chronic abutment. A large osteophyte is present at the inferior aspect of the humeral articular surface at the glenohumeral joint (arrow). *(B)* Oblique coronal T_2-weighted fast spin echo fat-suppressed magnetic resonance images. Fluid extends through the complete rotator cuff tear (arrowhead) into the subacromial/subdeltoid bursa. There is severe glenohumeral cartilage loss and marrow edema in the greater tuberosity and acromion related to the chronic abutment (arrows).

Osteoarthritis is also common at the first metatarsophalangeal joint, especially in people with hallux valgus. A developmentally squared morphology of the first metatarsal head may predispose to development of osteoarthritis; often large dorsal osteophytes develop, eventually causing pain and limitation of dorsiflexion, a condition called *hallux rigidus* or *hallux limitus* (Figure 3-25).

Erosive Osteoarthritis

There is a subset of patients with osteoarthritis who have a superimposed inflammatory component that causes intermittent swelling of the digits, usually of the DIP joints, and less often the PIP joints. In general, these patients are elderly, female, have had osteoarthritis for many years, and have been treated with NSAIDs. This entity is referred to as *erosive osteoarthritis* or *inflammatory osteoarthritis*. Radiographs of the hands show a typical distribution and appearance of primary osteoarthritis, but the finding that separates erosive osteoarthritis from conventional osteoarthritis is the presence of central erosions that appear as depressions in the central aspect of the proximal articular surface. This depression, in association with the overhanging osteophytes, creates the characteristic "seagull" shape

of the joint. In the later stages, affected joints may progress to ankylosis, although complete fusion is relatively rare.

PRIMARY SYNOVIAL PROCESSES AND RELATED DISORDERS

Inflammatory Disorders—Autoimmune

RHEUMATOID ARTHRITIS.   Rheumatoid arthritis is a common disorder and is the radiologic paradigm of inflammatory arthritis. Its occurrence, severity, and course appear to be related to a combination of genetic and environmental factors; family and twin studies suggest a heritable predisposition to the disease, related to histocompatibility antigens coded by the HLA-DRB1 allele. These antigens may resemble an exogenous antigen stimulating T-cell response against the body's own tissues, but the etiology appears to be more complex because no clearcut virus or other exogenous agent is strongly associated with development of the disease.

Rheumatoid arthritis affects females more often than males at a ratio of 2:1 to 3:1. Typically, adult-type rheumatoid arthritis is recognized at a young age, usually in the 20s to 40s; initial clinical manifestations may be seen rarely in the elderly. Symptoms

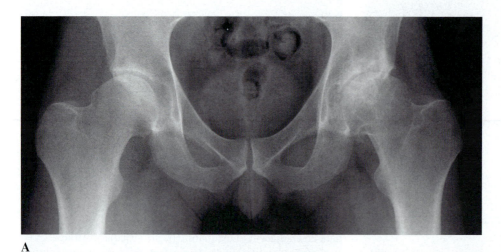

A

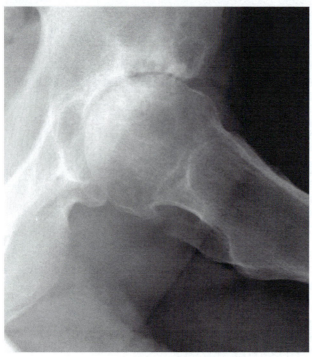

B

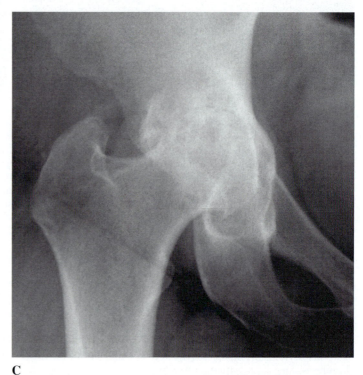

C

FIGURE 3-22. Osteoarthritis of the hips. *(A)* Anteroposterior and *(B)* frogleg lateral views of left hip show unilateral left hip joint narrowing, which asymmetrically involves the superior aspect of the joint; there is associated subchondral sclerosis, subchondral cystic change, and marginal osteophytes. Note improved visualization of the osteophytes on the lateral view. Also present is buttressing of the medial femoral neck, with cortical thickening compared with the right. *(C)* Anteroposterior view of a different patient with chronic rheumatoid arthritis and secondary osteoarthritis; note osteophyte formation and subchondral sclerosis. The diffuse joint narrowing and protrusio acetabula are characteristic of the underlying rheumatoid arthritis.

at presentation classically include joint stiffness, especially in the morning, with pain and swelling that is most commonly polyarticular and symmetric. Often the symptoms are insidious, with slow progression over months until treatment is sought. During this period intermittent arthralgias may occur in one joint or a few joints (monarticular or pauciarticular) and involvement can be asymmetric. Systemic manifestations include fatigue and weight loss. Clinical criteria for diagnosis include at least four of the following (criteria *a* through *d* must have been present for at least 6 weeks): (*a*) morning joint stiffness lasting at least 1 hour; (*b*) soft tissue swelling of at least three joints; (*c*) swelling of the PIP, MCP, or wrist joints; (*d*) symmetric involvement; (*e*) subcutaneous nodules; (*f*) positive rheumatoid factor; of (*g*) radiographic evidence of erosions of the joints of the hand or

wrist. Some patients have rapid progression of disease causing severe debilitation, but in many patients the disease becomes quiescent for long periods, with occasional flare-ups. Although most patients (approximately 85%) have positive rheumatoid factor, a small subset is factor negative but fulfills other criteria characteristic of rheumatoid arthritis rather than seronegative spondyloarthropathy. These patients subsequently may turn rheumatoid factor positive.

General Imaging Findings.   The basic pathology of rheumatoid arthritis is inflammation and proliferation of synovium (called the *pannus*), which leads to the various radiographic appearances. Periarticular swelling is due to a combination of

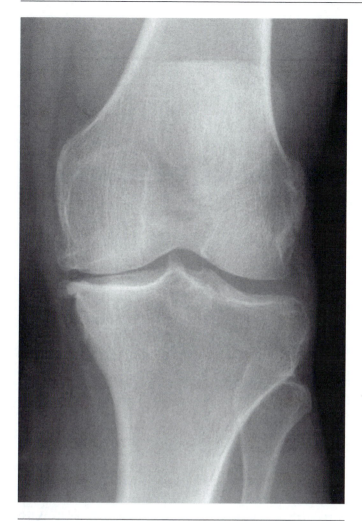

FIGURE 3-23. Osteoarthritis of the knee. Anteroposterior view shows medial compartment narrowing, subchondral sclerosis and cystic change at the tibial plateau, and large marginal osteophytes.

pannus and joint effusion. Fusiform soft tissue swelling is characteristic at the PIP joints of the hands, with focal soft tissue swelling at the MCP joints, at the dorsum of the wrist, and over the ulnar styloid. In the feet, soft tissue swelling is common at the MTP joints, especially the fifth. Rheumatoid arthritis can affect any synovial structure, including bursae and tendon sheaths. Bursitis can cause areas of ill-defined soft tissue planes or focal soft tissue prominence; this is most evident radiographically in the retrocalcaneal bursa and olecranon bursa. Tenosynovitis is evident radiographically as diffuse or longitudinally oriented soft tissue swelling, commonly involving the tendons of the wrist. Inflammatory nodular soft tissue lesions may occur, called *rheumatoid nodules*. Rheumatoid nodules occur in as many as 25% of all rheumatoid patients and appear as focal soft tissue masses, usually at sites of chronic friction, such as the olecranon (which can simulate olecranon bursitis) and the hands and feet.

Periarticular osteopenia is a classic radiographic feature, especially in early stages of rheumatoid arthritis of the hands and feet, although a generalized pattern of osteopenia can occur. The osteopenia is multifactorial, related to bone resorption from the markedly hyperemic synovium, decreased use of the painful

joints, steroid therapy, and propensity for osteoporosis in the population of affected females. A subset of patients has preservation of bone density but generally develops more severe articular destruction; this rare "robust" rheumatoid arthritis is most common in males with rheumatoid arthritis, especially laborers who continue to use the affected joints.

Involved joints generally demonstrate concentric, or uniform, joint narrowing related to diffuse cartilage loss; however, in weight-bearing joints there may be more severe narrowing at the weight-bearing surface. Axial migration can occur at the hips due to bone remodeling at the central portion of the acetabulum, with inward bowing of the acetabulum, medial to the iliopectineal line, called *protrusio acetabuli*.

Characteristic marginal erosions result from thickened, inflammatory synovial tissue (pannus) eroding the bone at the bare area adjacent to the margin of the articular cartilage.

Osseous proliferation is not a feature of rheumatoid arthritis; however, osteophyte formation can occur in longstanding rheumatoid arthritis as a result of superimposed secondary osteoarthritis.

Deformities of the hands and feet are common in rheumatoid arthritis for a variety of reasons: laxity and distention of the joint capsule; ligamentous laxity or disruption; tendinopathy or tendon tears; and altered muscle tone. These factors lead to a variety of deformities. The "swan neck" deformity is hyperextension at the PIP joint and flexion at the DIP joint. The *Boutonniere deformity* is flexion at the PIP joint and hyperextension at the DIP joint. These deformities result from imbalance of the flexor and extensor tendons. Subluxations at the MCP and MTP joints are also common; in general, the metacarpals slip in a volar direction. It is also common for the digits of the hands to deviate in an ulnar direction ("windswept hand" appearance). Hallux valgus is also common and may be severe, leading to overlap of the first and second toes. In the hands, the first CMC joints often sublux, with the first metacarpal slipping proximally. The carpal bones commonly erode, with ligamentous disruption and laxity causing carpal instability patterns. In more severe cases, this process of erosion and instability may reach a point at which there is carpal collapse with the metacarpal bases nearly apposed to the radius. The entire carpus and hand may slip in an ulnar direction, referred to as *ulnar translocation*. Carpal collapse and dissociation, in addition to mass effect from pannus, can cause impingement on the median nerve as it passes through the carpal tunnel, resulting in carpal tunnel syndrome.

Rheumatoid arthritis is most commonly recognized in the hands and feet; in fact, if there is a finding on a foot film that is of questionable significance, it is often useful to evaluate radiographs of the hands, and vice versa. Distribution in the hands is characteristically more proximal than distal, commonly involving the carpus and the MCP and PIP joints. In the feet and ankles, the distribution mimics that of the hands and wrists, with the MTP joints most commonly involved. Distribution is bilateral and symmetric; however, extent of involvement may not be the same from side to side. Moreover, "symmetric" involvement does not mean that the same digit on both sides is involved necessarily; rather, the joints of the digits, MCPs, MTPs, PIPs, and DIPs, are considered as separate groups; for example,

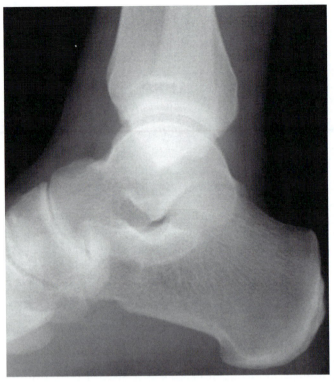 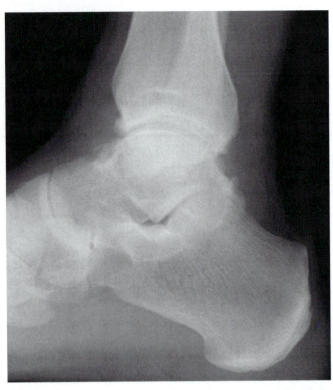

A   B

FIGURE 3-24. Osteoarthritis of the ankle. *(A)* Lateral view of the ankle of a patient with acute injury shows a normal joint space. *(B)* Lateral view of the same patient 5 years later (with persistent pain during that interval and more recent restriction of range of motion) shows development of secondary osteoarthritis, with marginal osteophytes limiting range of motion.

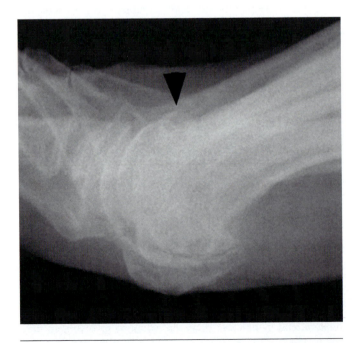

FIGURE 3-25. Hallux rigidus. Lateral view of the first metatarsophalangeal (MTP) joint shows dorsal spur formation (arrowhead). Also note the degenerative osteophyte formation at the metatarsosesamoid articulation.

there may be symmetric involvement in the PIP joints if the right third PIP and left second PIP joints are involved. In addition, symmetry only refers to involvement of the joint, not to the severity of involvement. Other circumstances can result in asymmetric involvement. Use of affected joints appears to lead to more severe involvement; conversely, lack of use of the joints may preserve the joints. Evidence for this is seen in patients with robust rheumatoid arthritis who continue to use the joints and can have more severe involvement, and asymmetric extent of involvement is seen in patients with unilateral paralysis or stroke who may have less severe destruction of the joints on the side less used. Large joints are also typically involved symmetrically, although not necessarily in extent. This is especially evident in the sacroiliac joints, which can be involved asymmetrically.

Imaging Findings in Specific Joints

HAND AND WRIST. The earliest radiographic manifestations of rheumatoid arthritis are typically seen in the hand and wrist (Figure 3-26). Earliest changes occur at the MCP joints; initially, soft tissue swelling is evident at the MCPs and/or PIPs. Soft tissue swelling is also commonly seen early on at the ulnar styloid due to pannus at the prestyloid recess and/or tenosynovitis of the extensor carpi ulnaris; subsequently, the dorsum of the wrist can become swollen from underlying carpal pannus or extensor tenosynovitis. Ganglia are commonly seen at the

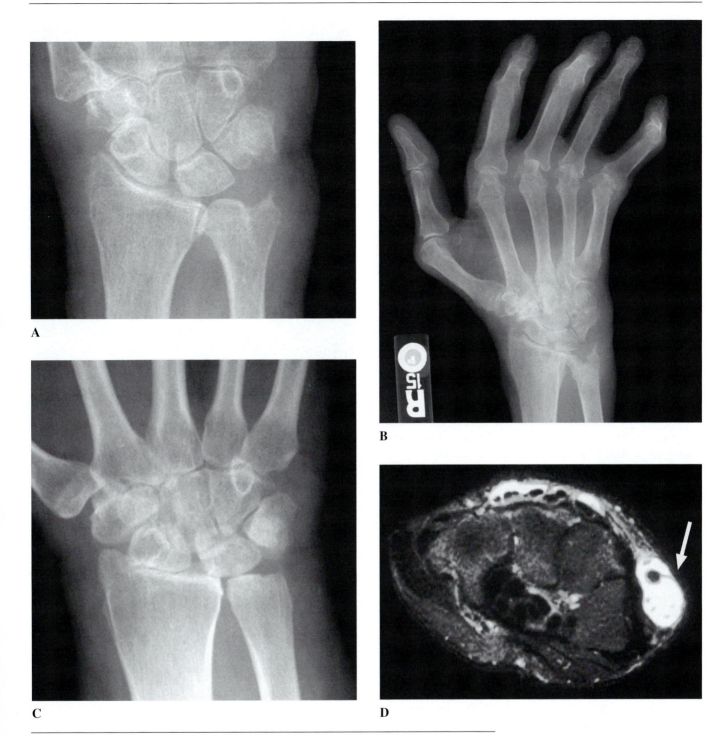

A

B

C

D

FIGURE 3-26.   Rheumatoid arthritis of the hand and wrist. *(A)* Early involvement on anteroposterior view of the wrist. There is soft tissue swelling at the ulnar aspect of the wrist, representing tenosynovitis, with an early adjacent erosion of the ulnar styloid. There is increased soft tissue density within the wrist joint, reflecting synovial proliferative disease. Note the separate erosion of the distal ulna from synovial disease in the wrist joint. *(B)* Anteroposterior view of the hand shows soft tissue swelling in the wrist similar to that shown in A, with more severe erosive change at the distal ulna. There is diffuse intercarpal joint narrowing, and there are erosions throughout the carpus. Soft tissue swelling and marginal erosive disease are present at the metacarpophalangeal joints, with severe joint narrowing. There is subluxation at the metacarpophalangeal joints with ulnar deviation of the digits (the "windswept hand"). Also note Boutonniere deformity of the digits. *(C)* Late involvement of the wrist with severe diffuse joint narrowing. Note ulnar translocation of the carpus due to erosion or laxity of the volar extrinsic ligaments. *(D)* Axial T_2-weighted fat-suppressed magnetic resonance image of the wrist shows chronic tenosynovitis of the extensors with "rice bodies" (arrow) (fibrous bodies resulting from chronic synovial inflammation).

wrist, extending into the subcutaneous tissues from the joints of the wrist or the tendon sheaths. Rheumatoid nodules are seen in some patients and are relatively common in the hands. Growth may be stimulated by methotrexate therapy. A small subset of patients has a condition called *benign rheumatoid nodulosis*, exhibiting numerous subcutaneous nodules with relative sparing of the joints. Periarticular demineralization is common, resulting from a combination of periarticular hyperemia and decreased use of the extremity. Joint narrowing is seen early on at the MCP joints and at the radiocarpal and intercarpal joints. Erosions without proliferative response form at the margins of these joints and may involve the PIP joints. The earliest locations to see erosions are at the ulnar styloid and at the MCP joints. Subchondral cysts are common at the distal radius and in the carpal bones and may grow to large size. More severe involvement can cause marked erosive changes at the carpus. Inflammatory synovium can erode the intrinsic and/or extrinsic ligaments, resulting in carpal instability, with scapholunate widening, dorsal intercalated segment instability (DISI) or volar intercalated segment instability (VISI) patterns, and SLAC. Silastic implants are occasionally used to correct deformities of the digits but often loosen, fragment, and incite particle disease or aggressive granulomatous response resulting in areas of bone lysis.

ELBOW. Rheumatoid involvement of the elbow causes displacement of the anterior and posterior fat pads, usually from pannus more than joint effusion. Large subarticular cysts are frequently seen (Figure 3-27). Marginal erosions are common and can progress to severe destructive arthropathy, with deformity and loss of range of motion. Rheumatoid nodules may form in the subcutaneous tissues of the olecranon and in the dorsal aspect of the forearm.

SHOULDER. Involvement of the shoulder is common in chronic rheumatoid arthritis. Pannus at the acromioclavicular joint often causes erosion of the distal clavicle. Synovial proliferation in the more capacious glenohumeral joint may not cause erosions until later in the disease process; when they occur, they tend to ring the anatomic neck of the humeral head and may simulate subchondral cysts. The inflammatory synovium causes erosion and eventual tearing of the rotator cuff; resultant instability and action of the dominant deltoid muscle then cause the humeral head to become high-riding or subluxed superiorly. Secondary osteoarthritis is commonly superimposed.

SPINE. A major site of serious musculoskeletal complications from rheumatoid arthritis is the cervical spine (Figure 3-28). The dens is surrounded by synovial tissue anteriorly at the junction of the dens with the anterior arch of C_1 and posteriorly at the transverse ligament, which extends across the C_1 lateral masses and helps hold the dens in place. Pannus at these synovial locations can cause laxity of the transverse ligament and erosion of the dens itself, leading to excessive motion and instability at C_1–C_2, defined as widening of the inferior margin of the predental space greater than 2.5 mm. The instability may not be apparent on a neutral lateral view; lateral views in

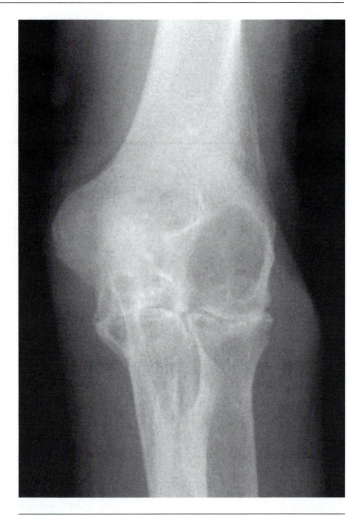

FIGURE 3-27. Rheumatoid involvement of the elbow. Anteroposterior view of the elbow demonstrates diffuse joint narrowing and large subchondral cysts.

flexion and extension are generally indicated to gauge the degree of instability, although the flexion and extension motion must be performed with great caution, always allowing the patients to flex and extend their neck voluntarily to determine their own limitations. If instability must be evaluated in an unconscious patient, it should be performed carefully by a trained physician under fluoroscopic observation. This instability is very important to identify in individuals at risk because relatively minor trauma in this setting can cause a high cervical cord injury. This is especially a concern in the preoperative setting because before and during surgery the unconscious patient's neck may be extended and flexed during intubation and anesthesia.

MRI is useful for determining extent of pannus formation and the degree of compromise of the spinal canal. Involvement of the other intervertebral levels is common, generally presenting radiographically as uniform disc narrowing at multiple levels, with disproportionately small endplate osteophytes and minimal multilevel spondylolisthesis. Erosions may occur at the facet joints and at the uncovertebral joints, although the latter are not true synovial joints. Spinal stenosis can occur at multiple levels related to spondylolistheses and disc bulges. Involvement of the thoracic and lumbar spine can occur but is less prominent.

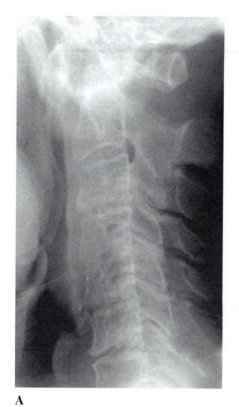

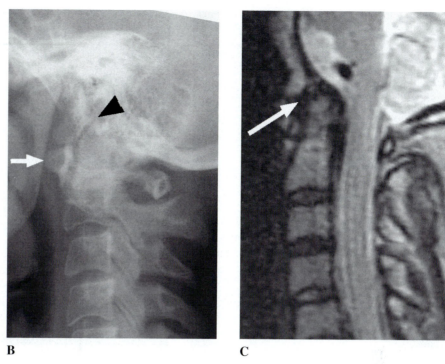

A

B   **C**

FIGURE 3-28.   Rheumatoid arthritis of the cervical spine. *(A)* Lateral view in flexion shows disc narrowing at multiple levels and erosion of the dens with atlantoaxial widening. *(B)* Lateral view of a different patient shows C_2 axial migration with basilar invagination of the dens. Arrow indicates anterior arch of C_1, which is abnormally positioned adjacent to the body of C_2. Note approximation of the base of the clivus with the dens (arrowhead). *(C)* Sagittal T_2-weighted magnetic resonance image of a different patient demonstrates close proximity of the dens and inferior clivus (arrow).

SACROILIAC JOINTS.   The sacroiliac joints are rarely involved, but when they are affected, the radiographic appearance is sacroiliitis with loss of the subchondral cortical line, erosions, especially at the synovial or anteroinferior aspect of the joint, with or without adjacent bone sclerosis. Although involvement is bilateral, the severity of involvement may be asymmetric and fusion is uncommon, unlike sacroiliitis from ankylosing spondylitis or inflammatory bowel disease.

HIPS.   The hip joints are commonly involved; joint narrowing is classically concentric (diffuse) or central, with axial migration of the femoral head. With more advanced disease, the iliopectineal line bows inward and the central acetabulum thins, an appearance called *protrusio acetabuli.* Erosions occur at the margins of the femoral neck and the acetabular rim, where the synovium attaches. Large subchondral cysts form in the femoral head and superior acetabulum because the articular cartilage is lost. Cysts may become so large that the articular surface becomes flattened, simulating collapse from avascular necrosis. Development of advanced secondary osteoarthritis is common after the cartilage is destroyed because the hips are weight-bearing joints. The end-stage hip may be so degenerated that it is difficult to determine the source of the initial insult without clinical information or evaluation of other joints.

KNEE.   When the knees are affected, radiographs show distention of the suprapatellar recess due to effusion and/or synovial proliferation. Soft tissue prominence in the popliteal fossa may represent a Baker cyst, which can be large and dissect up the thigh or down the calf. Uniform joint narrowing characteristically occurs, and large subchondral cysts are often seen. However, erosions are usually subtle and difficult to visualize except in severe involvement; this may be related to the large capacity of the knee joint, in which the pannus can float away from the margins of the joint, resulting in less "pressure effect" on the bare area.

ANKLE AND FOOT.   The ankle joint is analogous to the radiocarpal joint of the wrist, and the tarsal bones are analogs of the carpal bones; as such, involvement of the ankle joint and intertarsal joint is common. Uniform joint narrowing is seen; soft tissue prominence can be seen at the anterior and posterior margins of the ankle joint from underlying pannus and effusion. Erosions can be seen at the margins of the ankle joint and the distal tibiofibular syndesmosis, where this joint recess often fills with pannus.

The metatarsophalangeal joints are commonly involved (Figure 3-29); in fact, the earliest osseous manifestation of rheumatoid arthritis in the foot is usually found at the fifth metatarsophalangeal joint, where soft tissue swelling, slight joint narrowing, and loss of the cortical line at the bare area, or frank erosion are seen very commonly. Findings at this location often precede radiographic changes in the hands but are similar to those in the hands.

Tendinopathy of the foot, in particular the posterior tibialis tendon, is common in the rheumatoid population. Dysfunction

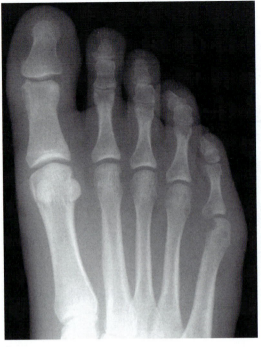
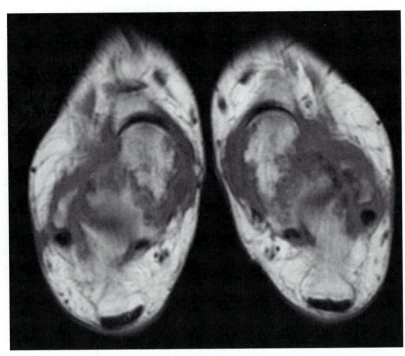

A   B

FIGURE 3-29. Rheumatoid involvement of the foot and ankle. *(A)* Anteroposterior view of the foot shows joint narrowing and marginal erosions at the fifth metatarsophalangeal (MTP) joint. Early involvement of the fifth MTP joint is characteristic. *(B)* Axial T_1-weighted image through the ankles shows symmetric synovitis at multiple joints, with erosive changes.

of the posterior tibialis tendon leads to flat foot and hindfoot valgus with abduction of the forefoot. As in the elbow and hand, rheumatoid nodules may form at the plantar aspect of the foot (Figure 3-30).

Associated Diseases. Systemic manifestations or disease of other organ systems can occur in association with rheumatoid arthritis. *Felty disease* is rheumatoid arthritis associated with splenomegaly and neutropenia; affected patients also experience weight loss, lymphadenopathy, and skin pigmentation and ulceration. *Caplan syndrome* is rheumatoid arthritis associated with pneumoconiosis, an association noted in coal miners; these patients have a high incidence of subcutaneous nodules similar to those seen in typical rheumatoid arthritis in addition to characteristic seropositive articular involvement.

Seronegative Spondyloarthropathy

The term *seronegative spondyloarthropathy* refers to a subset of inflammatory conditions of the joints of the extremities and spine that is typically rheumatoid factor negative. This group includes psoriatic arthritis, Reiter disease, ankylosing spondylitis, and arthropathy associated with inflammatory bowel disease.

PSORIATIC ARTHRITIS. Psoriatic arthritis is associated with the skin disease of the same name. An estimated 2 to 6% of patients with psoriasis have articular involvement, and most patients with articular disease have skin involvement. Most patients have the psoriatic rash for many years before onset of arthralgias. About

15% of patients experience simultaneous onset of the rash and arthritis, and in another 15% the arthritis precedes the skin manifestations. Peak age range of presentation with arthritis is 20 to 40 years, similar to that of rheumatoid arthritis. Unlike rheumatoid arthritis, most patients are rheumatoid factor negative. People with more severe skin involvement and pitting of the nails may be predisposed to articular disease. Patients may present initially with a single, few, or many joints involved. Distribution is the distal joints of the hands and feet, but large joints of the extremities and the sacroiliac joints and spine can also be involved. In the distal extremities, some rays may be involved severely, with sparing of other adjacent rays. Males and females are equally affected, but females predominate in cases of polyarticular disease and males predominate in cases of spinal disease.

Imaging Findings. Radiographically, the disease is characterized by erosions with bone proliferation, an appearance similar to Reiter disease (Figure 3-31). In fact, these two diseases can be difficult to differentiate on radiographs alone. One useful differentiating point is that psoriatic arthritis will commonly involve the hand, whereas Reiter disease does so rarely.

A pattern of diffuse joint narrowing is apparent. Subchondral cysts are not common.

Articular erosions occur at the bare areas of the joint margins. These erosions classically have a proliferative appearance, with a fluffy or whiskered quality identical to the erosions associated with Reiter disease. If the disease progresses, the erosions can become quite severe, with pencilling of the end of the bone, appearing as if it were put through a pencil sharpener. The articular

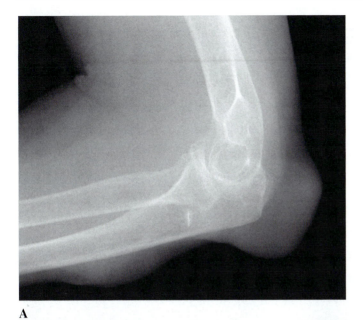

A

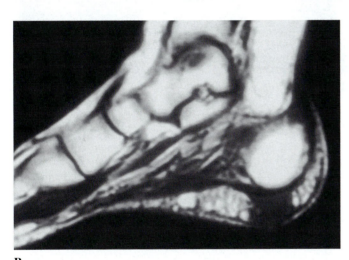

B

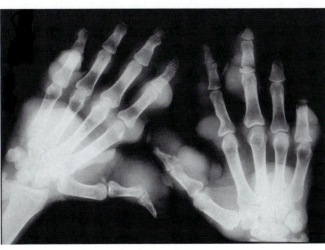

C

surface at the opposite side of the joint can become cupped, and there can be shortening of the digit from telescoping of one bone into the other. With severe involvement, the articular surfaces can undergo complete destruction, a pattern referred to as *arthritis mutilans*. Erosions also can occur at the entheses. Erosions can occur at the odontoid, resulting in atlantoaxial instability; however, this complication is very rare compared with rheumatoid arthritis. At the sacroiliac joints, there is early loss of the thin subchondral white line, which progresses to form discrete erosions, and surrounding reactive bone on both sides of the joint representing sacroiliitis. Sacroiliac involvement may be unilateral or bilateral but asymmetric.

Proliferation is a hallmark of psoriatic arthritis; in addition to proliferative-type erosions, there is often periostitis adjacent to an affected joint. Affected entheses commonly have a fluffy appearance. In the spine, rarely, paravertebral ossification occurs, resulting in osseous bridging between vertebral bodies or posterior elements. Classically, in the lumbar spine, this paravertebral ossification is lateral and asymmetric; multiple levels may be involved. The ossifications are large and prominent and protrude outward. Ankylosis can occur at any involved joint, but most commonly the interphalangeal joints, the sacroiliac joints, and the zygapophyseal joints of the spine are involved.

Distribution is characteristically within distal extremities, especially the interphalangeal joints, MCP and MTP joints of the hands and feet, the spine, and sacroiliac joints; however, other joints including the wrist, ankle, elbow, knee, and shoulder may be involved. Hip involvement is relatively uncommon. Unlike rheumatoid arthritis, involvement of the hand or wrist is more distal than proximal, and there can be dramatic differences in involvement of adjacent rays in psoriatic arthritis, unlike rheumatoid arthritis, where involvement tends to be more uniformly distributed. Asymmetry of involved joints also differentiates psoriatic arthritis from the classic symmetric distribution of rheumatoid arthritis.

Deformity related to psoriatic arthritis is generally limited to the digits of the hands, with subluxations and angular deformity. Fusiform soft tissue swelling occurs around the joints. With more severe involvement, the entire digit can become swollen, an appearance referred to as a *sausage digit* (Figure 3-32). Focal soft tissue swelling also can be seen at entheses due to inflammatory involvement and in periarticular tissues due to bursitis (Figure 3-33). Pitting of the nails occasionally may be seen on radiographs in more severe cases.

Bone mineralization is generally preserved, although early in the disease there may be some periarticular demineralization.

FIGURE 3-30. Rheumatoid nodules. *(A)* Lateral view of the elbow shows subcutaneous nodules at the olecranon and extensor surface. *(B)* Sagittal T$_1$-weighted magnetic resonance image shows a rheumatoid nodule in the subcalcaneal fat pad. *(C)* Benign rheumatoid nodulosis: Anteroposterior view of the hand shows diffuse involvement of the hands with subcutaneous nodules but relative sparing of the joints.

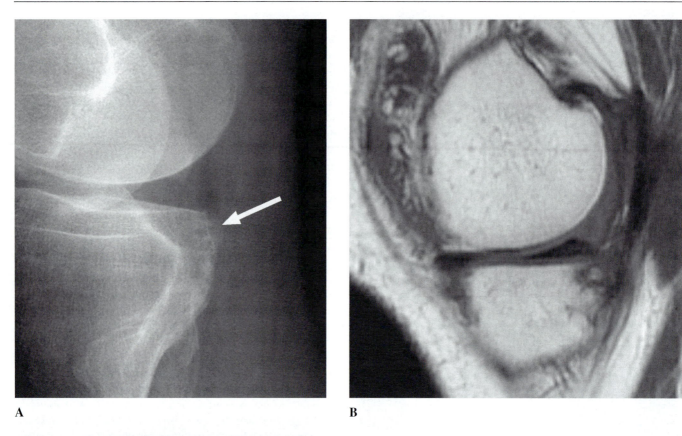

A

B

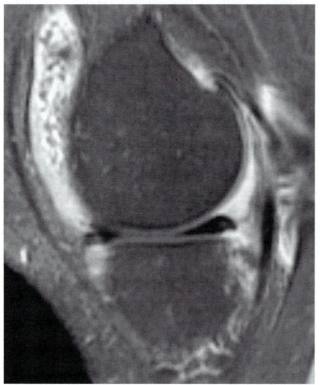

C

FIGURE 3-31.   Psoriatic arthritis: formation of proliferative erosion. *(A)* Magnified oblique view of the knee shows subtle proliferative erosion at the posterior margin of the tibial plateau. *(B)* Sagittal T$_1$-weighted and *(C)* T$_1$-weighted fat-suppressed post-gadolinium image of the same knee demonstrates marked synovial proliferation, with enhancing synovium eroding the margins of the tibial plateau.

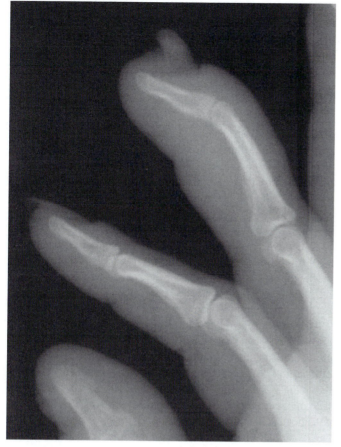

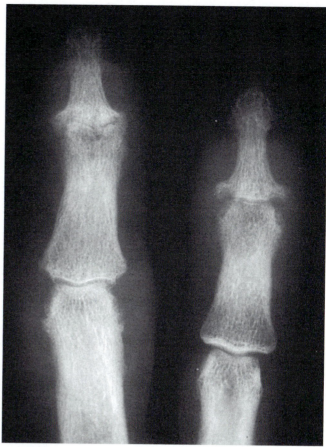

A

B

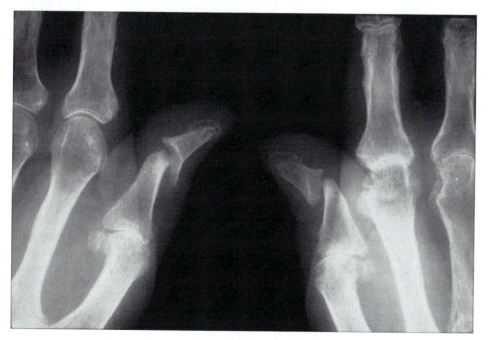

C

FIGURE 3-32. Psoriatic arthritis: hand involvement. *(A)* Lateral view of the digit shows diffuse swelling ("sausage digit") with deformity of the nail. *(B)* Anteroposterior view of the digits shows distal involvement, with proliferative erosions at the distal interphalangeal (DIP) and proximal interphalangeal (PIP) joints. *(C)* Views of both thumbs demonstrate arthritis mutilans.

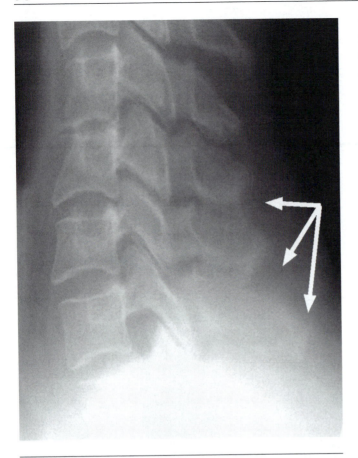

FIGURE 3-33. Psoriatic arthritis: enthesitis. Lateral view of the cervical spine shows fluffy enthesial proliferation of the posterior interspinous ligaments (arrows).

REITER DISEASE. Reiter disease, also known as *reactive arthritis*, is an oligoarticular arthritis and enthesopathy that follows an infectious condition, usually of the genitourinary or gastrointestinal tract. Age of onset varies from adolescence to middle age but peaks in the third decade. The clinical syndrome classically includes urethritis, conjunctivitis, and arthritis; however, frequently one of the first two is absent. The clinical symptoms usually begin within 1 month of the infection, which, if genitourinary, is typically *Chlamydia trachomatis*, and, if gastrointestinal, can be a number of organisms including *Shigella*, *Campylobacter*, or *Salmonella*. The arthritis related to genitourinary disease affects males approximately 9 times more commonly than females, whereas the syndrome following gastrointestinal disease is seen in males and females equally. White individuals make up approximately 80% of patients, and the HLA-B27 antigen is seen in more than 50% of people with the disease (rheumatoid factor is absent). Usually the disease follows a limited course, resolving within 1 year; however, about 15% of patients have chronic disease.

Imaging Findings. Oligoarticular involvement is most common, with an average of four joints involved. In addition to articular involvement, inflammation occurs at the entheses. Lower extremity joints, especially those in the ankle and foot, are usually affected. Joints of the upper extremities are rarely affected, but when they are, there is also involvement of the joints of the lower extremities. The sacroiliac joints are also commonly affected, causing an appearance of sacroiliitis similar to ankylosing spondylitis. However, unlike ankylosing spondylitis, involvement of the sacroiliac joints in Reiter disease is frequently asymmetric or even unilateral. Radiographic hallmarks of disease are diffuse joint narrowing, marginal erosions, and bone proliferation. The appearance can be indistinguishable from psoriatic arthritis; however, most patients with psoriatic arthritis have the characteristic skin rash of psoriasis or pitting of the fingernails. Also, psoriatic arthritis commonly involves the hand, whereas hand involvement is uncommon in Reiter disease.

Heel pain is very common in Reiter disease and is usually due to inflammation at the ankle entheses, especially the insertion of the Achilles tendon and the origin of the plantar fascia at the calcaneus. The enthesis becomes thickened, with poor definition of the adjacent fat planes. The retrocalcaneal bursa anterior to the Achilles tendon is also commonly distended with fluid and inflammatory synovium. With more chronic disease, this bursitis and enthesitis can cause erosions and bone proliferation to occur at the attachment sites on the adjacent calcaneus, resulting in a classic fluffy appearance (Figure 3-34). Enthesitis can occur at other locations in the foot and ankle (such as the base of the fifth metatarsal and the insertion of the peroneus brevis), but the calcaneus is the most common site. Diffuse soft tissue swelling can occur in a single or a number of the digits, causing a sausage digit (Figure 3-35).

As in psoriatic arthritis, distribution is usually distal, primarily involving the metatarsophalangeal and interphalangeal joints (although ankle involvement is not uncommon), and is characterized by proliferative, or fluffy, marginal erosions and joint narrowing; as in psoriatic arthritis, severe involvement may occur, with central erosions and a pencil-in-cup pattern of joint destruction or ankylosis. Periostitis with a whiskered appearance can also be seen at periarticular sites. The knee is less commonly involved; a joint effusion may be seen, with proliferative marginal erosions and diffuse joint narrowing. Hip involvement is uncommon, but proliferative enthesophytes can be seen at attachments of tendons and ligaments around the pelvis.

Sacroiliac involvement is common, and bilateral asymmetric or unilateral involvement distinguishes it from ankylosing spondylitis and inflammatory bowel disease. Early changes include loss of the subchondral line and erosions, especially at the anteroinferior aspect of the joint, with paradoxical "pseudo-widening" of the joint. Later changes include ill-defined reactive sclerosis of the subchondral bone, with occasional ankylosis (fusion is less common than in ankylosing spondylitis).

As with the other seronegative spondyloarthropathy types, the spine may be affected, although involvement is less common and different in appearance than in ankylosing spondylitis. Involvement tends to occur at the upper lumbar spine or thoracolumbar junction (unlike ankylosing spondylitis, which starts at the lumbosacral junction and progresses superiorly). Although bridging syndesmophytes can occur as in ankylosing spondylitis, more characteristic is paravertebral ossification, which forms

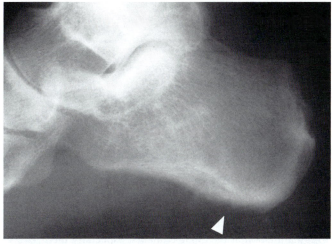

A

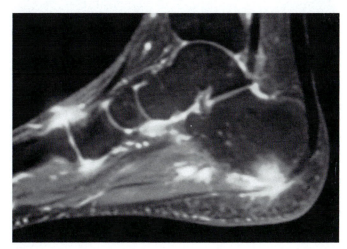

B

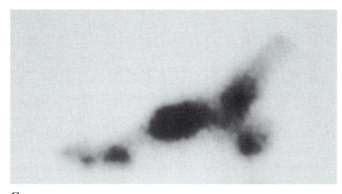

C

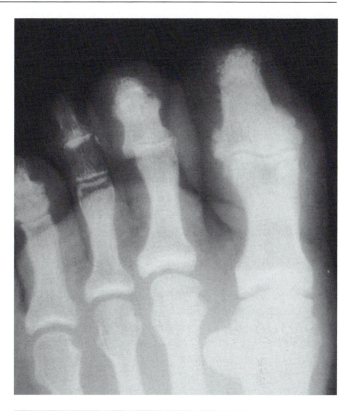

FIGURE 3-35. Reiter disease: involvement of the foot. Anteroposterior view of the toes shows diffuse swelling of the second digit, representing a "sausage digit." There are proliferative erosions at the first interphalangeal joint.

FIGURE 3-34. Reiter disease: enthesitis. (A) Lateral view of the calcaneus shows a proliferative enthesophyte at the origin of the plantar aponeurosis. (B) Sagittal T$_1$-weighted fat-suppressed post-gadolinium image shows enhancement of the enthesis and the tarsometatarsal (TMT) joint. (C) Delayed technetium 99m bone scintigraphic image shows uptake of tracer at these sites.

C-shape "claw-like" spurs laterally and which may eventually bridge the disc space. Asymmetric involvement is common, and the ossification can be seen at multiple adjacent levels. Because the underlying process is an inflammatory enthesopathy, the ossification may have a fluffy appearance, as in other involved entheses.

ANKYLOSING SPONDYLITIS. Ankylosing spondylitis is an inflammatory arthropathy and enthesopathy predominantly affecting the spine and pelvis. As with the other inflammatory arthropathies, onset peaks in young adulthood, ranging from 20 to 40 years of age. Males are more commonly affected than females at a ratio of approximately 3:1. There is a strong association with the HLA-B27 antigen, but the etiology remains unclear. Occasionally there is overlap with other arthropathies including Reiter disease, psoriatic arthritis, and inflammatory arthropathy associated with inflammatory bowel disease, and the disease may occur in a pediatric population (see Juvenile Chronic Arthritis).

Ankylosing spondylitis characteristically has an insidious onset, presenting as back pain and stiffness that may go on for months before the individual seeks medical attention. Pain is usually ill-defined, is worse in the morning or after periods of inactivity, and improves with exercise. Patients may attempt to alleviate symptoms by not bending over or twisting and instead performing activities with an intentionally straight posture. At this stage of the disease, there can be considerable improvement with NSAIDs and physical therapy. The disease can follow an intermittent course with recurrent flares. The hips and shoulders also can be involved, as can the entheses around the pelvis and heel. As the disease progresses, there is ankylosis of the spine and sacroiliac joints and fixed limitation of spinal range of motion. There is commonly thoracic kyphotic deformity that may be severe, making ambulation difficult. As ankylosis progresses, the pain associated with spinal motion subsides.

Imaging Findings.   Early radiographic changes in the spine include squaring of the anterior vertebral body; this can be very subtle, with loss of the normal concavity of the anterior vertebral margin. Enthesitis at the attachments of the anulus fibrosus to the anterior margins of the endplates causes erosion, irregularity (whiskering), and eventual reactive sclerosis, an appearance referred to as *shiny corners*. The anterior fibers of the anulus fibrosus and Sharpey fibers progressively ossify, leading to osseous bridging across the discs, called *syndesmophytes*. This causes a gradual undulating appearance of the vertebral margin on the frontal view (referred to as a *bamboo spine*), with a very straight margin of ossification of the anterior vertebral margin on the lateral view. The zygapophyseal, or facet, joints and the costovertebral joints also can become involved and may progress to fusion (Figures 3-36 and 3-37).

At the sacroiliac joints, initially there is poor definition of the subchondral white line and subsequently discrete erosions (see Fig. 3-5). Erosions occur initially at the iliac side (which has thinner cartilage) of the anteroinferior aspect of the joint, which is the synovial portion. Erosions may cause the joint to be paradoxically widened, called pseudo-widening. Later on, reactive bone at the margins of the joint causes a thick band of ill-defined sclerosis along the subchondral bone. Eventually the joint fuses and the reactive sclerosis may eventually subside. Synovial and ligamentous portions of the joint eventually fuse. Sacroiliitis in ankylosing spondylitis (and the look-alike arthropathy associated with inflammatory bowel disease) is characteristically bilateral and symmetric; sacroiliitis associated with psoriatic arthritis and Reiter disease can be unilateral or bilateral but asymmetric.

The osseous changes characteristically begin at the sacroiliac joints and lumbosacral junction and progress cranially to involve the entire lumbar spine, followed by the thoracic and then the cervical spine. However, occasionally the early radiographic findings are recognized initially at the thoracolumbar junction. Fusion also can occur at the facet joints and intervertebral ligaments of the posterior elements. The thoracic spine can be fixed with a prominent kyphotic deformity. Complications can occur as there is progressive fusion; stress from motion at the craniocervical junction with relative immobility of the cervical spine can lead to laxity of the transverse ligament of the dens and atlantoaxial instability. Trauma can result in spinal fractures with bizarre patterns, crossing obliquely through multiple vertebral levels. Fracture healing often progresses poorly, with resulting pseudarthrosis. Decreased respiratory function and respiratory infection can occur related to decreased mobility of the thoracic cage, particularly if the costovertebral joints are involved (Figure 3-38).

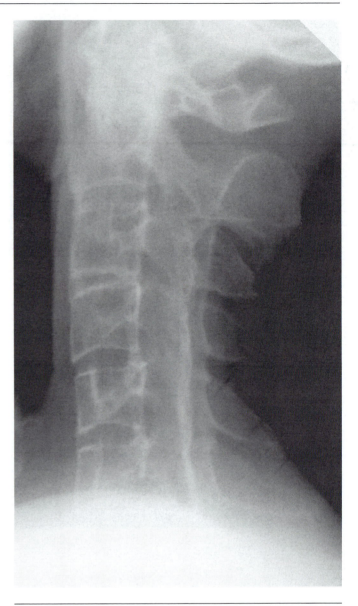

FIGURE 3-36.   Ankylosing spondylitis: cervical spine. Lateral view shows fusion of the zygapophyseal joints and syndesmophytes anteriorly.

In the appendicular skeleton, the hips are the most common sites of involvement, typically bilateral and symmetric, and can progress to ankylosis. Concentric bilateral joint narrowing with axial migration with minimal to no erosion is common, although a more erosive pattern with deformity of the femoral head can be seen before ankylosis. Involvement of the shoulders, knees, acromioclavicular joints, sternal articulations, or distal extremities occurs in 10 to 30% of cases and may result in joint fusion.

ARTHROPATHY ASSOCIATED WITH INFLAMMATORY BOWEL DISEASE. Arthritic symptoms are experienced by approximately 10 to 20% of patients with Crohn disease and ulcerative colitis; the etiology is unclear, but severity of peripheral arthralgia appears to be related to activity of the bowel disease. In fact, total colectomy in ulcerative colitis can result in resolution of the peripheral arthritis. However, progression of axial disease in the spine and sacroiliac joints tends to follow an independent

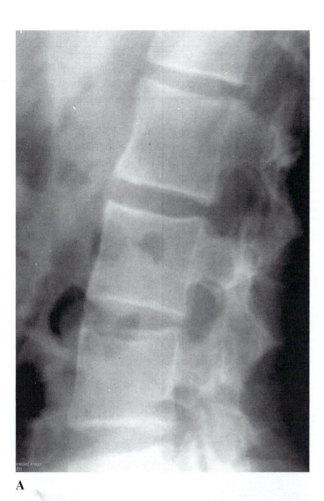

A

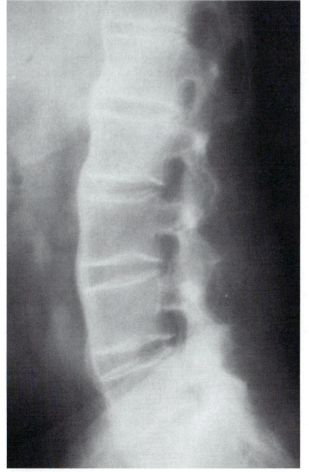

B

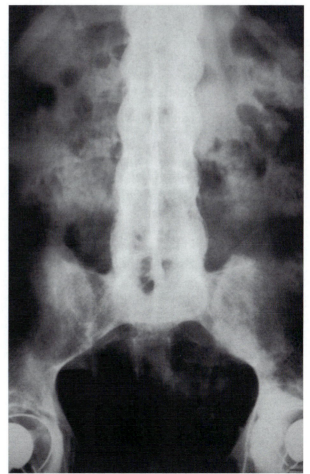

C

FIGURE 3-37. Ankylosing spondylitis: lumbar spine. *(A)* Early changes on a lateral view. Note erosion and sclerosis of the anterior endplates ("shiny corners"); early flat, bridging syndesmophytes; and flattening of the anterior vertebral body (compare with the relatively less involved upper vertebral body). Note also progression of disease from inferior to superior. Late changes on *(B)* lateral and *(C)* anteroposterior views: Bridging syndesmophytes, present throughout the lumbar spine, are flat on the lateral view and undulating on the anteroposterior view ("bamboo spine").

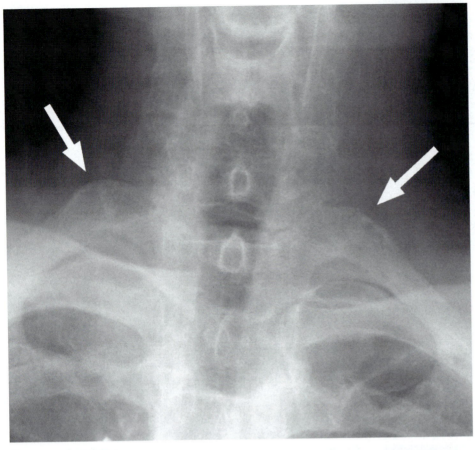

A

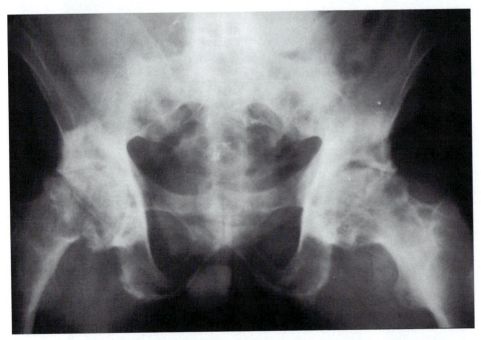

B

FIGURE 3-38. Ankylosing spondylitis: other commonly involved sites. *(A)* Anteroposterior view of the cervicothoracic junction shows ankylosis of the costovertebral joints. This can lead to respiratory compromise. *(B)* Anteroposterior view of the hips shows diffuse narrowing of the hip joints with severe secondary osteoarthritis.

course unaltered by bowel disease activity or treatment. The HLA-B27 antigen is found in approximately 50% of people with spinal involvement, although it does not appear to be related to the peripheral arthropathy. Spinal involvement is more common in males (approximately 3:1) with inflammatory bowel disease.

Imaging Findings. The radiographic appearance of arthropathy associated with inflammatory bowel disease is virtually identical to that of ankylosing spondylitis, with bilateral symmetric sacroiliitis and enthesitis of the spine resulting in syndesmophytes and fusion.

JUVENILE CHRONIC ARTHRITIS. Juvenile chronic arthritis (JCA) includes a number of subsets of articular disease presenting before adulthood. These subcategories include juvenile-onset adult-type (seropositive) rheumatoid arthritis, seronegative chronic arthritis (Still disease), juvenile-onset ankylosing spondylitis, psoriatic arthritis, arthritis associated with inflammatory bowel disease, and miscellaneous categories. All tend to occur in an adolescent population and mimic the manifestations of the adult-onset disease except Still disease, which typically occurs in younger children and is the most common form of JCA. People affected with JCA at a young age have certain manifestations on radiographic examinations related to chronic inflammation and hyperemia that occurs in growing joints; these manifestations are particularly associated with Still disease, likely in part related to the earlier age of onset of this disease.

Still disease (seronegative chronic arthritis) is the most common form of JCA, representing approximately 70% of cases. As the name indicates, serum rheumatoid factor is negative. The disease can present in a variety of forms: systemic (10%), polyarticular (40%), and pauciarticular or monarticular (50%). Onset of the systemic form is acute and often occurs before age 5 years. Systemic manifestations of the disease include fever, anorexia, rash, lymphadenopathy, hepatosplenomegaly, pericarditis or myocarditis, arthralgias and myalgias, and anemia or leukocytosis with increased sedimentation rate.

Patients may progress from the systemic form to the polyarticular form or may present initially with the polyarticular form, in which five or more joints are involved. Systemic manifestations also occur in the polyarticular form but are less pronounced than in the systemic form. Two subtypes are rheumatoid factor negative and positive; age of onset is later than in the systemic form, typically affecting patients older than 8 years. The seropositive form most closely resembles adult rheumatoid arthritis. Symmetric articular involvement is typical in the polyarticular form, with wrist joints, MCP and PIP joints of the hands, knee and ankle joints, intertarsal, MTP and interphalangeal joints of the feet, and the cervical spine articulations commonly involved.

A monarticular or pauciarticular (four or fewer joints involved) pattern is often seen initially, which may progress to the polyarticular form. There are early-onset and late-onset subtypes; early-onset may occur as early as 1 to 5 years of age. Joints commonly involved include the knee, ankle, elbow, wrist, and cervical spine. Systemic involvement is infrequent.

Imaging Findings. Some radiographic findings mimic the adult form of rheumatoid arthritis and include fusiform periarticular soft tissue swelling, periarticular osteoporosis, and concentric or uniform joint narrowing (although joint narrowing is typically seen only late in the disease course; Figure 3-39). However, unlike adult-onset rheumatoid arthritis, erosions are not a prominent feature. In addition, in Still disease there is often periostitis adjacent to affected joints, whereas proliferation is unusual in adult rheumatoid arthritis.

Because the disease affects growing joints, other radiographic characteristics become prominent. Hyperemia leads to overgrowth and a ballooned appearance of the epiphyses compared with the metaphyses and diaphyses. The hyperemic effect also can result in early fusion of the growth plate, causing an abrupt transition between the epiphysis and diaphysis. Early physeal fusion can cause growth disturbance, with bone shortening if the plate fuses uniformly or with deformity if the fusion affects only part of the growth plate. The diaphyses of affected extremities may be gracile, and the combination of thin diaphyses and epiphyseal overgrowth with abrupt transition results in an "over-tubulation" pattern.

JCA also causes joint ankylosis at a much higher frequency than does adult-onset rheumatoid arthritis. Any affected joints can fuse; in the cervical spine, fusion of the facet joints may lead to a growth disturbance of the vertebral bodies (Figure 3-40). Due to lack of space for the vertebral bodies to grow, they may become broad and flat or small and immature looking. Fusion of the carpal or tarsal bones is also common (see Fig. 3-39).

Overall, deformity rather than joint narrowing and erosion is the main feature of Still disease, thereby separating it from adult forms of inflammatory arthropathy. The deformity and effects of cartilage damage often result in development of early secondary osteoarthritis in affected joints, despite remission of the original inflammatory disease.

The rheumatoid factor positive polyarticular form of JCA tends to occur well after age 8 years and behaves like adult rheumatoid arthritis. It represents approximately 10% of all JCA cases. Females are affected more often than males. The wrist, MCP and PIP joints of the hands, the knees, and the MTP and interphalangeal joints of the feet are common sites of involvement. More than 50% of affected patients have severe destructive manifestation of their arthritis. As in adult rheumatoid arthritis, patients may have subcutaneous nodules.

Juvenile-onset ankylosing spondylitis, as in the adult form, is seen predominantly in males and is associated with the HLA B-27 antigen. Onset is typically between ages 10 and 12 years. Progressive involvement of the sacroiliac joints and spine, especially the thoracic and lumbar spine, mirror that of the adult-onset form, with early squaring of the vertebral bodies and sclerosis of vertebral corners (shiny corners) and late formation of syndesmophytes and sacroiliac ankylosis. As in the adult form, other joints may be involved. The joints of the lower extremities are commonly involved, including the hips, knees, ankles, and intertarsal joints.

Other manifestations of JCA include a pattern resembling psoriatic arthritis and a chronic arthropathy associated with inflammatory bowel disease. These forms of JCA are similar to the corresponding adult forms.

SAPHO SYNDROME. *SAPHO* is an acronym that stands for synovitis, acne, pustulosis, hyperostosis, and osteitis and is the preferred term to unify several different and likely related conditions that contain dermal and musculoskeletal manifestations ("skin and bones"). Patients with SAPHO are rheumatoid factor negative and may develop sacroiliitis and/or enthesitis. Therefore, it is felt that the SAPHO syndrome most likely reflects a type of seronegative spondyloarthropathy with features that are not as well established and may represent an undifferentiated form. SAPHO differs from the other seronegative disorders with respect to prognosis, which is favorable with an indolent course of symptoms that is usually self-limited. The imaging manifestations are important because they can suggest the diagnosis when the clinical presentation is confusing. The itemized features making up the acronym are present to a variable extent and are not necessarily concurrent findings. In addition, the severity and tempo of the listed features are variably present. Two of the more frequently encountered conditions that probably represent restricted forms of SAPHO are chronic recurrent multifocal osteomyelitis and sternocostoclavicular hyperostosis, both of which are frequently associated with skin conditions.

The pathogenesis is uncertain but may be related to a host response to the microorganism *Propionibacterium acne*. The musculoskeletal manifestations consist of synovitis, hyperostosis, and osteitis. The skin manifestations are severe acne and pustulosis, characteristically in a palmoplantar distribution.

Synovitis more frequently occurs in the axial skeleton especially the anterior chest wall and may involve the following articulations: sternoclavicular, costoclavicular, and sternomanubrial. Sacroiliitis, when present, may be unilateral. The peripheral arthropathy is pauci- or polyarticular but, compared with other seronegative spondyloarthropathy types, fewer joints are involved, the extent of destruction is not as great, and the

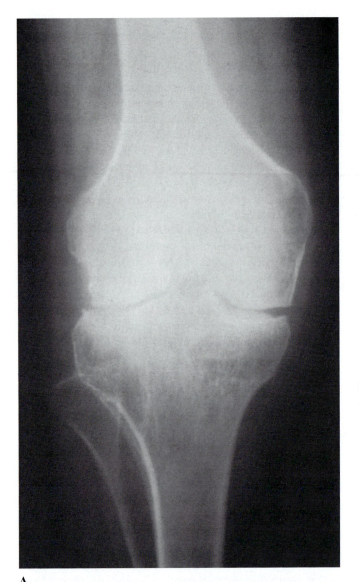

A

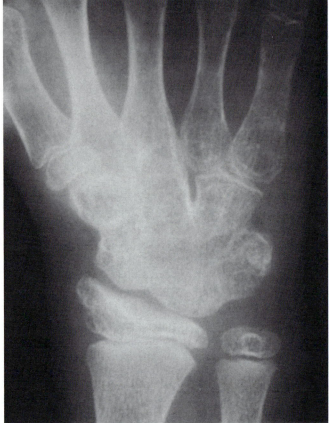

B

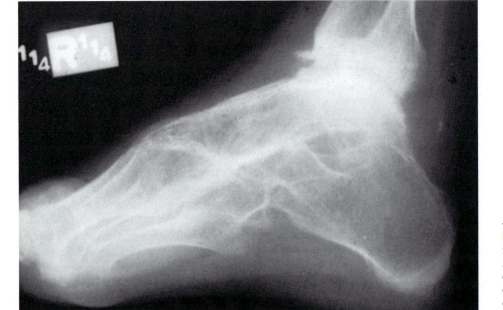

C

FIGURE 3-39. Still disease: late effects in the appendicular skeleton. *(A)* Anteroposterior view of the knee shows diffuse joint narrowing and overgrowth of the epiphyses without erosions. Secondary osteoarthritis is evident, with marginal osteophytes. *(B)* Anteroposterior view of the wrist and *(C)* lateral view of the ankle demonstrate intercarpal and intertarsal fusion.

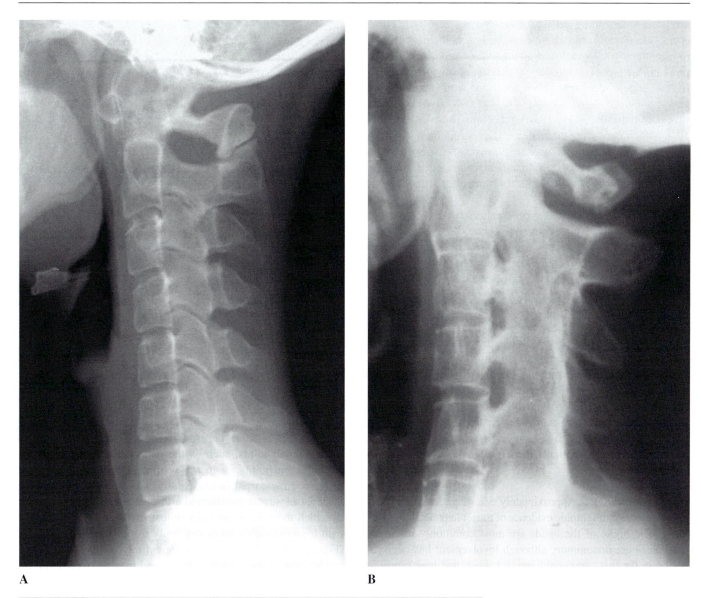

A   B

FIGURE 3-40. Still disease: cervical spine. *(A)* Lateral view shows deformity of the vertebral bodies with prominent height and associated overgrowth of the facets without fusion. *(B)* Lateral view of a different patient shows fusion of the facet joints with deformity of the vertebral bodies.

frequency of involvement is lower. *Hyperostosis* refers to increased osteogenesis, which may occur in periosteal, endosteal, or enthesial locations. Findings in the tubular bones consist of cortical thickening and sclerotic opacity, with mature (not aggressive) periosteal new bone and a diminished medullary canal. The distribution is predominantly of the anterior thorax and axial skeleton. *Osteitis* is inflammation of bone and mostly refers to cortical involvement without marrow involvement and is due to an inflammatory cell infiltrate. The area is usually symptomatically painful and tender to palpation.

Other Inflammatory Disorders

SARCOIDOSIS. Sarcoidosis is a granulomatous disease of uncertain etiology that can involve multiple organ systems, with the pulmonary system being most common. Males and females are affected with approximately equal frequency. Typically, the early manifestations of the disease are recognized in young adults between ages 20 and 40 years. Black individuals are most commonly affected, with a prevalence approximately 10 times greater than in whites in the United States; however, the disease is also relatively common in northern Europe, especially Sweden.

Acute and chronic forms are recognized clinically; pulmonary involvement is very common, occurring in as many as 90% of patients. Other organ systems are often involved, resulting in variable patterns of adenopathy, hepatosplenomegaly, ocular abnormalities (iritis and uveitis), and erythema nodosum. Less commonly, involvement of the heart, nervous system, and musculoskeletal system may occur. Symptoms include cough, dyspnea, fever, malaise, anorexia, arthralgia,

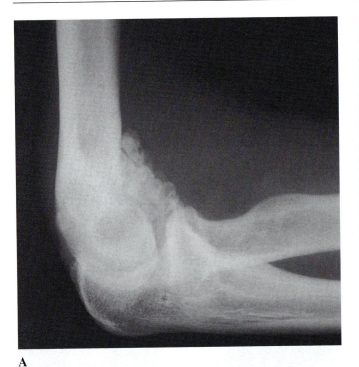
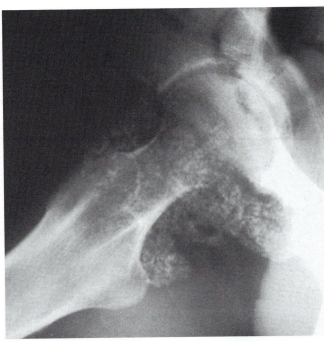

A   B

FIGURE 3-43. Synovial osteochondromatosis. *(A)* Lateral view of the elbow shows numerous intraarticular bodies in the anterior humeral recess and the olecranon recess, without osteoarthritis. *(B)* Frogleg lateral view of the hip shows innumerable tiny intraarticular bodies throughout the distended hip joint, with thinning of the femoral neck due to erosion.

from the underlying arthritis and from body formation and include pain, crepitus, and locking.

Imaging Findings. Radiographically, increased soft tissue opacity is present, representing synovial proliferation or an associated joint effusion. Intraarticular bodies are calcified or ossified in 70 to 95% of cases and are approximately equal in size (Figure 3-43). The osseous structures of the joint demonstrate normal mineralization. The articular cartilage is preserved until late in the course of the disease; therefore, the joint space is typically normal at initial presentation. Erosions may occur in articulations with tight capsules (eg, the hip). No periosteal reaction is associated with uncomplicated synovial osteochondromatosis. Deformity occurs only when secondary degenerative joint disease ensues. The disorder may involve only a portion of the synovium (localized form) or may be diffuse. Bodies that form are usually adherent to the synovium but may break loose and collect in recesses.

Cross-sectional imaging is a useful adjunct to radiographs especially when there are no calcified or ossified bodies (Figure 3-44). CT arthrography (double contrast or air alone) is excellent for demonstrating erosions and determining whether an opacity is intra- or extraarticular when radiography is indeterminate. MRI findings depend on the composition of the bodies. The typical MR appearance is a lobulated intraarticular mass with signal intensity that follows the signal intensity of hyaline cartilage (low to intermediate signal intensity of T1W and hyperintensity on T2W) and may have punctate signal voids due

to mineralization that is not apparent radiographically. Calcified bodies, if present, have low signal intensity on T1W and T2W images. Ossified bodies have fatty marrow centrally and follow fat signal intensity on all pulse sequences; the outer margin, however, is cortical bone represented by a signal void. When conventional MRI is indeterminate, intravenous gadolinium assists in differentiating synovitis, hyperplasia, or bodies from a simple joint effusion. Intraarticular gadolinium is helpful for evaluating the location, size, and number of bodies. Chondrosarcomatous degeneration is suggested by extension beyond the confines of the joint capsule.

Secondary synovial osteochondromatosis typically demonstrates intraarticular bodies that are fewer and more variable in size than in the primary form. The joint also manifests findings of the underlying disorder (eg, osteoarthritis, osteonecrosis, rheumatoid arthritis, crystal associated arthropathy, or osteochondral fracture).

When evaluating a joint with intraarticular bodies, the first consideration is to decide whether it is a primary process or a secondary manifestation of a joint abnormality. An absence or paucity of arthritic findings and monoarticular involvement are the features that suggest primary synovial osteochondromatosis.

PIGMENTED VILLONODULAR SYNOVITIS. Pigmented villonodular synovitis (PVNS) is a benign proliferative synovitis of unknown etiology, occurring as a diffuse form (common) or as a localized form (uncommon), denoted as such as with the

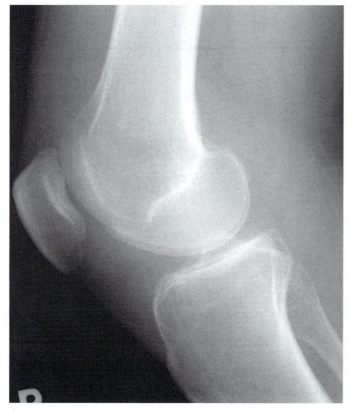

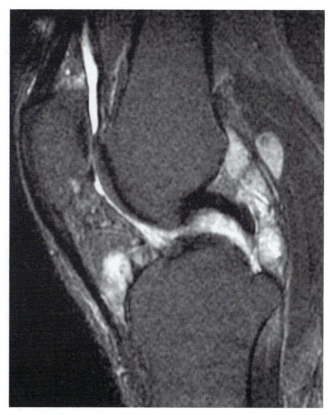

A   B

FIGURE 3-44.   Synovial chondromatosis. *(A)* Lateral view of the knee shows no calcified or ossified intraarticular bodies. *(B)* Sagittal T_2-weighted fat-suppressed fast spin echo magnetic resonance image demonstrates lobulated synovial thickening, which has a high signal on T_2 but a heterogeneous and lower signal than fluid.

prefix D or L, respectively. When this disorder occurs in the extraarticular form, it is as a focal process involving a tendon (common) or a bursa (uncommon). It is most appropriate to name these extraarticular lesions *pigmented villonodular tenosynovitis* and *pigmented villonodular bursitis*, respectively. Pigmented villonodular tenosynovitis is also known as *giant cell tumor of the tendon sheath* or *localized nodular tenosynovitis*. There is no relation to giant cell tumor of bone.

The extraarticular localized form is about four times more common than the intraarticular diffuse form, which has an incidence of approximately 2 per million.

Although the exact cause of PVNS is uncertain, it may be neoplastic (more likely) or a reactive monocyte response to an unknown stimulus (less likely). At gross inspection the synovium has an orange-yellow to red-brown appearance. Microscopically, synovial cell hyperplasia and surface proliferation are present. This proliferation manifests as two types of villous formation: coarse and fine. The confluence of fine villi form discrete nodules. Hyperplastic synovium invades into the subchondral bone producing cysts. There is also subsynovial accumulation of hemosiderin-laden macrophages, multinucleated giant cells, and fibroblasts. Hemosiderin deposition occurs extracellularly and intracellularly and is secondary to recurrent synovial hemorrhage. Lipid-laden ("foamy") macrophages are

also present histologically. The extraarticular localized form has the same histology but usually contains less hemosiderin than the articular counterpart.

The intraarticular form commonly occurs as a diffuse process (Figure 3-45) and uncommonly occurs as a focal process involving only a small portion of the synovium (Figure 3-46). Diffuse PVNS (DPVNS) presents as a monoarticular arthropathy with insidious onset of symptoms, most frequently encountered in one of the large joints of the lower extremity, in the following order: knee (80%), hip, and ankle. The age of presentation is broad but is typically in the range of 20 to 40 years, with no sex predilection. Arthrocentesis may demonstrate serosanguineous fluid. The presence of a bloody effusion in the absence of trauma suggests PVNS. Treatment consists of synovectomy, which may be supplemented with intraarticular radioisotope treatment using a beta emitter.

Pigmented villonodular tenosynovitis (localized nodular tenosynovitis) most commonly presents as an extraarticular soft tissue mass or focal swelling, typically in the hand or foot and usually related to a flexor tendon. The age of presentation is older than that with intraarticular PVNS, occurring in the fifth to sixth decades of life, with a female predilection. It is the second most common soft tissue lesion of the hand after a ganglion.

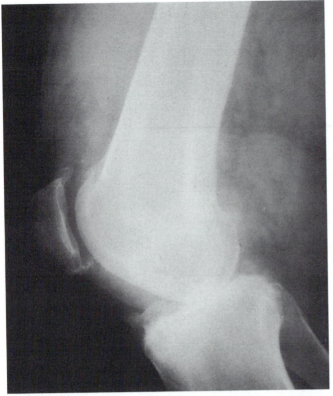

A

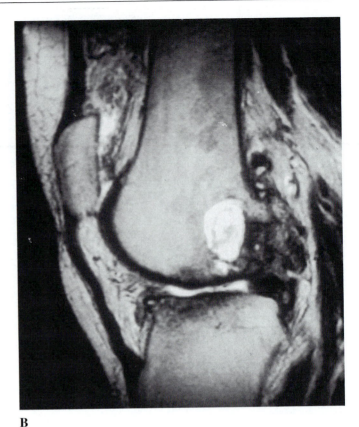

B

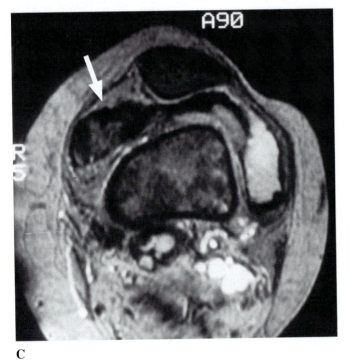

C

FIGURE 3-45.   Pigmented villonodular synovitis: diffuse form. *(A)* Lateral view of the knee shows what appears to be a massive joint effusion but with relatively high density. No calcifications are present. *(B)* Sagittal T_2-weighted fast spin echo magnetic resonance image shows that the "effusion" suspected radiographically represents marked synovial proliferation. Note low T_2 signal of the synovium, representing hemosiderin deposition. *(C)* Axial gradient echo magnetic resonance image at the level of the suprapatellar pouch shows low signal of the synovium, which is more prominent than on the T_2-weighted image, representing magnetic susceptibility ("blooming") artifact from hemosiderin deposition (arrow).

Imaging Findings: Intraarticular.   DPVNS appears as increased soft tissue density on radiography similar to hemophilia. The soft tissue component does not calcify, and there is no osseous proliferation, periosteal reaction, or demineralization associated. The osteocartilaginous changes are inversely proportional to the joint capacity. In a "tight" joint, the findings are

multiple subchondral lucencies and pressure erosions on intracapsular cortices, which are often marginal, simulating erosions of an inflammatory arthropathy. Gradual cartilage loss and joint narrowing occur over time, progressing to development of osteoarthritis. The differential diagnosis of multiple well-defined subchondral lucent lesions includes osteoarthritis, rheumatoid

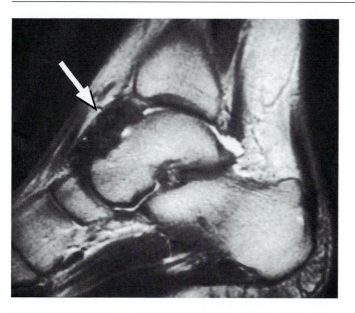

FIGURE 3-46. Pigmented villonodular synovitis: localized form. Sagittal T$_2$-weighted magnetic resonance image of the ankle shows a synovial mass of low signal at the anteromedial joint margin (arrow). Otherwise, the joint is unaffected.

arthritis, amyloid, hemophilia, chronic infection such as tuberculosis, and synovial chondromatosis in addition to DPVNS. In a capacious joint such as the knee, erosions are less common but, because of the synovial proliferation widening of the intercondylar notch, may occur similarly to hemophilia and JCA. Conventional arthrography demonstrates multiple irregular nodular filling defects.

Imaging Findings: Extraarticular. Pigmented villonodular tenosynovitis (localized nodular tenosynovitis), or giant cell tumor of the tendon sheath, has a prevailing soft tissue component causing scalloped pressure-type erosions on the cortex of an adjacent bone, which may be near to or somewhat remote from a joint. This form most commonly is encountered in the hands or feet and most often is related to a flexor tendon about the phalanges. The subjacent bone typically demonstrates no periostitis or proliferation because PVNS is slow growing. However, substantial osseous remodeling and erosions do occur because the lesion is often situated in a confined area between the tendon and the underlying bone. The differential diagnosis for these findings in the hand (or foot) includes a ganglion, epidermoid inclusion cyst, tophaceous gout, nerve sheath tumor, or juxtacortical neoplasm with an indolent growth pattern (benign, such as chondroma, or malignant, such as synovial cell sarcoma).

Cross-Sectional Imaging. CT has limited use but can demonstrate erosions from hyperattenuating or, less commonly, hypoattenuating masses (with respect to muscle) and can differentiate extrinsic from intrinsic joint lesions. Grayscale ultrasound typically shows an echogenic mass and power Doppler may reveal hyperemia. However, ultrasound is probably most useful for dynamically evaluating the relation of a tendon sheath to the subjacent lesion.

MRI reflects the pathoanatomic substrate of hemosiderin, lipid, fibrosis, and synovial proliferation. DPVNS shows diffuse synovial thickening, with signal characteristics that strongly suggest the diagnosis. Hemosiderin appears markedly hypointense (virtually without signal) with respect to muscle on T1W and T2W images. These areas of signal void appear larger when imaged with gradient echo pulse sequences secondary to the increased susceptibility artifact from hemosiderin. This phenomenon has been termed *blooming.* Uncommonly, PVNS may have intermediate signal intensity with respect to muscle on T1W or proton density (PD)-weighted pulse sequences and fluid signal intensity on T2W pulse sequences, which is felt to be related to areas of loculated fluid collections. The other forms of PVNS have a variable amount of hemosiderin and may show only a peripheral ring of low signal intensity or may demonstrate uniform low signal similar to DPVNS (Table 3-15).

LIPOMA ARBORESCENS. Lipoma arborescens is a rare disorder of unknown etiology characterized by proliferation of lipomatous tissue within the synovium. It may result from a chronic inflammatory synovitis with resultant hyperplasia of the fatty subsynovial tissue, but often there is no recognized history of previous arthropathy. It presents as chronic mass-like enlargement of the joint and most commonly affects the knee. MRI shows mass-like synovial proliferation that has signal characteristics of fat, with numerous frond-like excrescences (Figure 3-47).

COLLAGEN VASCULAR DISEASES ASSOCIATED WITH ARTHROPATHY

Scleroderma

Systemic sclerosis (scleroderma) is a rare, idiopathic disorder that consists of vasculopathy and fibrosis occurring in various parts of the body, most noticeably the skin and smooth muscle. Musculoskeletal involvement typically manifests as arthralgias and myalgias. Radiography may show acroosteolysis secondary to pressure erosions from skin contractures and soft tissue calcifications. A true arthritis occurs in 50%, which is similar to rheumatoid arthritis and may be related to development of an overlap disorder or mixed connective tissue disease. CREST

TABLE 3-15

Dark Synovium on Magnetic Resonance Imaging: Differential Diagnosis

Hemorrhage
    Pigmented villonodular synovitis
    Hemophilia
    Synovial hemangioma
    Rheumatoid arthritis (occasionally)
    Repetitive trauma/surgery
Synovial osteochondromatosis (if synovium is calcified)
Amyloid
Gout
Tuberculosis arthritis (occasionally)

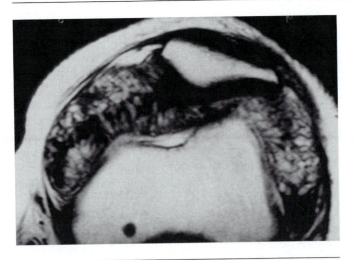

FIGURE 3-47. Lipoma arborescens. Axial T$_1$-weighted magnetic resonance image of the knee shows frond-like lipomatous proliferation in the synovium, markedly distending the joint. *(Courtesy of Dr. Timothy Sanders.)*

syndrome is a limited form of scleroderma. The acronym stands for calcinosis (soft tissue calcification), Raynaud phenomenon, esophageal dysmotility, sclerodactyly, and skin telangiectasias (Figure 3-48). In CREST only the face and hands are usually involved with fibrosis.

Systemic Lupus Erythematosus

SLE is an autoimmune disease that has familial aggregations among first-degree relatives and manifests positive antinuclear antibody. It usually occurs in a younger population (15 to 40 years old), with a predisposition for females (5:1 over males). The musculoskeletal manifestations are arthralgias and arthritis. The arthritis is a nonerosive but deforming disease characterized on radiography by subluxations without erosions (Figure 3-49). The differential diagnosis of this finding is Jaccoud arthropathy, which is a post rheumatic fever arthropathy that develops in a small percentage of patients (approximately 4%) with a history of rheumatic heart disease. Patients with SLE may also have large soft tissue masses of flocculent calcification.

Mixed Connective Tissue Disease and Overlap Syndromes

Mixed connective tissue disease (MCTD) is an admixture of scleroderma, SLE, and polymyositis and may be considered a

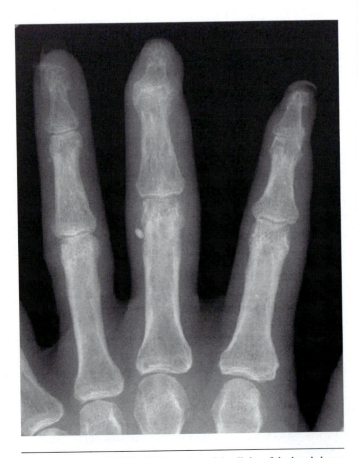

FIGURE 3-48. CREST. Oblique view of the digits of the hand shows coarse soft tissue calcification and acroosteolysis, with whittling of the soft tissues distally.

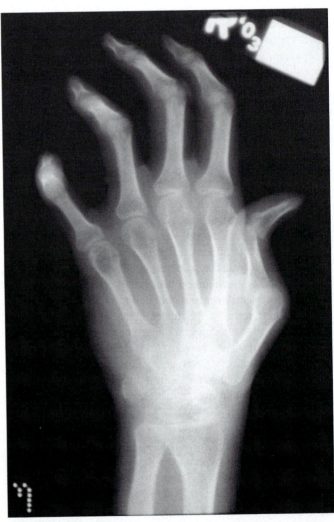

FIGURE 3-49. Systemic lupus erythematosus. Anteroposterior view of the hand shows subluxation at multiple joints without erosive disease.

variant of SLE. MCTD and "overlap syndromes" are separate entities. Overlap syndromes simultaneously satisfy criteria of more than one disease and tend to occur in specific combinations such as SLE and rheumatoid arthritis, scleroderma and rheumatoid arthritis, scleroderma and SLE, and scleroderma and polymyositis. Further, MCTD and overlap syndromes should be distinguished from undifferentiated connective tissue syndromes that do not satisfy criteria for any specific diagnosis. Over time an undifferentiated syndrome may develop additional signs or symptoms that satisfy the criteria for a specified syndrome and in this sense is an early incomplete presentation of that disorder.

MCTD affects many body systems including musculoskeletal, gastrointestinal, pulmonary, renal, cardiovascular, and neurologic (central and peripheral). This population of patients has an increased frequency of Raynaud phenomenon. There is an overwhelming female preponderance, with a 15:1 ratio of involvement. Musculoskeletal symptomatology consists of polyarthralgia (90 to 100%) and myalgias or myositis (50%). The arthropathy includes development of erosions with a rheumatoid arthritis–like pattern.

Laboratory evaluation often reveals a distinctive pattern of serology. Patients with MCTD are positive for antinuclear antibody (95%) and rheumatoid factor (50%). A unique feature is the presence of autoantibodies to the ribonucleic protein of two distinct extractable nuclear antigens (nRNP and/or U1RNP). Hypergammaglobulinemia (immunoglobulins G and M), and elevated sedimentation rate are frequently present. MCTD patients do not exhibit autoantibodies to smooth muscle, and there is a decreased frequency of hypocomplementemia.

Imaging Findings. The soft tissues demonstrate swelling with a sausage digit pattern. Calcinosis is common. The bone mineralization is decreased, which may be juxtaarticular or more diffuse. Joint narrowing representing loss of articular cartilage occurs as part of the inflammatory arthropathy. Erosions develop in two patterns: distal phalangeal tuft erosions (25 to 70%) and synovial marginal erosions. Osseous proliferation is not a feature. Flexion deformities and subluxations contribute to malalignment. Ankylosis is a late finding typically occurring at the metacarpophalangeal and interphalangeal joints. The distribution of MCTD favors small joint involvement.

DIFFERENTIAL DIAGNOSIS. By definition, several connective tissue diseases share the individual findings of MCTD, thus confounding the imaging differential diagnosis. The diagnosis of an overlap syndrome is facilitated when the constellation of "classic" findings of two different connective tissue disorders exists in a single patient. However, because MCTD is not necessarily the full expression or a complete combination of more than one disorder, atypical patterns predominate and the following discriminators may be useful. The distribution of involvement of MCTD includes distal interphalangeal joints versus "pure" rheumatoid arthritis where these articulations are uncommonly affected. In addition, although MCTD is a bilateral process, it tends to be asymmetric with a more haphazard distribution than rheumatoid arthritis. Synovial type erosions are uncommon in "pure" scleroderma and SLE. Scleroderma has frequent calcinosis, whereas

only occasional soft tissue calcifications occur in uncomplicated SLE. The presence of calcinosis and synovial type "marginal" erosions should raise the possibility of an overlap syndrome, MCTD, or a rheumatic disorder complicated by end-stage renal disease with an elevated calcium phosphate product level (secondary hyperparathyroidism).

DEPOSITION DISEASES

Crystal-Associated Disorders

Different crystals have been associated with arthritis and other articular manifestations. Three types of crystals are the most commonly encountered and clinically relevant: monosodium urate monohydrate (MSUM), CPPD, and HA, also known as basic calcium phosphate (BCP). The diagnosis is usually made by crystal analysis after arthrocentesis or characteristic imaging findings in the appropriate clinical setting. Although these crystals are associated with joint changes, an actual causal relationship has not definitely been established for each type of crystal. There is no single unified theory to explain crystal-associated arthritis, so each is considered separately.

The mechanism of crystal deposition may be related to one or more of the following factors: local or global metabolic changes that increase solute concentration, surfaces that facilitate crystal nucleation (such as degenerated cartilage), or loss of inhibitory regulation for crystal growth. The associated inflammatory component may be induced by a rapid rate of change of concentration (not necessarily absolute concentration) or actual crystal shedding into a joint. Inflammation is initiated by the adsorption of multiple protein molecules onto the surface of the crystal, thus activating the immune system and neutrophilic phagocytosis ensues. Because crystals are not readily degraded by lysosomes, cell death occurs, and leaked lysosomal proteolytic enzymes cause articular cartilage destruction. MSUM crystal is the most membranolytic, and this may be related to the relatively large size or shape and to the chemical composition. Chemotaxis attracts additional neutrophils, which amplifies the inflammatory response and propagates synovitis. The symptoms of an acute febrile illness are derived from the release of additional inflammatory mediators that have systemic effects. Colchicine blocks the release of chemotactic factors for neutrophils and mononuclear cells and can be an effective therapy.

The pathologic-etiologic relationship between crystals and arthritis is complex and may be broadly divided as causal or coincidental. The deposition of MSUM is a true cause-and-effect relationship producing gout. Pyrophosphate is probably a manifestation of chondrocyte repair, and HA found in the intraarticular form may simply be a degradation product ("bone dust") from a destructive arthropathy. Therefore, the difference between CPPD arthritis and HA arthritis may be a reflection of host response to degenerative joint disease. The inability of an articulation to sustain normal biomechanical forces or function (joint failure) may induce a robust response (hypertrophic osteoarthritis) associated with CPPD crystals or may be manifested by a wearing away response (atrophic osteoarthritis) with HA.

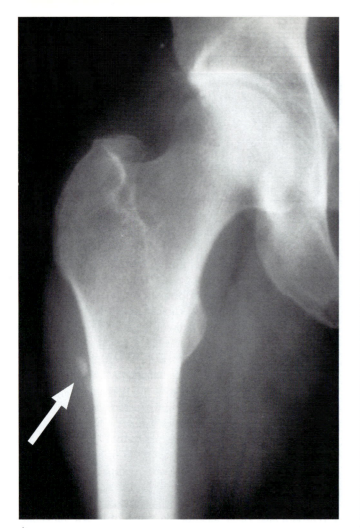

A

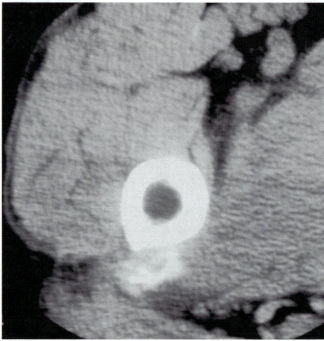

B

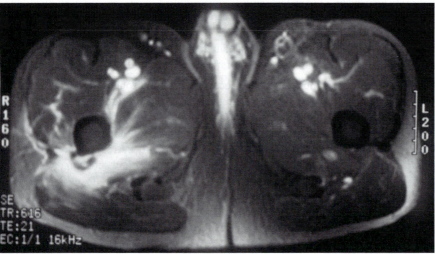

C

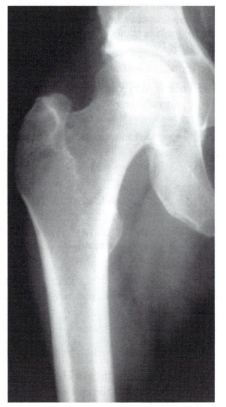

D

FIGURE 3-54. Hydroxyapatite deposition disease: acute presentation by a 55-year-old febrile male with mild leukocytosis, increased sedimentation rate, rapid onset of tenderness, swelling, and erythema at the posterior aspect of the upper thigh. The clinical diagnosis was cellulitis, and the patient was referred for cross-sectional imaging to rule out osteomyelitis. *(A)* Anteroposterior view of the femur shows a small focus of calcification adjacent to the femoral shaft (arrow). *(B)* Axial computed tomographic image of the same area demonstrates focal calcification in the soft tissues at the insertion of the gluteus maximus muscle on the linea aspera. *(C)* Axial T_1-weighted fat-suppressed post-gadolinium magnetic resonance image shows marked enhancement in the surrounding tissues, with a low signal focus in the center representing the area of calcification. Based on these findings, the patient was diagnosed with acute hydroxyapatite deposition disease and was treated with nonsteroidal antiinflammatory drugs. Symptoms resolved completely within 48 hours. *(D)* Anteroposterior view 1 week later shows disappearance of the hydroxyapatite deposit.

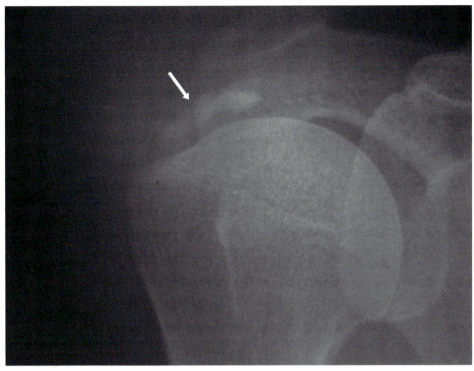

A

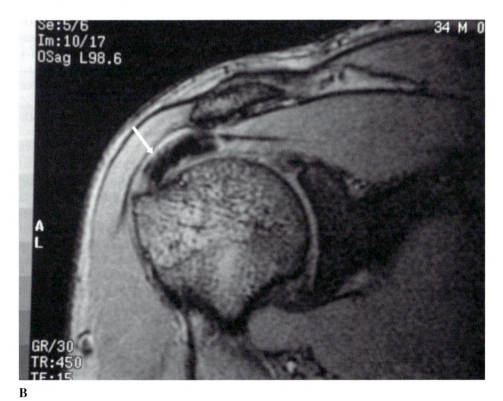

B

FIGURE 3-55. Hydroxyapatite deposition disease: shoulder. *(A)* Anteroposterior radiograph shows a large focus in the supraspinatus tendon (arrow). *(B)* Corresponding oblique coronal gradient echo image shows the large, low signal intensity focus (arrow).

locations are involved. One notable area is the cervical spine, which is not commonly encountered but may be misdiagnosed clinically and radiographically as infection and is known as *retropharyngeal tendinitis*. Treatment may be conservative, with systemic agents such as NSAIDs, or with local aspiration and corticosteroid injection. The aspirate typically has a chalky, toothpaste quality, so a large gauge needle (16 or 18 gauge) may be required.

Imaging Findings. Radiographically, there is periarticular amorphous calcific opacity. The size and shape typically have no relation to the presence of symptomatology. In an acute symptomatic presentation, crystals may extrude from the tendon into adjacent soft tissues such as a bursa, causing acute bursitis. Over time (days to months), a well-defined homogeneous calcification in tendons may transform into a faint diffuse calcification in the bursa or may become ill defined, smaller, and disappear (dissolve). Resorption of the HA crystal is due to inflammation and hyperemia.

Normal bone mineral density is exhibited. Erosions are not a usual feature; however, there are two important areas where enthesial erosions may be apparent: the pectoralis major tendon insertion on the humerus and the portion of the gluteus maximus tendon insertion on the linea aspera of the femur. When present, this finding should not be mistaken for a focally destructive neoplasm. In the periarticular form of HADD, there is no osseous proliferation and no joint deformity.

The shoulder is the most commonly involved joint, most often in the supraspinatus tendon, which may extend into the subacromial or subdeltoid bursa (Figure 3-55). The wrist is a common area, demonstrating a solitary focus in the extensor carpi ulnaris or flexor carpi ulnaris tendons or around the metacarpal phalangeal or interphalangeal joints. Retropharyngeal tendinitis characteristically appears as prevertebral soft tissue swelling associated with calcific opacities of the longus colli tendons usually present at the level of C_2 just below the arch of C_1. Pelvic

The frequency of the joints affected is in the following order: shoulder, hip, elbow, wrist, and knee. The initial presentation of severe pain and loss of function gradually resolves over days to weeks. Confounding presentations occur when atypical

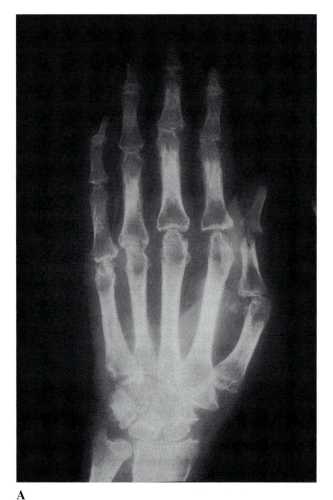

A

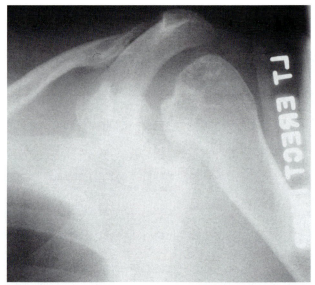

B

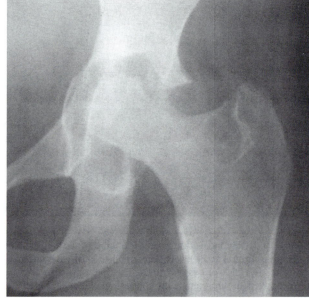

C

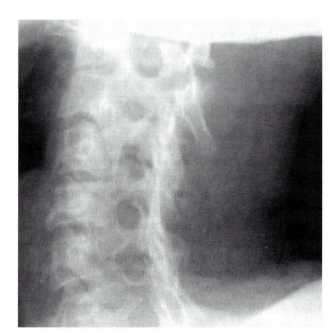

D

FIGURE 3-61. Multicentric reticulohistiocytosis: polyarticular involvement mimicking rheumatoid arthritis. *(A)* Anteroposterior view of the hand shows severe diffuse marginal erosive disease. *(B)* Anteroposterior view of the shoulder demonstrates a high-riding humeral head consistent with rotator cuff tear. There are erosions of the humeral head and the distal clavicle. *(C)* Anteroposterior view of the hip shows severe erosion of the femoral head. *(D)* Oblique view of the cervical spine shows cutaneous nodules representing deposits of lipid-laden macrophages. Unlike nodules seen in rheumatoid arthritis, these are small, are not confined to the extremities, and are also found in the mucosal tissues.

TABLE 3-17

Neuropathic Arthropathy

LOCATIONS	ASSOCIATED ETIOLOGY
Hand/wrist	Leprosy, syrinx
Elbow	Syrinx, idiopathic
Shoulder	Syrinx, idiopathic
Spine	Paralysis, syrinx, tabes dorsalis
Pelvis/hip	Tabes dorsalis
Knee	Tabes dorsalis, amyloid, sensory neuropathies
Ankle	Amyloid, tabes dorsalis, sensory neuropathies
Foot	Diabetes (TMT, IT, MTP), myelomeningocele (IT, MTP), alcoholism (IT, MTP), leprosy, sensory neuropathies (IT, MTP, IP)

ABBREVIATIONS: IP = interphalangeal, IT = intertarsal, MTP = metatarsophalangeal, TMT = tarsometatarsal.

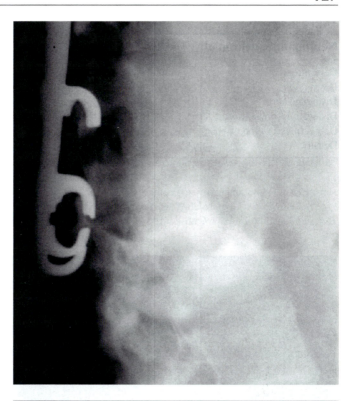

margins. Proliferative response and bone repair is absent, but the remaining bones are normally mineralized. A large portion of bone may be absent, with swelling (edema) and debris filling in the region. This very aggressive appearance may be mistaken for an infection, neoplasm, or other destructive arthropathy (eg, rapidly destructive hip osteoarthritis). Useful discriminators are that neoplasm only infrequently involves both sides of an articulation and infection does not produce a well-defined sharp transition (ie, "surgical margin").

The atrophic pattern is customarily seen in non–weight-bearing joints such as in the upper extremities and is commonly associated with a spinal cord syrinx (Figure 3-62). The hypertrophic form appears as a robust osteoarthritis, with severe joint narrowing, extensive osteophytosis, new bone production, and fragmentation (Figure 3-63). There is virtual disintegration of the articular margins and subluxation. Extensive subchondral sclerosis is often present.

FIGURE 3-63. Neuropathic arthropathy: hypertrophic pattern (spine). There is destruction of the disc spaces, increased density of the involved vertebrae, debris, and disorganization of the thoracolumbar spine in this patient with spinal cord injury who underwent fusion to stabilize the thoracic spine.

The mixed form has elements of resorption and production present. This pattern of neuropathic arthropathy has been summarized as the Ds based on the radiographic appearance (destruction, debris, preserved bone density, disorganization, and dislocation; Table 3-18). This pattern is characteristically found with diabetic foot neurarthropathy (Figure 3-64). The most

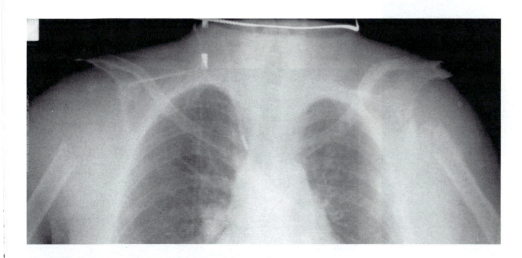

FIGURE 3-62. Neuropathic arthropathy: atrophic pattern. Frontal view of the chest shows severe osteolysis of the proximal humeri bilaterally related to a syrinx.

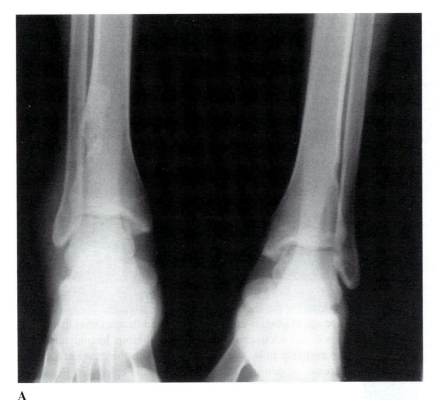

A

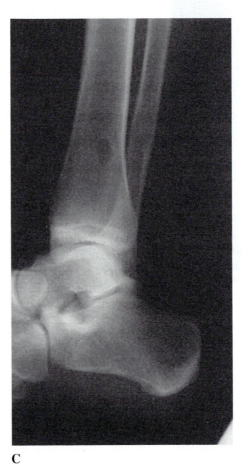

B   C

Tumors in the long bones are typically metaphyseal, with extension to the epiphysis seen more commonly in adults. Lesions are radiographically lytic, demonstrating a geographic pattern of bone destruction and cortical thinning (Figure 4-16). The transition zone is narrow, and a sclerotic rim is characteristically absent. Most lesions will demonstrate internal residual bony trabeculae. Disruption of the cortex with infiltration into the soft tissues has been reported to occur in about 50% of cases and is best appreciated on cross-sectional imaging. The extent of cortical thinning and disruption and the presence of residual intralesional trabeculation are best demonstrated by CT. CT also shows soft tissue infiltration. Recently described MRI features of desmoplastic fibroma include areas of low to intermediate signal intensity on T_2-weighted spin echo images and a substantially heterogeneous pattern of contrast enhancement within the same tumor, varying from no to minimal enhancement to areas of intense enhancement. The low signal intensity observed on the T_2-weighted spin echo images is attributed to the dense fibrous matrix that characterizes this tumor and to its hypocellularity.

Patients are generally treated with wide surgical excision because a high recurrence rate is associated with curettage alone.

OSSIFYING FIBROMA.   Sometimes called *osteofibrous dysplasia*, this benign fibro-osseous skeletal lesion closely resembles fibrous dysplasia pathologically and radiographically. More than 90% of lesions occur in the tibia, generally presenting in patients younger than 7 years. A slight predilection for males has been reported. About 50% of all patients present with a hard painless mass involving the anterior cortex of the tibial shaft associated with anterior bowing of the tibia. A small percentage of patients will present with a pathologic fracture. Radiographic manifestations are that of a well-defined, elongated, mixed sclerotic and lytic lesion with a well-defined sclerotic margin involving the anterior tibial cortex. Most lesions resolve spontaneously and do not require treatment. Sometimes surgery is performed when anterior tibial bowing persists after the lesion has resolved.

FIBROUS DYSPLASIA.   Initially discovered in patients between ages 3 and 15 years, this relatively common disorder has been attributed to malfunctioning bone-forming mesenchymal tissue. A slight predilection for females is associated with this disorder. Fibrous dysplasia may be monostotic or polyostotic. When solitary, the most common location is the femur, followed by

FIGURE 4-14.   Fibrous cortical defect and nonossifying fibroma in a 17-year-old boy. *(A)* Frontal and *(B, C)* lateral views of the lower legs show a small, fibrous, cortical defect and a contralateral, large, nonossifying fibroma. Note that they are cortical, well marginated, and vertically oriented.

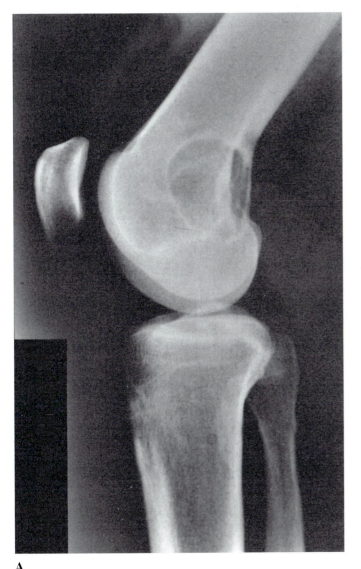

A

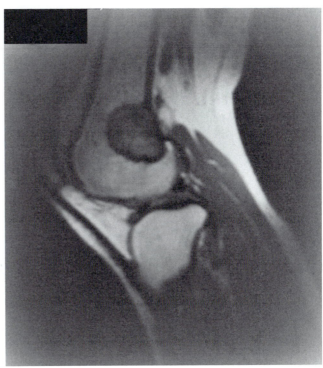

B

FIGURE 4-15. Benign fibrous histiocytoma. *(A)* Radiograph and *(B)* sagittal T$_1$-weighted spin echo magnetic resonance image show a well-marginated, slightly expansile, lytic lesion in the distal femur with a well-defined sclerotic rim. This lesion is typically isointense to muscle on T$_1$-weighted spin echo magnetic resonance imaging. *(Courtesy of Dr. Bernard Ghelman.)*

the ribs and mandible. Additional sites are other long bones, the skull, pelvis, spine, and, uncommonly, the tubular bones of the hands and feet. Polyostotic fibrous dysplasia can occur anywhere and can be associated with endocrine abnormalities (*McCune-Albright syndrome*) and intramuscular myxomas (*Mazabraud syndrome*). Aside from the monostotic lesions that are discovered incidentally on imaging studies performed for other reasons, patients present with pain secondary to minor injuries causing cortical infractions. With each injury, progressive skeletal deformities develop.

The radiographic appearance of fibrous dysplasia varies. An early solitary lesion may present as an intramedullary radiolucency with a smoked-glass appearance (Figure 4-17). With increasing mineralization, increasing density develops, giving some lesions a mixed lytic and sclerotic appearance. Mature lesions typically demonstrate a thick, dense, sclerotic rim, termed the *rind sign*. Lesions in the long bones may cause bony expansion with cortical thinning and endosteal scalloping. Periosteal reaction is not a feature of fibrous dysplasia. With repetitive fracture, bowing deformities result. Multiple fractures to the

proximal femur with secondary alteration in the shape of the affected area can give rise to the *shepherd's-crook deformity*. Lesions in the innominate bones tend to appear lobulated and cyst-like. The presence of well-defined, thick, sclerotic margins should establish the diagnosis of fibrous dysplasia. Lesions in the skull are generally lytic when affecting the convexities of the cranium and sclerotic when affecting the floor of the anterior fossa. The term *leonine facies* is used to describe cranial asymmetry caused by fibrous dysplasia of the anterior fossa and maxilla. *Cherubism* may result when fibrous dysplasia is confined to the maxilla and mandible. Lesions in the ribs tend to be lytic, with thinning of the overlying cortex and bony expansion (Figure 4-18). Rib lesions, however, also can be mixed, with lytic and sclerotic areas, and, occasionally, purely sclerotic. Spinal lesions are unusual and tend to show lytic and sclerotic foci.

With the exception of fracture, most cases of fibrous dysplasia do not cause cortical destruction. Occasionally, however, a more aggressive form of fibrous dysplasia is encountered, where well-defined cortical perforations occur. Frequently, such findings on T_2-weighted images. In such cases, malignant lesions, such as metastatic disease, multiple myeloma, and lymphoma, must be considered in the differential diagnosis. Even more confusing is when an atypical hemangioma is associated with extraosseous extension into the spinal canal. Lesions involving the neural arch are often expansile and lytic and without coarse trabeculae, thus simulating aneurysmal bone cyst or osteoblastoma. Lesions in the skull, which are multifocal about 15% of the time, manifest as lucent areas containing radiating striations, likened to a "sunburst" or "cartwheel" pattern. Solitary hemangiomas of the extremities have more variable radiographic manifestations (Figure 4-23). They may demonstrate a permeative trabecular pattern or a reticular or lace-like pattern. Although most lesions of the appendicular skeleton are intramedullary in location, nearly 33% are periosteal and about 10% are intracortical.

Symptomatic spinal hemangiomas have been treated successfully by CT-guided percutaneous intralesional injection of ethanol and by percutaneous vertebroplasty.

EOSINOPHILIC GRANULOMA. The presence of a solitary eosinophilic granuloma is the commonest and mildest manifestation of Langerhan's cell histiocytosis. Most cases of eosinophilic granuloma occur in children and adolescents but exceptions to this rule are not unusual, and patients have presented with eosinophilic granuloma in middle age. Most of these lesions are found in the skull, mandible, spine, ribs, pelvis, and long bones. A male predilection exists. Although most lesions are solitary, about 20% are multiple but do not necessarily develop at the same time. Patients may complain of localized pain, tenderness, and swelling. Eosinophilic granuloma also can present as an incidental radiologic finding. On occasion, patients will present with a pathologic fracture. The absence of significant constitutional complaints helps to distinguish eosinophilic granuloma from the more aggressive forms of histiocytosis and from Ewing tumor. Histologically, it is considered one of the "round cell" lesions (Table 4-9).

The radiographic manifestations of solitary eosinophilic granuloma are those of a central, well-circumscribed lytic lesion. When the appendicular skeleton is involved, the lesions tend to be located in the diaphysis or in the metaphysis. Occasionally, lesions in the long bones are poorly defined and

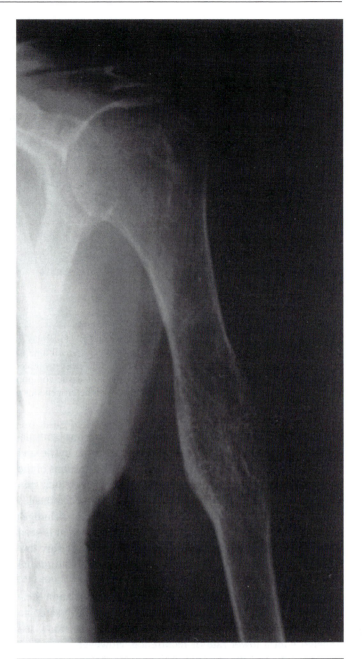

FIGURE 4-23. Hemangioma. Anteroposterior view of the humerus shows an expansile lucent lesion with coarse linear striation.

TABLE 4-9

Round Cell Lesions

Benign
    Osteomyelitis
    Eosinophilic granuloma
Malignant (from childhood to adulthood)
    Retinoblastoma metastasis
    Neuroblastoma metastasis
    Leukemia
    Ewing disease
    Primitive neuroectodermal tumor
    Osteosarcoma
    Lymphoma
    Myeloma

demonstrate a permeative trabecular pattern that can be mistaken for osteomyelitis, lymphoma, or Ewing tumor, particularly when periosteal reaction is present due to cortical erosion (Figure 4-24). At other times, eosinophilic granuloma can present as a bubbly expansile lesion. Lesions in the flat bones, particularly those located in the skull, may demonstrate beveled edges with or without sclerotic margins due to asymmetric destruction of the inner and outer cortices or the inner and outer tables of the skull (Figure 4-25). At times, a central sclerotic focus is seen with involvement of the skull, a finding known as a *button sequestrum*. Involvement of the mandible is a cause of "floating" teeth. Spinal involvement in children manifests as progressive anterior vertebral body wedging, leading to complete flattening (*vertebra plana*), which usually improves over time.

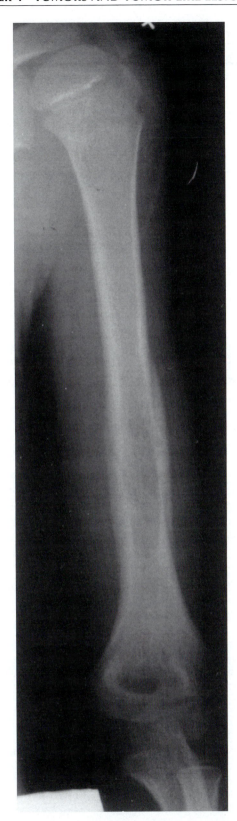

FIGURE 4-24. Eosinophilic granuloma. Anteroposterior view of the humerus in this child shows an ill-defined permeative lytic lesion with periosteal reaction in the humeral shaft. This appearance is similar to that of Ewing tumor and osteomyelitis.

INTRAOSSEOUS LIPOMA. This extremely rare tumor can occur at any age and usually is discovered as an incidental radiologic finding. There is a slight predilection for males. Most lesions occur in the long bones and are metaphyseal in location. They also have been reported in the small bones of the hands and feet; in these locations, the lesion appears to have an affinity for the calcaneus. Lesions also have been reported in the skull, mandible, ribs, and sacrum.

Lesions are typically lytic and well-defined. Residual trabeculae within the lesion may give rise to a loculated pattern. Amorphous central calcification or ossification may be demonstrated (Figure 4-26). When intraosseous lipoma occurs in a thin bone, such as the rib or fibula, bony expansion is common. There is no known tendency for malignant transformation.

LIPOSCLEROSING MYXOFIBROUS TUMOR. This benign fibro-osseous tumor is characterized histologically by a combination of fatty, fibrous, cystic, necrotic, ossific, myxomatous, and occasionally cartilaginous elements. The most common location is the intertrochanteric region of the femur, which accounts for about 90% of these tumors, followed by the femoral shaft, the ilium, and the humerus. About 50% of patients complain of pain, with the remaining lesions discovered as incidental radiologic or scintigraphic findings. About 10% of patients present with pathologic fractures.

Radiographically, liposclerosing myxofibrous tumor presents as a well-defined lytic lesion with a sclerotic margin (Figure 4-27). The degree of marginal sclerosis can be quite extensive. Although most lesions are not associated with alteration in the contour of the affected bone, mild expansile remodeling has been reported in about one-third of cases, with more extensive remodeling reported in a minority of cases. Mineralization occurs in nearly 75% of cases. The extent of marginal sclerosis and the presence of mineralization of the matrix are best demonstrated by CT. Few reports of the MRI characteristics of liposclerosing myxofibrous tumor have appeared in the literature. Among those reported, however, MRI depicts a thick rind of low signal intensity that appears to correlate with the sometimes dramatic sclerotic rim seen on plain films. The non-mineralized portions of this tumor are isointense to muscle on T_1-weighted spin echo images and generally show mild to moderate heterogeneous increased signal intensity on T_2-weighted spin echo images.

Unlike the benign fibrous lesions discussed in this section, a significant potential for malignant transformation exists with liposclerosing myxofibrous tumor of bone. The reported prevalence of malignant transformation ranges from 10 to 16%. Osteosarcoma and MFH have been reported in association with this tumor.

MALIGNANT

Bone Forming

OSTEOSARCOMA. Osteosarcoma, a tumor of mesenchymal origin derived from osseous connective tissue, is the third most common malignancy in children and adolescents. Several types of osteosarcoma have been described. The classic type is referred to as *conventional osteosarcoma*.

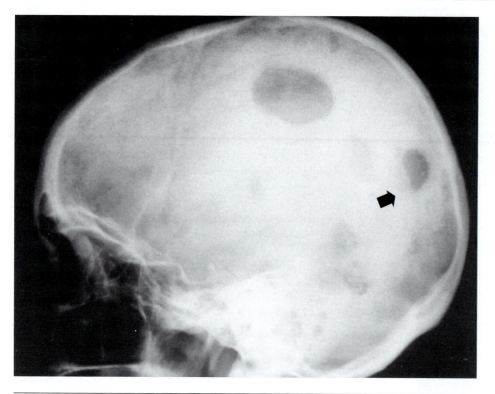

FIGURE 4-25. Eosinophilic granuloma. Lateral view of the skull shows multiple lytic lesions in a 50-year old woman, demonstrating multiple well-circumscribed lytic lesions. Note the beveled edge in the occipital lesion (arrow).

primary osteosarcomas can occur in patients between ages 40 and 70 years.

Most patients present with a dull, aching pain of several weeks' or even months' duration. An acute episode of increased pain may reflect penetration of the cortex, with irritation of the periosteum or a pathologic fracture. Nocturnal pain causing the child to wake is not uncommon and should not be mistaken for growing pains. On physical examination, localized tenderness, swelling, mass, or deformity, with limited range of motion of the nearby joint, are encountered. Regional lymphadenopathy is rare and should suggest the diagnosis of osteomyelitis rather than of osteosarcoma. Approximately 50% of patients have an elevated serum alkaline phosphatase. Approximately 80% of patients do not exhibit evidence of metastatic disease at the time of presentation. The most common site of metastatic disease is the lung, followed by the bones. Patients presenting with a pathologic fracture have a more guarded prognosis and are more likely to have pulmonary metastases at the time of presentation.

Conventional osteosarcoma has a strong predilection for the metaphysis and diametaphysis of the long bones around the knee and for the proximal portion of the humerus. However, this tumor can arise within any bone. Most patients are between ages 10 and 25 years, with few cases occurring after age 30. The male predominance is attributed by some to the longer growth period that exists in boys as compared with that of girls. Although most osteosarcomas discovered in older patients represent malignant transformation from Paget disease or radiation-induced osteosarcoma,

Initial imaging evaluation consists of conventional radiography. The different amounts of malignant bone, cartilage, osteoid, and/or fibrous tissue determine the radiographic appearance of the tumor. Typically, conventional osteosarcoma of a long bone is diametaphyseal in location and demonstrates a focal lesion with a mixture of osteolytic and osteosclerotic elements, a wide zone of transition, and disorganized periosteal reaction (Figures 4-28 and 4-29). The growth plate generally acts as a barrier

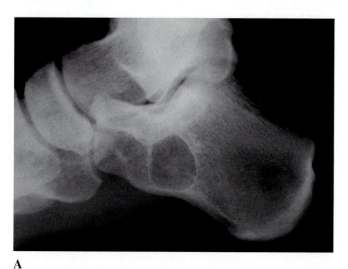

A

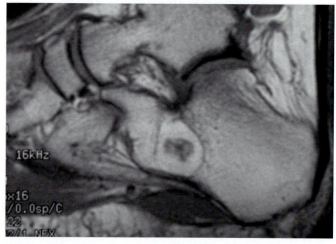

B

FIGURE 4-26. Intraosseous lipoma. *(A)* Lateral radiograph of the calcaneus shows an oval lucency with a thin sclerotic rim and faint central mineralization. *(B)* Sagittal T_1-weghted spin echo image shows the high signal intensity lipoma, with the central low signal intensity due to mineralization.

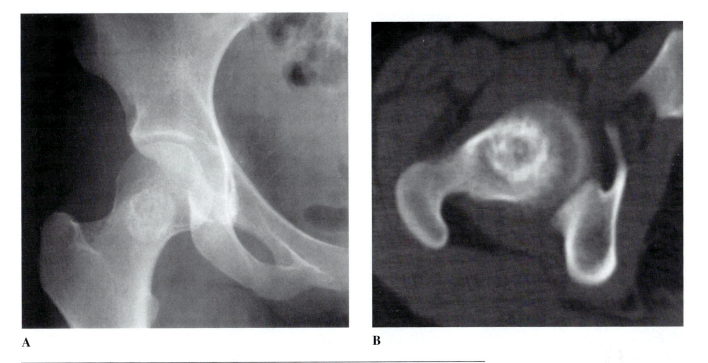

FIGURE 4-27. Liposclerosing myxofibrous tumor. *(A)* Radiograph and *(B)* computed tomographic image show a liposclerosing myxofibrous tumor of the femoral neck. Note the well-defined sclerotic margin and the mineralized matrix.

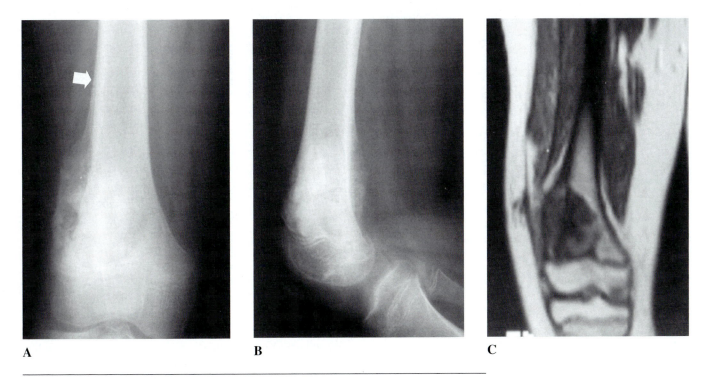

FIGURE 4-28. Osteosarcoma. *(A)* Frontal and *(B)* lateral radiographs and *(C)* coronal T_1-weighted spin echo magnetic resonance image in a 9-year-old girl show a conventional osteosarcoma of the distal femoral metaphysis. Note the mixed lytic and sclerotic elements of this tumor, with periosteal reaction and a Codman triangle (arrow). Sparing of the epiphysis is demonstrated by magnetic resonance imaging.

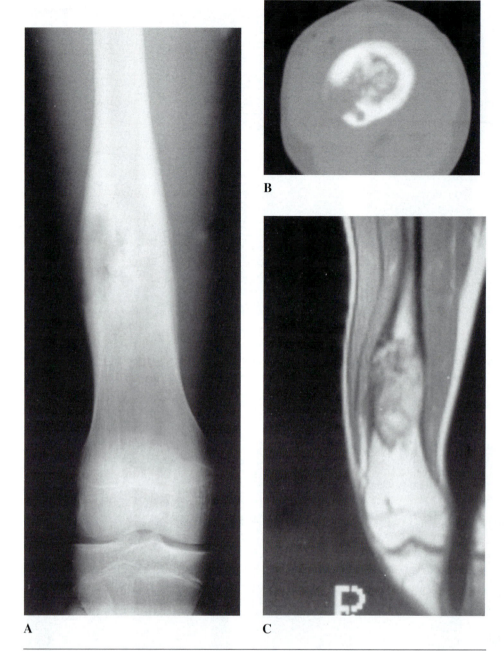

FIGURE 4-29.   Osteosarcoma. *(A)* Frontal view of the femur in a 16-year-old boy shows a mixed lytic and sclerotic lesion in the femoral shaft with periosteal reaction. *(B)* Cortical destruction is best demonstrated by computed tomography, which also shows soft tissue extending beyond the cortex. *(C)* The lesion is delineated more precisely by magnetic resonance imaging, which shows heterogeneous signal intensity on the T_1-weighted spin echo image.

osteolytic components and areas of cortical destruction. The development of increasing ossification of the tumor and a calcified rim around the tumor indicate a positive response to chemotherapy, as does decreased size. CT of the chest is performed routinely at the time of presentation and every 3 to 6 months for the first 2 years after surgery to evaluate for pulmonary metastases. Ossification of pulmonary metastases is a worse prognostic sign than nonossified metastases.

MRI is the single most important imaging modality for staging musculoskeletal tumors. MRI shows the full extent of the intraosseous and extraosseous components of the tumor, its relation to the nearby neurovascular bundle, involvement of muscle compartments, and detection of joint involvement. This information is imperative for selecting the appropriate surgical procedure. Limb salvage surgery can be performed regardless of whether the tumor extends to the joint. When the tumor is confined to the shaft, surgical resection of the affected bone is undertaken, with preservation of the joints. When the joint is involved and cannot be preserved, a biological osteoarticular allograft or an endoprosthesis is used. Combined arthroplasty, consisting of bone allografts to treat the skeletal defect and a conventional prosthesis cemented into the allograft, is another option. Advantages of osteoarticular allografts include restoration of bone stock and their ability to provide attachment sites for soft tissue structures. Disadvantages are the long period of protective weight bearing required for this procedure and the 20 to 30% incidence of late complications that include infection, joint instability, nonunion, fracture, and articular collapse. Endoprostheses provide immediate joint stability, with return to function sooner than with osteoarticular allografts. Fewer late complications are associated with endoprostheses, with long-term loosening, reported in up to 25% of patients at 5-year follow-up, being the primary disadvantage. Preoperative imaging with MRI always should include the entire bone, from joint to joint, because skip lesions may occur.

against extension of the tumor to the epiphysis. The sclerotic portion represents tumoral and reactive bone. The rapidly growing tumor may cause abrupt elevation of the periosteum at the upper or lower margins of the lesion, resulting in a Codman triangle. A "sunburst" or "sun-ray" pattern of periosteal reaction is rare. The focal nature of the lesion and the absence of a purely permeative destructive pattern differentiate conventional osteosarcoma from Ewing tumor and lymphoma.

CT and MRI are used to assess the extent of disease in the bones and soft tissues. CT is helpful in delineating the full extent of the mineralized matrix of the tumor and depicting the

Radionuclide imaging is performed routinely to evaluate for osseous metastases and for the possibility of multifocal osteosarcoma. Patients with osseous metastases have a poor prognosis.

Pathologically, the dominant element is neoplastic osteoid, which is responsible for the osteolytic appearance seen on radiographs and CT. Tumoral mineralization of the neoplastic osteoid is responsible for the osteosclerosis. Although most lesions contain osteolytic and osteosclerotic components, occasionally a lesion may be purely one or the other.

The differential diagnosis includes osteomyelitis, fracture, and other malignant neoplasms of bone. With regard to pyogenic osteomyelitis, clinical presentation and location are not helpful distinguishing factors because both entities occur in the metaphysis and present with swelling, pain, and fever. Radiologically, osteomyelitis and osteosarcoma demonstrate bone destruction, periosteal reaction, and a wide zone of transition. However, the presence of a sequestrum and the presence of diffuse rather than of circumscribed soft changes favor the diagnosis of infection rather than of neoplasm. In addition, infection tends to blur the surrounding fat planes, while tumor tends to displace them.

A healing fracture can be mistaken for osteosarcoma radiologically when there is abundant periosteal reaction and callus formation but no discrete fracture line. In such cases, CT performed with thin, 1-mm slices may be helpful in establishing the diagnosis by demonstrating the fracture line. MRI can be misleading by demonstrating abnormal signal intensity due to extensive bone marrow edema extending significantly proximally and distally to the fracture, thereby simulating a pathologic fracture through a bone lesion. To further complicate matters, the pathologist may have difficulty distinguishing a healing fracture from an osteosarcoma, since new bone formation is a feature of both.

Differentiation from other primary bone tumors, including the various types of osteosarcoma, can be difficult. Distinguishing osteosarcoma from Ewing tumor deserves special attention because these two entities occur in the same age group and can be quite similar radiographically. Even though Ewing tumor generally is located in the diaphysis and osteosarcoma is generally metaphyseal, exceptions to both rules do occur. In addition, purely lytic and predominantly sclerotic osteosarcomas have the appearance of osteolytic and osteoblastic metastases, respectively. In such cases, knowledge of the age and clinical findings should prevent an erroneous diagnosis.

Establishing the diagnosis of osteosarcoma relies on bone biopsy. This procedure can be performed by percutaneous needle biopsy or open biopsy. The use of preoperative and adjuvant chemotherapy is responsible for the longer survival rates reported in recent years. Reduction in the size of the tumor has contributed to easier surgical resection and improvement of limb salvage surgery technique. Long-term survival and cure currently are reported to occur in up to 80% of patients who present with localized disease.

Additional varieties of osteosarcoma include parosteal (also known as juxtacortical), periosteal, high grade surface osteosarcomas, multifocal, telangiectatic, and soft tissue osteosarcomas.

Parosteal osteosarcomas, also known as *juxtacortical osteosarcoma*, comprise fewer than 4% of osteosarcomas. These tumors arise from the periosteum or the parosteal connective tissue. Unlike conventional osteosarcoma, more than 50% of

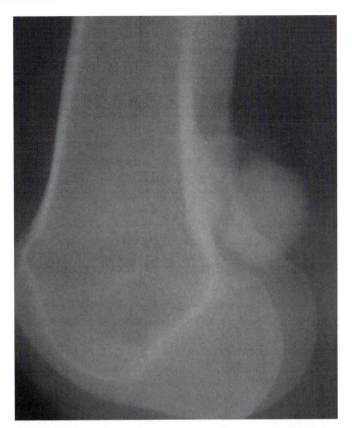

A

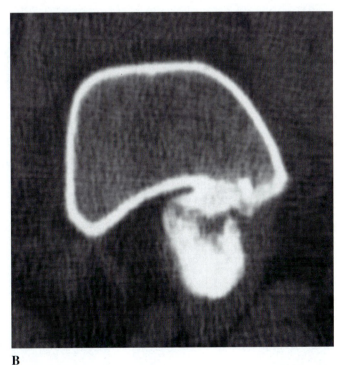

B

FIGURE 4-30. Parosteal osteosarcoma. *(A)* Lateral radiograph shows a dense mass adjacent to the posterior cortex of the distal femur. *(B)* Axial computed tomographic image shows the cortical origin of the tumor. The linear lucency represents an area of non-mineralized tumor.

cases occur after age 30 years and have a slight predilection for females. This tumor occurs most commonly in the metadiaphysis of the long bones around the knee, in particular the posterior aspect of the distal femoral metaphysis, and the proximal humerus. Locations in other long bones and in the flat bones have been reported but are exceedingly uncommon. Parosteal osteosarcomas initially demonstrate a dense plaque of new periosteal bone (Figure 4-30). With continued growth, the tumor extends circumferentially to encase the bone from which it arises. Parosteal osteosarcomas have a better prognosis than conventional osteosarcomas as long as the cortex is not breeched and the medullary cavity not entered. Once the tumor involves the medullary cavity, it has access to the venous system and can metastasize. A linear zone of lucency separates the tumor from the bone of origin in the early stages. With continued growth, this linear lucency becomes obliterated, and as the inner portion of the tumor becomes denser and the periphery of the tumor becomes relatively less dense, the *zonal sign* is created. The zonal sign is useful in distinguishing parosteal osteosarcomas from myositis ossificans, with the latter being denser in the periphery than it is centrally. In addition to posttraumatic myositis ossificans, the differential diagnosis includes osteochondroma. Osteochondromas should be distinguishable from parosteal osteosarcomas on conventional radiography. However, sometimes, CT must be performed to identify the continuity of the cortex and medullary canal of the parent bone with that of the osteochondroma.

Periosteal osteosarcoma is distinguished from conventional and parosteal osteosarcomas by its predominantly cartilaginous matrix, its involvement of the cortex and periosteum, with sparing of the medullary cavity. Radiologically, this lesion is characterized by calcified spicules of bone extending perpendicularly to the cortex (Figure 4-31). This tumor also occurs predominantly in the lower extremities and is usually diaphyseal.

High grade surface osteosarcoma arises from the surface of the bone, most often developing from the diaphysis of the femur and tibia. The tumors demonstrate dense, fluffy ossifications with a broad cortical attachment. Unlike parosteal osteosarcomas, the presence of a cleavage plane is rare, and the high-surface osteosarcoma is histologically more aggressive. Unlike periosteal osteosarcomas, periosteal bony spicules located perpendicular to the bone are rare and the high grade surface osteosarcomas are histologically identical to conventional osteosarcomas, whereas periosteal osteosarcomas are mainly cartilaginous tumors.

The rare multicentric osteosarcoma is generally purely osteoblastic and initially is symmetrical in distribution and of similar size. By definition, these osteosarcomas present without pulmonary metastases. These tumors are aggressive and rapidly extend proximally and distally into the ossification centers and through the cortex into the adjacent soft tissues. Unlike the parosteal and periosteal osteosarcomas, the prognosis of the multicentric type is worse than that of the conventional osteosarcoma.

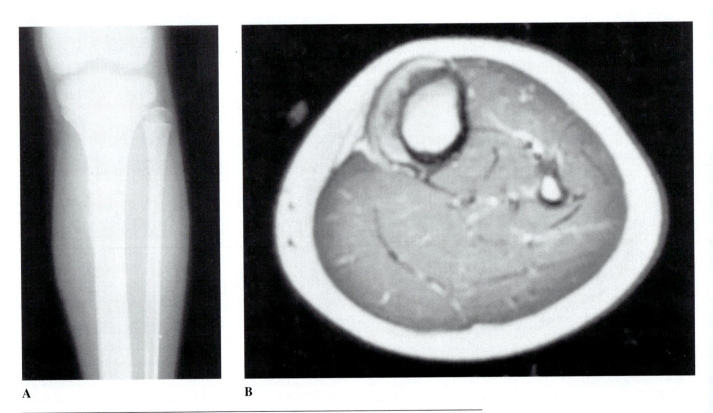

A   B

FIGURE 4-31.   Periosteal osteosarcoma. *(A)* Frontal view of the leg shows aggressive, disorganized, new bone formation perpendicular to the proximal tibial diaphysis. *(B)* T$_1$-weighted spin echo image shows the low signal intensity tumoral bone perpendicular to the tibia and a soft tissue mass without involvement of the medullary cavity.

The most aggressive form of osteosarcoma is the telangiectatic type, characterized by rapid bony destruction and little or no mineralization. The age and location of this tumor are similar to those of conventional osteosarcoma, although its occurrence in flat bones is much less common. An expansile lytic pattern of bone destruction is associated with a rapidly enlarging soft tissue mass. The radiographic appearance and the pathologic finding of multiple blood-filled spaces can cause confusion between this type of osteosarcoma and an aneurysmal bone cyst, particularly on cross-sectional imaging, since both disorders may demonstrate fluid-fluid levels.

Extraosseous osteosarcoma is extremely rare. As the name implies, these tumors arise from the soft tissues and not from bone. On plain films, they are virtually indistinguishable from other soft tissue sarcomas. They tend to occur in elderly, rather than young, people.

Cartilaginous Lesions

CHONDROSARCOMA. This generally slow-growing neoplasm of cartilaginous origin occurs most commonly in patients between ages 30 and 60 years. Approximately two-thirds of chondrosarcomas arise de novo and are referred to as *primary* chondrosarcomas. Those tumors arising from preexisting benign cartilaginous lesions, such as osteochondromas, enchondromas, and periosteal chondromas, are called *secondary* chondrosarcomas. Secondary chondrosarcomas also may arise from pagetic and irradiated bone. The most common preexisting benign chondroid lesion from which chondrosarcomas arise is the osteochondroma. Although the risk of malignant transformation from a single osteochondroma or a single enchondroma is low, the risk is increased in patients with multiple osteochondromatosis and with Ollier disease. The risk of malignant transformation in patients with Maffucci disease is the highest.

Chondrosarcomas are further categorized as central or peripheral, with the former referring to tumors in the central or medullary portion of the bone and the latter referring to tumors on the surface of the bone or in the juxtacortical region and demonstrating a mass protruding away from the bone. Several forms of chondrosarcoma are recognized histologically. The most common type of chondrosarcoma is the conventional, or medullary, form. Other types of chondrosarcoma are periosteal chondrosarcoma, clear cell chondrosarcoma, mesenchymal chondrosarcoma, dedifferentiated chondrosarcoma, and extraosseous chondrosarcoma.

Conventional chondrosarcoma is a particularly slow-growing, well-differentiated tumor that can be easily mistaken for a benign cartilaginous lesion histologically unless several blocks of tissue are examined. For this reason, correlation of the biopsy specimen with the radiologic findings is essential to avoid an erroneous diagnosis. In contrast, poorly differentiated lesions are diagnosed more readily histologically.

Most patients with conventional or central chondrosarcoma present in the fourth, fifth, or sixth decade of life with pain and swelling of the affected area. There is no sex predilection. Although most tumors occur in the long tubular bones, central chondrosarcomas have been reported in the pelvis, the ribs, the skull, the maxilla, the sternum, the calcaneus, the patella, and the hyoid bone. Most central chondrosarcomas arising in the long tubular bones are metadiaphyseal in location.

No useful clinical laboratory data exist to aid in establishing the diagnosis of chondrosarcoma, and evaluation of the patient relies heavily on conventional radiography. Typically, radiographs demonstrate a lytic lesion arising from the medullary cavity. The zone of transition varies from a clear line of demarcation to a wide transitional zone. The presence of a mineralized matrix, which can vary from amorphous, punctate, curvilinear, comma shape, or ring-like and circular, to fluffy or "popcorn" like, is the key to arriving at the diagnosis of a cartilaginous tumor. The slow growth of central chondrosarcomas contributes to the smooth, endosteal scalloping and the fusiform shape of the affected bone frequently observed on radiography. Although periosteal reaction can be a feature of chondrosarcoma, unlike the case with osteosarcoma and Ewing tumor, the periosteal reaction seen with conventional chondrosarcoma is generally smooth and organized, another feature emphasizing slow growth. Disorganized periosteal reaction, cortical destruction, periosteal elevation, and a permeative trabecular pattern are late radiographic features of central chondrosarcoma.

CT is helpful in demonstrating the mineralized matrix seen with this tumor and demonstrating areas of cortical destruction and periosteal reaction. The noncalcified portion of the tumor and its extraosseous extension are best demonstrated by MRI, where there is high signal intensity on T_2-weighted spin echo and gradient echo images, often with discrete lobulations of cartilage. Peripheral, septal, and nodular enhancement is seen on MRI after the administration of contrast. Areas of calcification or ossification demonstrate foci of signal void on all imaging sequences. In addition to demonstrating the full extent of the lesion, MRI is used to assess for recurrence of tumor after surgery.

Distinguishing central chondrosarcoma from enchondroma by imaging studies presents a serious challenge to radiologists. Frequently, this distinction cannot be made and the radiologist can offer little beyond recommending close observation. However, there are subtle differences between these two disorders. For example, while endosteal scalloping is a feature of enchondromas and chondrosarcomas of the appendicular skeleton (excluding the hands and feet), a statistically significant difference exists in the extent and depth of the endosteal scalloping: When the longitudinal extent of the endosteal scalloping involves greater than two thirds of the longitudinal extent of the lesion, and when the depth of endosteal scalloping is thicker than two thirds of the cortex, the possibility of a chondrosarcoma should be raised. Tumoral size is also important. Enchondromas tend to be less than 5 cm in size, and chondrosarcomas tend to be larger than that. Neither the degree of CT attenuation nor the MR signal intensity of the non-mineralized portion of the tumor is helpful in distinguishing enchondromas from central chondrosarcomas. Further, neither the degree nor the pattern of contrast enhancement observed on MRI serves to differentiate these two lesions. Frank cortical destruction and/or an associated para-osseous soft tissue mass indicate chondrosarcoma. Bone scintigraphy may help differentiate enchondromas from central chondrosarcomas in the appendicular skeleton. Although both lesions show increased activity on bone scans, lesions demonstrating activity greater than that seen in the anterior superior iliac spine are reportedly more likely to be malignant. The presence or absence of pain is not a useful clinical discriminator.

Juxtacortical or *peripheral* chondrosarcomas occur most commonly between ages 20 and 30 years and usually develop within the cartilaginous cap of an osteochondroma (Figure 4-32). Continued growth of an osteochondroma after skeletal

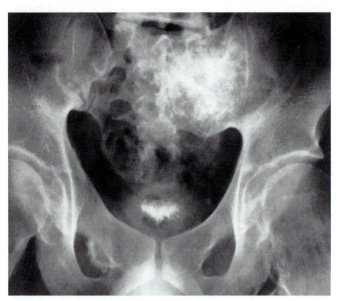

A

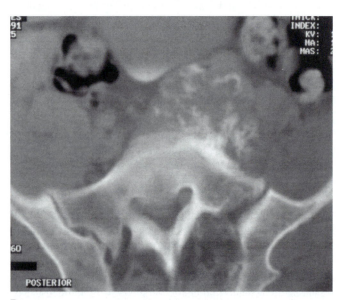

B

FIGURE 4-32.   Chondrosarcoma. *(A)* Radiograph and *(B)* computed tomographic image show malignant transformation of a sacral exostosis into a chondrosarcoma in a 35-year-old man with multiple hereditary exostoses. Note the dispersed flocculent calcification within the soft tissue mass anterior to the sacrum.

maturity and sonographic or MRI evidence of a cartilaginous cap thicker than 1.5 cm should be considered suspicious for malignancy. The male-to-female ratio reported for juxtacortical chondrosarcoma is about 7:4. Peripheral chondrosarcomas occur most commonly in the pelvis, proximal femur, scapula, and the proximal humerus. Compared with central conventional chondrosarcomas, they are recognized more readily radiographically by their predominantly extraosseous location and heavily calcified exophytic component. Although CT will visualize the calcifications associated with this tumor, it is not reliable for evaluating the thickness of the cartilaginous cap or the extent of the soft tissue component. On MRI, the cartilaginous cap of an osteochondroma is readily distinguished from the adjacent soft tissue structures, demonstrating high signal intensity on T_2-weighted spin echo and gradient echo images. Low grade peripheral chondrosarcomas tend to lobulated, demonstrating low signal intensity septae within lobulated areas of high signal intensity. High grade chondrosarcomas tend to be less lobulated and demonstrate intratumoral areas of necrosis on MRI. Histologically, peripheral chondrosarcomas do not differ from conventional chondrosarcomas.

CT is useful in demonstrating the mineralized chondroid matrix of these tumors and demonstrating areas of cortical destruction. MRI is essential for evaluating the full extent of the osseous component of the tumor and the soft tissue component and its relation to adjacent soft tissue structures, in particular the neurovascular bundle. For this reason, MRI is the preferred modality for staging of the tumor and preoperative planning.

The term *periosteal chondrosarcoma* is used when the tumor arises from the bone surface, with no associated underlying osteochondroma. This lesion is extremely rare and can be confused with periosteal osteosarcoma radiographically. Clinically, periosteal chondrosarcoma is less aggressive in its growth, and patients present with less symptomatology. Identification of "popcorn-like" calcification should prevent an erroneous diagnosis of periosteal osteosarcoma. Another distinguishing factor is that periosteal chondrosarcoma is generally metaphyseal in location, whereas periosteal osteosarcoma is generally in the diaphysis. Conventional radiography demonstrates a juxtacortical cartilaginous mass with scattered calcifications. The cortex may be thickened due to reactive bone formation or may show erosion.

Clear cell chondrosarcoma is exceedingly rare, accounting for no more than 2% of all chondrosarcomas. This tumor is of low grade malignancy and may be mistaken radiologically for a benign cartilaginous tumor or fibrous dysplasia due to its narrow zone of transition and frequently present sclerotic rim (Figure 4-33). Histologically, clear cell chondrosarcoma demonstrates chondrosarcomatous tissue with clear cells, chondroblast-like cells, and evidence of osseous metaplasia. Clear cell chondrosarcoma is an end-of-bone lesion, a feature it shares with chondroblastoma. Clear cell chondrosarcoma presents in an older group, with a mean age of 35 years at presentation, compared with chondroblastoma, which is a lesion of childhood. Clear cell chondrosarcoma is found almost exclusively in the femoral and humeral heads, followed by the pelvis. Plain film findings include a lytic expansile lesion with deceptively

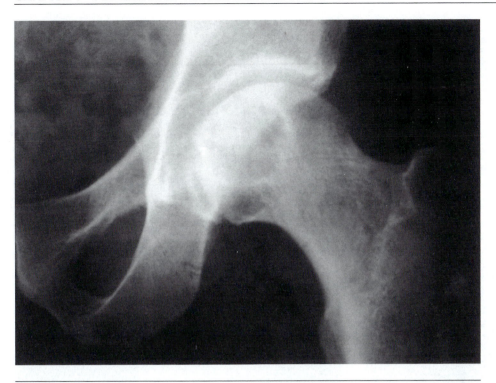

FIGURE 4-33. Clear cell chondrosarcoma. Radiograph of the hip shows a deceptively benign-appearing lytic lesion in the femoral epiphysis. The well-defined sclerotic rim is not an unusual finding associated with this slow-growing malignancy. *(Courtesy of Dr. Bernard Ghelman.)*

can occur at the site of a previously resected chondrosarcoma. In addition to imaging the lesion for staging and surgical management, bone scintigraphy and chest CT should be used to evaluate metastatic spread of this lesion, known for its widespread dissemination. Preoperative chemotherapy is followed by wide surgical resection, sometimes necessitating amputation. The 5-year survival rate is reportedly about 10%, with patients succumbing to widespread metastatic disease within 1 year of diagnosis.

Extraosseous or soft tissue chondrosarcomas are extremely rare, demonstrating a predilection for the soft tissues of the lower extremity. Radiographically, a lobulated pattern of soft tissue calcification is demonstrated. In addition to the lower extremities, this low grade chondrosarcoma has been described in the thyroid and cricoid cartilage and in the abdominal viscera.

benign-appearing margins and usually without mineralization. The appearance of this lesion is quite similar to that of conventional central chondrosarcoma, with the end-of-bone location being a major exception. The benign appearance of this tumor is responsible for the all too frequent delay in diagnosis. Patients are treated surgically.

Even more rare than clear cell chondrosarcoma is the *mesenchymal* type, accounting for about 1% of all chondrosarcomas. As its name indicates, this lesion derives from primitive mesenchymal cartilaginous cells. Most patients are in the third decade of life. This tumor is found most frequently in the lower limbs and in the skull, where it has shown a predilection for the maxilla and mandible. Conventional radiography depicts a lytic lesion with focal areas of mineralization and well-defined margins without a sclerotic rim. Mesenchymal chondrosarcomas are more aggressive than conventional chondrosarcomas, and treatment consists of wide surgical resection with chemotherapy and radiation.

The presence of a high grade chondrosarcoma juxtaposed with a low grade chondrosarcoma is called the *dedifferentiated* type of chondrosarcoma. The histologic appearance is that of two separate neoplasms with an abrupt line of demarcation between the low grade chondrosarcoma and the much more malignant tumor. Dedifferentiated chondrosarcoma demonstrates a predilection for the proximal ends of the femur and humerus. Most dedifferentiated chondrosarcomas arise from central rather than from peripheral chondrosarcomas, but they can arise from either and have been reported in patients with Ollier disease and in patients with multiple osteochondromatosis. This lesion also

Fibrous Lesions

MALIGNANT FIBROUS HISTIOCYTOMA. Malignant fibrous histiocytoma (MFH) is an unusual neoplasm that occurs far more commonly in the soft tissue than in the bone. About 10 to 20% of those tumors arising from bone develop in areas of abnormal bone, including osteonecrosis, irradiated bone (particularly in the flat bones of the pelvis after radiation for gynecologic malignancies), Paget disease, chronic osteomyelitis, giant cell tumor, and after hip replacement. The true incidence of this tumor is unknown because several tumors diagnosed as intraosseous fibrosarcomas are thought by some pathologists to have been MFHs, and, because in those cases in which substantial intraosseous and soft tissue components exist, it is sometimes difficult to establish the point of origin. MFH of the soft tissue can secondarily invade bone, and intraosseous lesions can develop prominent soft tissue extensions. Regardless of its true incidence, this tumor occurs far less commonly than osteosarcoma and is considered one of the more unusual malignant tumors of bone, believed by some investigators to represent only 5% of all primary malignant bone tumors.

Patients of all ages can be affected, although a predilection exists for the fourth decade of life. A male-to-female predominance of 2:1 has been reported. Patients complain of pain and swelling of the affected area, with about 20% of patients presenting with a pathologic fracture. Most lesions are in the long bones, with the distal femur the most commonly affected site. Lesions of the axial skeleton account for approximately 20% of cases. The metaphysis is the most commonly affected

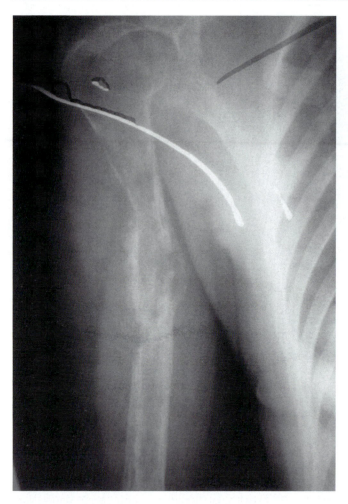

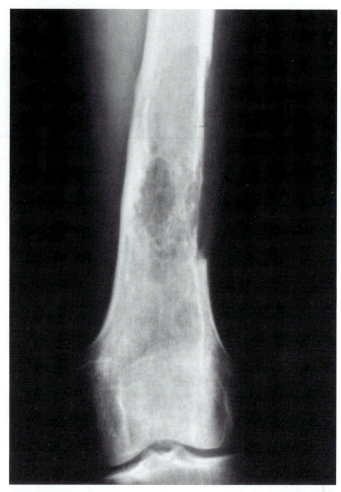

FIGURE 4-34. Malignant fibrous histiocytoma. Frontal view of the humerus demonstrates a poorly marginated, destructive, lytic lesion with multiple areas of cortical destruction and periosteal reaction in the diaphysis. *(Courtesy of Dr. Bernard Ghelman.)*

FIGURE 4-35. Fibrosarcoma. Frontal view of the femur shows an elongated, poorly marginated, ill-defined, destructive lytic lesion in the distal femoral metaphysis. *(Courtesy of Dr. Bernard Ghelman.)*

area when lesions are found in the long bones, followed by the metadiaphysis, the epi-metaphysis, and, less commonly, the diaphysis.

The radiographic features of MFH are those of an aggressive, non-mineralized, poorly marginated lytic lesion with a wide zone of transition and cortical destruction (Figure 4-34). In a small number of cases, associated features such as bony expansion, reactive sclerosis, and periosteal reaction are also present. The extent of bony destruction is better appreciated on CT than on conventional radiography. CT also shows soft tissue extension, a common feature of this disorder not necessarily suggested by plain films alone. The full extraosseous extent of the tumor is best illustrated by MRI. On MRI, these tumors demonstrate signal intensity that is isointense to or lower than that of muscle on T_1-weighted spin echo images and inhomogeneous, and high signal intensity on T_2-weighted spin echo images. A heterogeneous, nodular pattern of contrast enhancement has been described on contrast-enhanced T_1-weighted images. As with all bone and soft tissue tumors, MRI plays a vital role in demonstrating the full extent of disease and the relation of the tumor to the neurovascular bundle, knowledge of which is essential for patient management and surgical planning. Most

patients are treated with chemotherapy and wide surgical resection that occasionally requires limb salvage techniques or amputation. In some cases, postoperative radiation treatment is also used. The prognosis for MFH is poor and recurrence is common.

FIBROSARCOMA. This rare malignant tumor of bone occurs even less commonly than MFH. Although this tumor has been reported in patients of almost all ages, a predilection for the fourth and fifth decades of life has been demonstrated. According to some investigators, up to 30% of fibrosarcomas are associated with preexisting disorders, including longstanding bone infarcts, radiation therapy, Paget disease, fibrous dysplasia, chronic osteomyelitis, chronic tuberculosis, and tropical ulcer. Most tumors are found in the long bones, about the knee, and in the pelvis. Lesions are typically metadiaphyseal when located in the long bones. Rarely, fibrosarcoma can present with multifocal disease. Patients generally complain of increasing pain.

The radiographic manifestations are those of a highly destructive lytic lesion with a wide zone of transition or that of a permeative or moth-eaten trabecular pattern similar to that seen with round cell tumors (Figure 4-35). Characteristically, an associated soft tissue mass is present. Disorganized periosteal reaction and Codman triangles are common associated features. When fibrosarcoma arises in previously irradiated bone, cortical thickening, areas of sclerosis, and a thick coarsened trabecular pattern within the destructive lesion are seen. The vast majority of lesions are intramedullary in origin.

Miscellaneous Lesions

EWING TUMOR.   This round cell sarcoma of uncertain origin was first described in 1921 by James Ewing. Ewing sarcoma is one of a group of malignant round cell tumors of bone that include peripheral neuroectodermal tumor (PNET), neuroblastoma, primary lymphoma of bone, and small cell osteosarcoma (Table 4-9). Many of the clinical and imaging features of Ewing sarcoma are similar to those of other small cell tumors. Ewing tumor occurs far less commonly than osteosarcoma and chondrosarcoma, although it is more common than osteosarcoma in the first decade of life and is the second most common malignant bone tumor of childhood and adolescence. This tumor usually develops between ages 5 and 30 years. A male predilection exists.

Ewing sarcoma generally develops in areas of active red marrow production, favoring the proximal diaphysis and proximal diametaphysis of the major long bones, in particular the femur, and the pelvis. Additional sites of involvement are the ribs, spine, and sacrum. Less commonly, Ewing tumor has been reported in the tubular bones of the hands and feet, the occipital bone, the temporal bone, and the clavicle.

Initially, most patients complain of intermittent pain and swelling related to strain or minor trauma, with absence of nocturnal symptoms. In such instances, patients are frequently misdiagnosed with tendonitis. As the pain and swelling become increasingly severe, constitutional symptoms consisting of fever, increased sedimentation rate, leukocytosis, and anemia develop. A soft tissue mass is frequently palpated on physical examination in patients with lesions of the appendicular skeleton and the rib. Patients with Ewing tumor involving the spine may present with back pain or sciatica.

Conventional radiography typically depicts a predominantly lytic, permeative, or moth-eaten destructive lesion arising from the medullary cavity with a wide zone of transition, irregular cortical destruction, and a soft tissue mass (Figures 4-36 and 4-37). Periosteal reaction is an early radiographic feature. With time, the initial lamellar periosteal reaction develops spiculation. The classic "onion skin" type of periosteal reaction described in patients with Ewing tumor actually occurs relatively

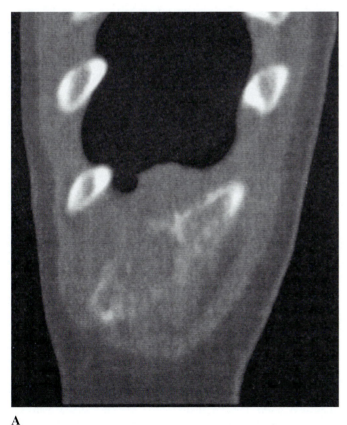

A

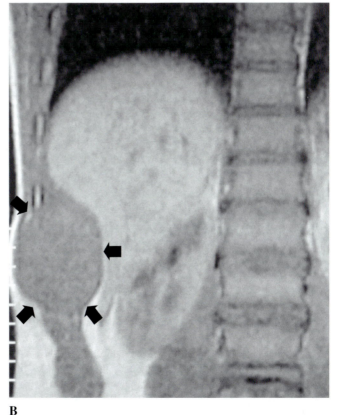

B

FIGURE 4-36.   Ewing tumor. *(A)* Sagittal reformatted computed tomographic image of a 12-year-old boy complaining of chest wall pain shows an expansile, destructive lesion of the rib associated with a large soft tissue mass. *(B)* The soft tissue component (arrows) is best appreciated on this T_1-weighted spin echo coronal magnetic resonance image, where it is causing extrinsic compression on the liver. This patient also presented with intermittent fever and an erythrocyte sedimentation rate of 60. *(Courtesy of Dr. Jerald Zimmer.)*

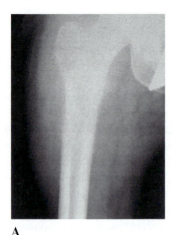

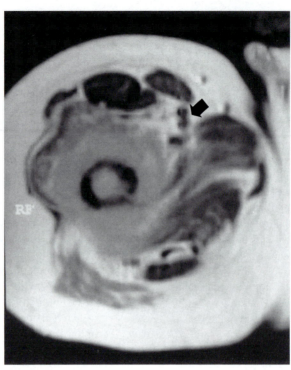

FIGURE 4-37. Ewing tumor. *(A)* Anteroposterior view of the femur shows a permeative trabecular pattern with disorganized periosteal reaction in the proximal femoral shaft in a 34-year-old man with Ewing tumor. *(B)* The soft tissue component and its relation to the neurovascular bundle (arrow) are well delineated on this axial proton density magnetic resonance image.

infrequently. Codman triangles are commonly observed. The elongated appearance of Ewing tumor helps to distinguish this malignancy from osteosarcoma, which generally manifests as a shorter focal lesion. There is often a large soft tissue component, best appreciated by MRI. Radiographic features of spinal involvement that have been reported include vertebra plana and spondylolisthesis.

Less commonly observed radiographic features described with this tumor are minimal involvement of the medullary cavity and a predominantly sclerotic appearance. Pathologic studies of those cases in which a predominantly sclerotic radiologic appearance is demonstrated have shown that the sclerotic bone represents reactive or dead bone and not the tumoral bone seen with osteosarcoma. When the lesion is primarily juxtacortical in location, with only slight involvement of the medullary cavity and minimal cortical destruction, "saucerization" of the outermost cortical surface may be seen. This frequently subtle finding represents subperiosteal extension of the tumor and is an early radiologic feature of Ewing sarcoma. At this stage, the tumor may be mistaken for osteomyelitis. In addition, the saucerization defect can be mistaken for pressure erosion due to an adjacent soft tissue sarcoma, lymphadenopathy, aneurysm, pigmented villonodular synovitis, or an adjacent infectious process. The saucerization defect also resembles the "cookie-bite" or "cookie-cutter" defect described with cortical metastases from bronchogenic carcinoma.

After the diagnosis of Ewing tumor is suggested by conventional radiography, further evaluation by bone scan and chest CT is performed to evaluate for additional occult osseous lesions and pulmonary metastases. These studies are followed by biopsy that can be performed percutaneously or by an open procedure.

Consultation with the oncologic surgeon before percutaneous core needle biopsy by the radiologist is advisable to avoid compromising the patient's surgical management. The biopsy track should be positioned in such a way that it is easily resected with the specimen at the time of definitive surgery and should not cross anatomic compartments. If an open biopsy is performed, an incisional biopsy is preferable to an excisional biopsy because the former results in less tissue contamination.

Once the diagnosis is established, cross-sectional imaging is used to evaluate the full extent of the lesion, particularly regarding skip metastases or epiphyseal involvement. This knowledge is imperative for surgical planning of limb salvage procedures. MRI provides excellent demonstration of the osseous and extraosseous components of Ewing sarcoma; for this reason, the surgeon depends on MRI for determining excisional margins. Although attempts have been made to differentiate peritumoral edema from tumor, this is of less importance to the surgeon because the edema is considered part of the reactive zone surrounding the tumor and must be removed en bloc with the specimen to ensure an adequate result.

CT and MRI also provide a pretreatment baseline of the extent of the disease, thus permitting measurement of chemotherapeutic response. Contrast-enhanced MRI can distinguish recurrent tumor from tumoral necrosis and from postsurgical fluid collections.

MRI features are essentially nonspecific with regard to the osseous and extraosseous components, demonstrating low signal intensity on T_1-weighted spin echo images and homogeneous or heterogeneous increased signal intensity on T_2-weighted spin echo images. Contrast enhancement is generally heterogeneous. Areas of consistently low signal intensity on T_1- and T_2-weighted images probably represent reactive bone or, in the case of the soft tissue component, dystrophic calcification due to therapy.

A rarely occurring subtype of the conventional or medullary form of Ewing sarcoma is the periosteal type. By definition, this form of Ewing tumor is subperiosteal in location and "never" invades the bony medulla. This tumor consists of a subperiosteal mass extending longitudinally along the periosteum, causing excavation of the cortex (a large saucerization defect), and periosteal reaction resulting in Codman triangles. Identification of extension of the tumor into the cancellous bone on CT or MRI alters the diagnosis to that of conventional Ewing tumor. The clinical presentation is similar to that of conventional and extraosseous Ewing tumors, with patients complaining of pain and swelling and possibly a mass. The male predominance of periosteal Ewing is even stronger than that of the medullary form of this tumor. Two important additional distinguishing factors are the greater predilection for involvement of the proximal portions of the extremities and the absence of metastatic disease at the time of presentation with the periosteal form. As with conventional Ewing tumor, there is distinct absence of mineralized matrix. However, calcification may develop after radiation therapy. Periosteal Ewing has a better prognosis than the medullary form, a theme that appears to be common to periosteal osteosarcoma in relation to conventional osteosarcoma and periosteal chondrosarcoma in relation to conventional chondrosarcoma. Because there are no histopathologic features to distinguish periosteal Ewing from medullary or soft tissue Ewing tumor, CT and MRI are essential for establishing the absence of involvement of the cancellous bone and the contiguity of the periosteum. The generally uninterrupted periosteal reaction seen with periosteal Ewing tumor is quite distinct from the onion-skin pattern of periosteal reaction occasionally seen with the conventional form of this tumor. The MRI features are similar to those described for conventional Ewing tumor. After biopsy for purposes of establishing the diagnosis, patients are treated with chemotherapy before surgical excision of the tumor and then with radiation therapy.

The prognosis for Ewing sarcoma has improved considerably because patients are no longer treated primarily by radiation. The use of adjuvant or neoadjuvant chemotherapy combined with surgical excision with wide margins has significantly reduced recurrence and increased survival. The reduction in the use of radiation treatment also has resulted in less morbidity that previously consisted of limb-length discrepancies, joint ankylosis, and radiation-induced sarcomas. Limb salvage surgery has become the standard of care for osteosarcoma and Ewing tumor, regardless of whether the lesions are of low or high grade malignancy.

PRIMITIVE NEUROECTODERMAL TUMOR OF BONE. Histologically and radiographically similar to Ewing sarcoma, and affecting the same age group, PNET arises more often in the soft tissues than in bone. PNET, in addition to Ewing sarcoma, small cell osteosarcoma, lymphoma, and neuroblastoma, belongs to the group of lesions classified as malignant round cell tumors of bone. Characteristic of round cell tumors, PNET arises centrally from the medullary cavity and usually is found in the metadiaphysis or diaphysis of long bones and in the flat bones of the pelvis (Figure 4-38). Histologically, positive staining for neurone-specific enolase or S100 protein distinguishes PNET

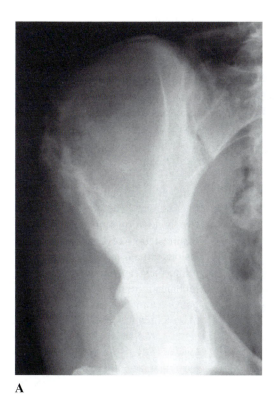

A

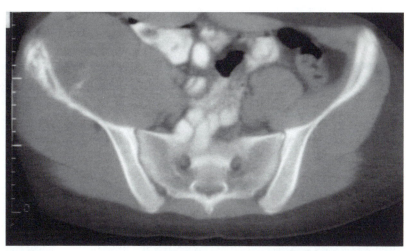

B

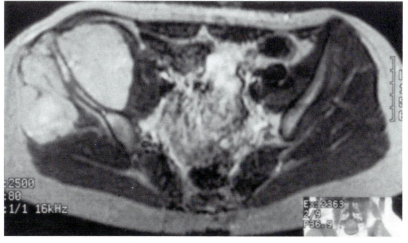

C

FIGURE 4-38. Primitive neuroectodermal tumor of bone in a 14-year-old girl who complained of right-side pelvic wall pain. *(A)* Radiograph shows an ill-defined, mixed lytic and sclerotic lesion in the right iliac bone with an associated soft tissue mass. Bony detail, including periosteal reaction, and the soft tissue mass are better demonstrated by *(B)* computed tomography, whereas *(C)* the T$_2$-weighted magnetic resonance image clearly defines the size and extent of the lesion.

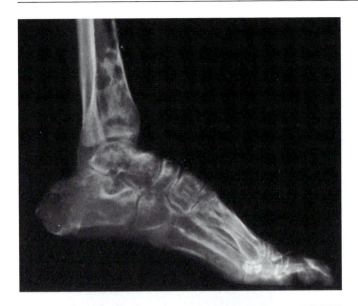

FIGURE 4-43. Angiosarcoma. Lateral radiograph of the foot shows multiple, well-defined lytic lesions throughout the distal tibia, ankle, and foot. *(Courtesy of Dr. Bernard Ghelman.)*

heterogeneous hyperintense signal on T_2-weighted images. Less commonly, chordomas show low signal intensity on T_2-weighted images. Typically, chordomas enhance after intravenous contrast administration.

Although chordomas rarely metastasize, the prognosis is poor due to their locally severe destructive behavior.

ADAMANTINOMA. This rare, locally aggressive malignancy of adolescents and young adults generally occurs in the diaphyseal portion of long bones and has demonstrated a marked affinity for the tibia. Patients usually present with persistent aching pain sometimes associated with a palpable tender swelling. Rarely, patients present with a pathologic fracture. Inadequate local excision renders recurrence inevitable with this radiation-insensitive tumor. It is therefore essential for the radiologist to demonstrate the full extent of the tumor to achieve adequate treatment.

Typically, the radiographic findings consist of a large round or elongated lytic lesion located centrally in the diaphysis of a long bone (Figure 4-42). This locally aggressive tumor frequently demonstrates a rather nonaggressive radiologic picture, with a narrow zone of transition and, not infrequently, a sclerotic margin. Not uncommonly, a loculated soap-bubble appearance is demonstrated. At other times, however, the zone of transition may be wide, and some lesions demonstrate wide and narrow transitional zones with sclerotic margins simultaneously.

TABLE 4-10

Ivory Vertebra

Hodgkin disease
Osteoblastic metastasis
Radiation
Paget disease
Sclerotic myeloma (rare)

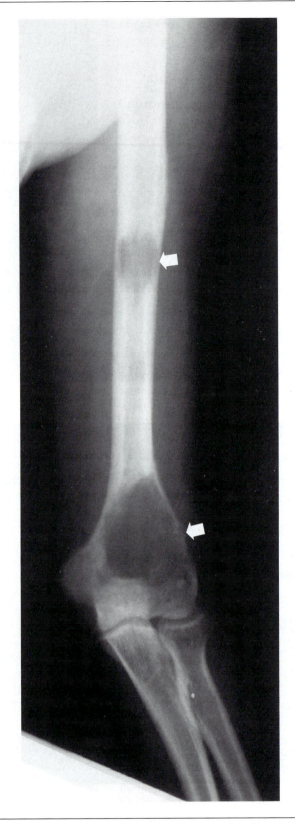

FIGURE 4-44. Multiple myeloma. Radiograph of the humerus in a patient with multiple myeloma shows two discrete lytic lesions (arrows). The lesion in the distal humerus shows cortical thinning and is in danger of fracture.

Cortical expansion and thinning are characteristic. Lesions that are eccentric rather than central in location are more likely to be associated with cortical destruction, particularly when located on the anterior aspect of the tibia. Cortical saucerization also has been reported with adamantinoma. Demonstrating the full extent of this tumor is greatly aided by cross-sectional imaging. Cortical detail is best illustrated by CT, whereas MRI shows the full extent of the osseous and soft tissue components. MRI should include the entirety of the affected bone because skip lesions are common. Successful treatment depends on complete removal of the tumor with wide surgical excision.

ANGIOSARCOMA. This rare malignant tumor of bone, also called *hemangioendothelial sarcoma*, can present at any age, although it is generally found in patients in the third, fourth, and fifth decades of life. A male predilection has been described. Patients present with local pain and swelling. Lesions in the cranium and spine are associated with headaches, backaches, and neurologic deficits. Patients also may present with pathologic fractures. Multicentric disease has been reported in up to 50% of cases, with separate lesions occasionally occurring in a single bone or multiple bones of the same extremity. Involvement of paired long bones is also characteristic. Angiosarcomas also have been described in association with preexisting disorders such as chronic osteomyelitis, osteonecrosis, and neoplastic disease.

Most lesions are found in the diaphysis or metaphysis of the long bones, in particular the tibia, femur, and humerus. Less frequently, angiosarcomas are found in the skull, pelvis, ribs, and vertebrae, although they have been reported in the sternum, clavicle, scapula, radius, patella, and small bones of the hands and feet.

One of the radiographic characteristics of angiosarcoma is a regional distribution in the involved bone consisting of multiple lytic lesions of different sizes (Figure 4-43). The lesions may be localized to the cortex or the medullary portion and may be well defined or poorly marginated. Cortical thinning or even bony expansion may be associated radiographic features. Periosteal reaction is unusual. In addition to metastatic disease, the multiple lytic lesions resemble multiple myeloma, the histiocytoses, cystic angiomatosis, Kaposi sarcoma, and fungal or tubercular disease.

After surgical excision for well-differentiated angiosarcoma, the prognosis is favorable. For high grade angiosarcomas of bone, the prognosis is dismal.

MULTIPLE MYELOMA AND PLASMACYTOMA. This disorder of bone marrow, characterized histologically by the neoplastic proliferation of abnormal plasma cells and overproduction of immunoglobulins, is the most common primary malignancy of bone, but it is a malignancy of the marrow elements, not of the bone itself. Plasmacytoma, the solitary form of multiple myeloma, has been reported in patients ranging from adolescence to older than 80. In general, however, patients with multiple myeloma are older than 40. A significant predilection for males has been reported, particularly with solitary plasmacytoma. Patients present with pain and swelling, frequently secondary to pathologic fracture. The propensity for involvement of the axial skeleton results in a clinical presentation of gradually increasing back pain or acute onset of pain due to sudden vertebral body collapse. Constitutional manifestations, including weakness, weight loss, fever, and anemia, also may constitute presenting complaints.

The radiographic manifestations can range from completely normal to widely disseminated, focal, destructive lytic lesions of the axial and appendicular skeleton. Sometimes, the only radiographic abnormality is severe osteopenia. In the case of solitary plasmacytoma, the typical radiographic appearance is that of a large, expansile, lytic lesion. The zone of transition can vary from narrow to wide. Occasionally, a plasmacytoma will have a thin sclerotic rim, in which case the lesion will appear benign. Very rarely, a solitary plasmacytoma will present as a sclerotic lesion. When this occurs in the spine, the result is an ivory vertebra indistinguishable from that seen with Hodgkin disease, osteoblastic metastasis, and metastatic carcinoid (Table 4-10). Associated soft tissue masses are typical with solitary

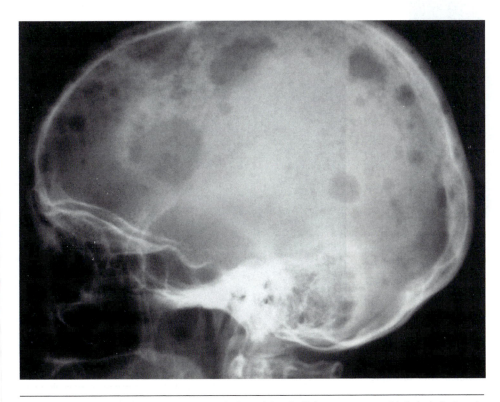

FIGURE 4-45. Multiple myeloma. Lateral view of the skull demonstrates multiple lytic lesions in a patient with multiple myeloma.

CHAPTER 5

SOFT TISSUE TUMORS

The imaging analysis of soft tissue masses is a common task for radiologists. Every imaging modality can be used to evaluate soft tissue tumors, but radiographs always should be performed first because they may give a clue to the underlying diagnosis. For example, a radiolucent mass indicates a fatty tumor, the presence of phleboliths indicates a vascular malformation, and peripheral calcification suggests myositis ossificans. Computed tomography (CT) can be helpful for the evaluation of suspected faint calcification, and, with the combination of multidetector scanners and powerful workstations, multiplanar reconstructed images are possible in a fraction of the time that it takes to perform a magnetic resonance (MR) examination. However, soft tissue contrast of CT does not equal that of MR imaging (MRI).

MRI is the workhorse for the evaluation of soft tissue masses. Its anatomic delineation and soft tissue contrast are unequaled, and it is therefore the preferred modality for preoperative staging. Because many soft tissue tumors have a nonspecific appearance of low to intermediate signal intensity on T_1-weighted sequences and high signal intensity on T_2-weighted sequences, intravenous gadolinium contrast may be necessary to distinguish solid masses from cystic masses such as ganglia.

Dynamic contrast enhancement, in which the degree of enhancement over time of a particular region of tumor, can be performed to determine the vascularity of a solid soft tissue mass or to monitor the chemotherapeutic response of a known malignant soft tissue tumor. It cannot reliably distinguish benign from malignant masses because of the overlap of vascularity between tumor types.

Sonography is excellent for determining whether a mass is cystic or solid. Power Doppler sonography should be used in the evaluation of a solid soft tissue mass because malignant soft tissue tumors have a greater percentage of internal vascularity than do benign tumors, and the morphology of the neo vascularity tends to be tortuous. Resistive indices, however, are not helpful for distinguishing benign from malignant masses.

Positron emission tomography scanning can be used for the evaluation of lymphoma and melanoma and is being investigated in the evaluation of other soft tissue masses. It may not be able to assist in a diagnosis but may be able to distinguish benign from malignant tumors based on degree of metabolic activity.

Even though some soft tissue tumors do have characteristic imaging appearances, such as a benign lipoma, a hemangioma, or a vascular malformation with phleboliths, it is often not possible to make a specific diagnosis or to distinguish benign from malignant conditions. Nonetheless, certain information may help in the imaging diagnosis of a soft tissue mass:

1. Location. Some masses have typical locations. For example, a small mass on the plantar aspect of the foot is most likely a plantar fibroma; a small mass around the wrist, hand, and fingers is most likely a ganglion cyst; a mass near the scapula is most likely an elastofibroma; masses around the knee are most likely meniscal cysts or bursae; masses around the shoulder are perilabral cysts or ganglia; and masses around the ankle are ganglia or distended joint recesses. In addition, some tumors have predilections for certain anatomic compartments, such as subcutaneous (malignant fibrous histiocytoma [MFH], lipoma, nodular fasciitis, and nerve sheath and dermal tumors), intermuscular (synovial sarcoma, nerve sheath tumors, and myositis ossificans), and intramuscular (MFH, liposarcoma, rhabdomyosarcoma, and lipoma).

2. Clinical history. A history of blunt trauma suggests myositis ossificans or hematoma formation; a history of anticoagulation and rapid development suggests hematoma formation; and a history of gout suggests tophus formation.

3. Physical examination. Some masses are soft, such as lipoma or hemangioma; some are firm, such as fibromas; some characteristically feel larger on examination than on imaging, such as fibromas; and some are painful, such as nodular or proliferative fasciitis and nerve sheath tumors.

Regardless of being able to make a specific diagnosis or even a distinction between benign and malignant, the radiologist's role is to stage the mass and aid preoperative planning by telling the surgeon the anatomic compartment or location of the mass, the size of the mass, involvement of adjacent neurovascular structures, and any bone or joint involvement.

Benign soft tissue tumors are more common than malignant ones, but the radiology and pathology literature differ on the exact proportions of each.

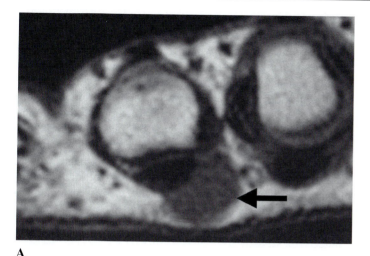

A

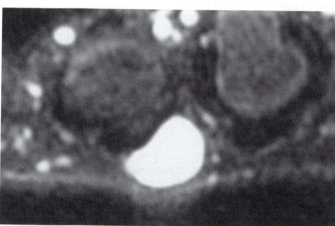

B

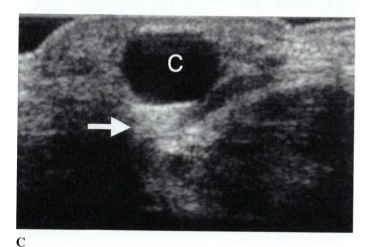

C

FIGURE 5-1. Ganglion cyst. Coronal T_1-weighted magnetic resonance image *(A)* through the distal metatarsals shows a well-circumscribed and homogeneous low signal intensity mass in the plantar subcutaneous tissue (arrow), which becomes uniformly high signal intensity on the corresponding fat-suppressed fast spin echo T_2-weighted magnetic resonance image *(B)*. *(C)* Corresponding sonogram shows the anechoic cyst with a thin well-defined wall and posterior acoustic enhancement (arrow). C = cyst.

BENIGN

Ganglion Cyst

Ganglion cysts are the most common benign soft tissue mass and are usually encountered around the wrist, hand, and fingers, and ankle or foot. When superficial, they can present as firm masses. They tend to arise near tendons and may represent a focal degenerative or posttraumatic process of the tendon sheath. Histologically, they have a thin fibrous wall lined with flat cells. Radiographs can show a bump in the contour of the affected region because the cyst has the same water density as muscle. Similarly, CT may show a water density mass that may be difficult to distinguish from muscle. MRI shows a well-defined mass that is uniformly low signal intensity on T_1-weighted sequences and homogeneously high signal intensity on T_2-weighted sequences (Figure 5-1), but intravenous gadolinium is necessary to reveal its cystic nature. It is usually round or oval but may be elongated and may insinuate itself between tendons or small bones of the hands and feet.

Sonography is the preferred method of evaluation of suspected ganglia because it is rapidly performed and can immediately distinguish a cystic from a solid mass. The cyst should be completely anechoic, with a thin wall and posterior acoustic enhancement (see Fig. 5-1). Moreover, dynamic scanning can be performed during flexion and extension of the digits, if the ganglion is located in a finger or toe, and can demonstrate whether the mass is tethered to the tendon.

Ganglia sometimes can be clinically occult, meaning that they are not palpable or visible on physical examination. These occult ganglia usually occur around the wrist or in the foot and can be a cause of pain. MRI and sonography can demonstrate these cysts, but sonography has the additional benefit of being able to guide percutaneous aspiration. However, MRI can provide a more global assessment of the wrist and foot and is able to evaluate other potential causes of the patient's symptoms.

Sometimes ganglia are imaged because they have recurred after aspiration and decompression. Such ganglia may not have the typical homogeneous fluid signal intensity on MRI or anechoic appearance sonographically because of fibrosis and hemorrhage after the needle puncture (Figure 5-2). Similarly, superficial ganglia are easily traumatized and may have a more heterogeneous and atypical appearance.

Lipoma

Lipoma is one of the most commonly encountered soft tissue masses. Although histologically identical to typical subcutaneous or deep fat, it is a neoplastic process that is separated from the body's metabolic regulation of fat. Thus, even an emaciated person can have a lipoma, and no matter how much weight one loses, the lipoma will remain unchanged in size. Lipomas are typically soft, painless, and located in the subcutaneous fat, but can occur within or between muscles. Radiographs and CT demonstrate a mass with fatty (radiolucent) density or attenuation (Figure 5-3). Sonographically, it is a well-demarcated

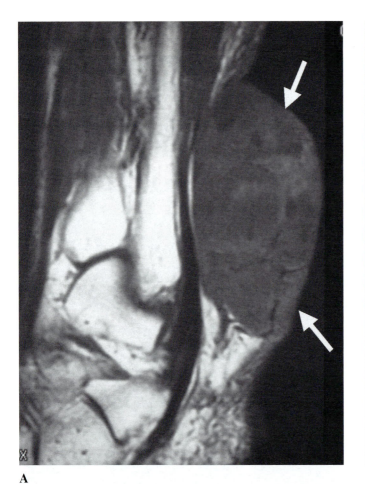

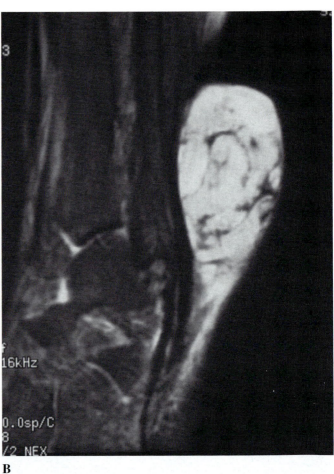

A   B

FIGURE 5-21. Malignant fibrous histiocytoma. *(A)* Sagittal T_1-weighted magnetic resonance image shows a large heterogeneous soft tissue mass in the posterolateral aspect of the ankle (arrows). *(B)* Corresponding sagittal fat-suppressed fast spin echo T_2-weighted sequence shows the heterogeneity and thick internal septation. *(Courtesy of Dr. Frieda Feldman.)*

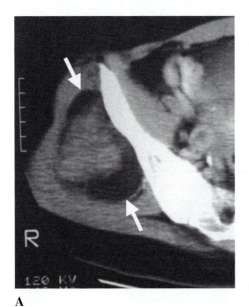

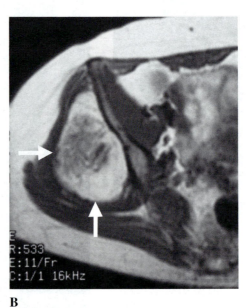

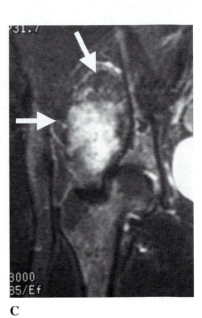

A   B   C

FIGURE 5-22. Liposarcoma. *(A)* Axial computed tomography through the pelvis shows a large fat-containing mass (arrows) with internal higher density mesenchymal tissue. *(B)* Corresponding axial T_1-weighted magnetic resonance image shows the fatty mass (arrows) with internal low signal intensity mesenchymal tissue. *(C)* Corresponding coronal fat-suppressed T_2-weighted magnetic resonance image shows the mass (arrows) with suppression of the fatty element and high signal intensity within the mesenchymal element. *(Courtesy of Dr. Frieda Feldman.)*

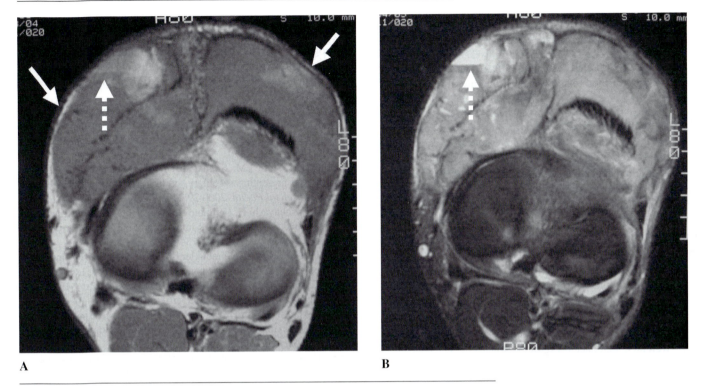

A   B

FIGURE 5-23.   Synovial sarcoma. *(A)* Axial T$_1$-weighted image at the level of the femoral condyles shows a large extra articular mass (solid arrows) with irregular and thick septations and a fluid level (dashed arrow). *(B)* Corresponding fat-suppressed fast spin echo T$_2$-weighted image shows the lobulated mass and the fluid level (arrow). *(Courtesy of Dr. Marcia Blacksin.)*

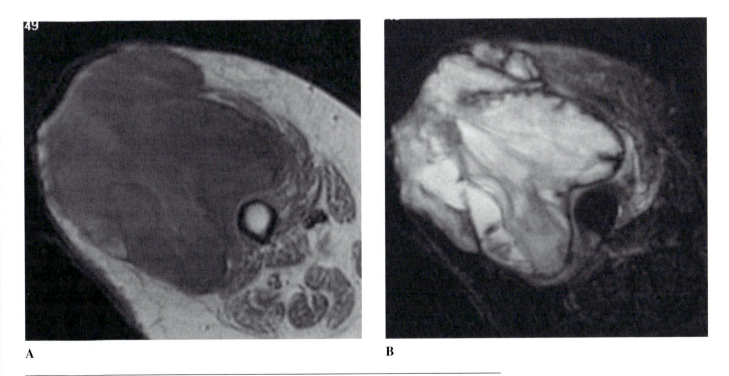

A   B

FIGURE 5-24.   Recurrent rhabdomyosarcoma in an adult. *(A)* Axial T$_1$-weighted magnetic resonance image shows a large lobulated exophytic mass arising from the vastus lateralis muscle. *(B)* Corresponding fat-suppressed fast spin echo T$_2$-weighted image shows the heterogenicity and lobulation.

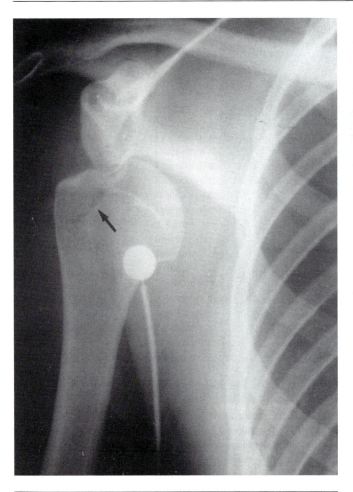

FIGURE 6-19. Anteroposterior radiograph of an anterior dislocation shows the impaction of the superolateral aspect of the humeral head against the inferior rim of the glenoid with production of a nondisplaced fracture of the greater tuberosity (arrow).

due to the stress incurred on this apophysis during throwing. In adults, distal humeral fractures are usually intercondylar, with an intraarticular T or Y shape.

Fractures of the proximal radius are the most common adult elbow injury. Radial head fractures are classified according to Mason: type I are most common, consisting of approximately one half of all radial head fractures, and are nondisplaced; type II fractures are seen in about one third of cases and have 2 mm or more of displacement (Figure 6-25); type III fractures are angulated or dislocated; and type IV fractures are any radial head fracture combined with an elbow dislocation.

Sometimes, fractures about the elbow are occult or subtle. A clue to their presence is a joint effusion, representing the hemarthrosis of an intraarticular fracture. The effusion is seen on a lateral radiograph as visibility of the normally unseen posterior fat pad and elevation of the normally visible anterior fat pad ("sail" sign; Figure 6-26).

Isolated proximal ulnar fractures typically involve the olecranon, secondary to excessive triceps tension, or involve a chip fracture of the coronoid process.

One must always keep in mind that fractures of a long bone may also involve the joint proximal or distal to that fracture, and this relationship is particularly true in the forearm.

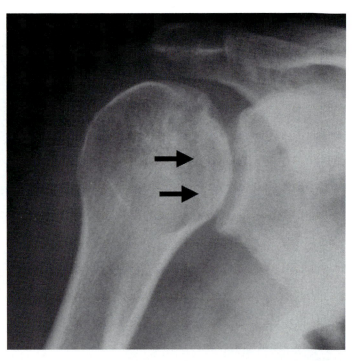

FIGURE 6-20. Posterior dislocation. Anteroposterior radiograph shows the trough sign (arrows) and internal rotation of the humeral head. Note that the glenohumeral joint space appears normal.

The combination of radiocapitellar dislocation and fracture of the proximal third of the ulna is called a *Monteggia fracture-dislocation* (Figure 6-27), and a fracture of the mid to distal radius with dislocation of the distal radioulnar joint is called a

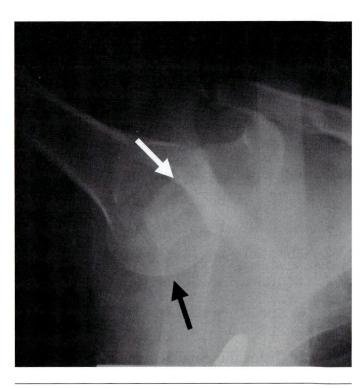

FIGURE 6-21. Anteroposterior radiograph shows the abducted position of the humerus typical for luxatio erecta. The humeral head (black arrow) has been levered out of the glenoid (white arrow).

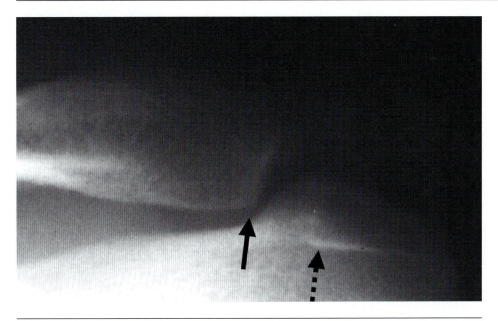

FIGURE 6-22.   Anteroposterior radiograph of the acromioclavicular joint shows a grade II separation with mild stepoff of the undersurfaces of the distal clavicle (solid arrow) and acromion (dashed arrow).

Galeazzi fracture-dislocation (Figure 6-28). An *Essex-Lopresti fracture-dislocation* consists of a displaced fracture of the radial head and dislocation of the distal radioulnar joint.

A *nightstick* fracture is a transverse fracture through the distal third of the ulna, so named because this is the type of fracture that ruffians and ne'er-do-wells used to sustain when putting up their arms to protect themselves from being hit over the head by a policeman's nightstick.

Wrist Fractures

Falls on an outstretched arm are responsible for a wide variety of fractures and dislocations about the wrist, despite the common mechanism of injury.

A *Colles fracture* is a dorsally angulated fracture of the distal radius. It is much more common in women than in men, in particular elderly women, because of osteoporosis. Sometimes,

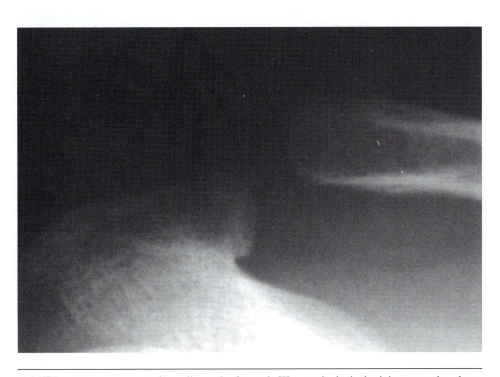

FIGURE 6-23.   Anteroposterior radiograph of a grade III acromioclavicular joint separation shows complete displacement of the AC joint.

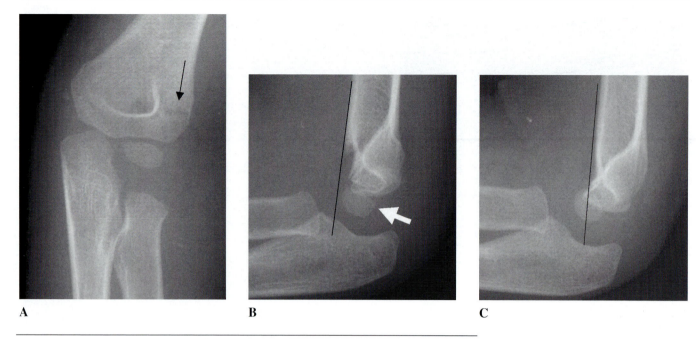

A   B   C

FIGURE 6-24. Supracondylar fracture in a child. *(A)* Anteroposterior radiograph of the elbow shows only a portion of the faint fracture line (arrow). *(B)* Lateral radiograph of this patient shows the posterior displacement of the capitulum (arrow). A line drawn along the anterior cortex of the humerus should intersect the middle third of the capitulum. *(C)* Lateral radiograph of the patient's contralateral elbow shows the anterior humeral line intersecting the normal capitulum.

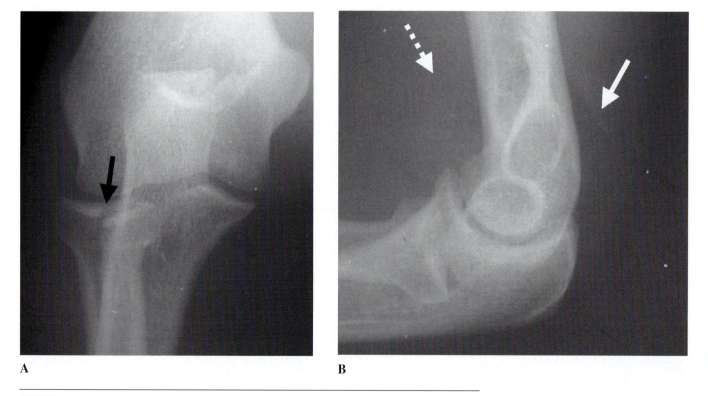

A   B

FIGURE 6-25. Fracture of the radial head. *(A)* Vertical fracture of the radial head with approximately 2 mm of stepoff (arrow). *(B)* Corresponding lateral radiograph shows the displaced anterior (dashed arrow) and posterior (solid arrow) fat pads.

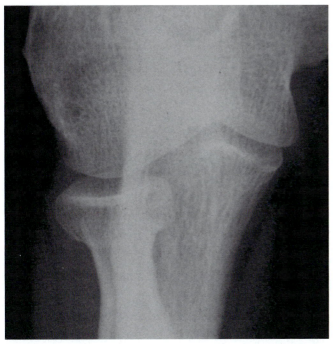

A

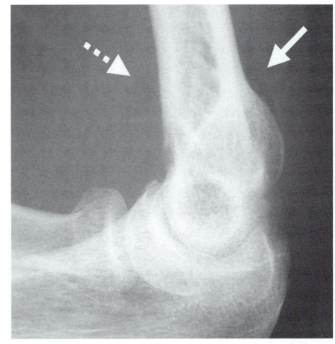

B

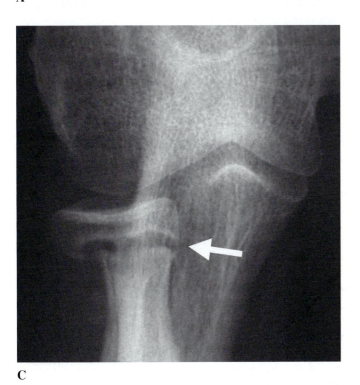

C

FIGURE 6-26.   Occult fracture of the radial neck. *(A)* Anteroposterior radiograph shows no discrete fracture. *(B)* Lateral radiograph shows elevation of the anterior fat pad (sail sign; dashed arrow) and demonstrates the posterior fat pad (solid arrow). These elevated fat pads indicate a joint effusion that is a secondary sign of fracture. *(C)* The patient was lost to follow-up but returned 6 months later complaining of elbow pain, and the anteroposterior radiograph shows the nonunion of the surgical neck fracture (arrow).

the actual fracture line is not visible as a lucency because the fracture is impacted; the clue to diagnosis is loss of the normal volar tilt of the distal radius articular surface on a lateral radiograph. Ten degrees to 15° of volar tilt is normal (Figure 6-29), and anything less than this, even as innocuous appearing as neutral position, is considered dorsally angulated (Figure 6-30). The lateral radiograph also may show volar soft tissue swelling, with bulging of the pronator fat pad, but this fat pad sign is unreliable.

On the AP radiograph, there may be increased radial inclination (tilt of the distal articular surface of the radius toward the ulna); normally, it is approximately 30°. There is often foreshortening of the radius with resultant positive ulnar variance.

Colles fractures are often associated with ulnar styloid fractures. The classification of Colles fractures is by Frykman and has 8 types. All even numbers have involvement of the ulnar styloid; Frykman types I and II have no articular extent, types

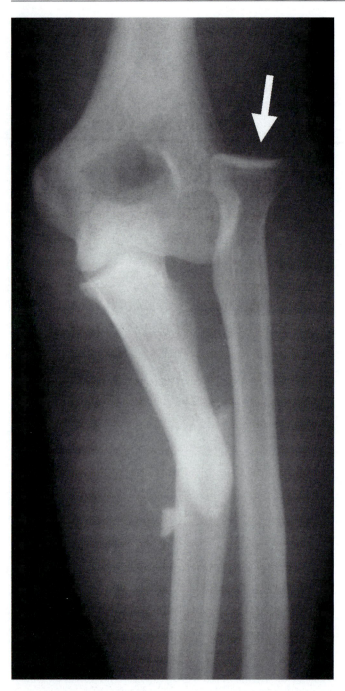

FIGURE 6-27. Anteroposterior radiograph shows a Monteggia fracture with a comminuted angulated and overriding fracture of the proximal third of the ulna and dislocation of the radial head (arrow).

III and IV extend into the distal radioulnar joint, types V and VI extend into the radiocarpal joint, and types VII and VIII extend into the radiocarpal and distal radioulnar joints.

The *Smith fracture* is a reverse Colles fracture; there is excessive volar angulation of the distal radius. This is also typically an osteoporotic injury.

A *Barton fracture* is an oblique fracture of the distal radius that extends to the dorsal articular rim; a reverse Barton involves the volar rim. Of note, the carpus and the hand remain articulated with the distal fracture fragment and may be significantly

displaced away from the shaft of the radius, mimicking a carpal dislocation.

A *chauffeur's fracture* is an isolated fracture of the radial styloid due to a direct blow. It gets its name from the early days of automobile use, when the chauffeur would have to crank the engine by hand to start it, and a back-firing crankshaft would strike the chauffeur's wrist.

The most frequently fractured carpal bone is the scaphoid, seen in 60 to 70% of all wrist fractures (see Chapter 11). Most of these scaphoid fractures involve the waist (Figure 6-31). Nonunion and avascular necrosis are complications of scaphoid fractures. The more proximal the fracture, the greater the risk of avascular necrosis.

The second most commonly fractured carpal bone is the triquetrum, occurring in approximately 20% of carpal fractures. The fracture is usually an avulsion of the dorsal ulnotriquetral ligament from the dorsal tubercle and is best seen on lateral or slightly off-lateral radiographs (Figure 6-32). This fracture has little clinical significance.

Fractures of the hamate can involve the dorsal aspect or the hook; fractures of the hook are due to a direct blow, often associated with holding a golf club or racket, and may have associated injury of the adjacent ulnar nerve. Fractures of other carpal bones are extremely uncommon.

Wrist Dislocations

Carpal dislocations are not rare. The diagnosis of carpal dislocation can be made on the AP radiograph and confirmed on the lateral view.

Dislocations disrupt the *arcs of Gilula*, which are imaginary lines conforming to the contours of the carpal rows. The first arc contains the proximal cortices of the proximal carpal row. The second arc follows the distal cortices of the proximal carpal row. The third arc follows the proximal aspect of the hamate and capitate (Figure 6-33). Slight offset of these arcs implies instability, whereas frank disruption of an arc implies dislocation. On a normal lateral radiograph, the distal radius, the lunate, the capitate, and the third metacarpal should line up (see Fig. 6-33), and the carpal bones should not extend volarly or dorsally to the volar and dorsal rim of the distal radius.

Failure of the extrinsic and intrinsic ligaments of the wrist occurs in a predictable pattern, leading to three types of carpal dislocations, which are, in order of increasing severity, perilunate, midcarpal, and lunate dislocations. Perilunate dislocations are the most common form and occur because of a normal weakness in the dorsal joint capsule at the level of the lunocapitate joint, called the *space of Poirier*. The distal carpal row dislocates, almost always dorsally, around a normally positioned lunate, appearing as overlapping bones and loss of the normal second and third arcs on an AP radiograph (Figure 6-34). Scaphoid fractures are often associated, at which point the injury is termed a *transscaphoid* perilunate dislocation. Midcarpal dislocation involves dorsal subluxation of the distal carpal row and mild volar subluxation of the lunate, but without frank dislocation of either. Lunate dislocation is the most severe of these injuries and involves frank dislocation of the lunate from its articulations with

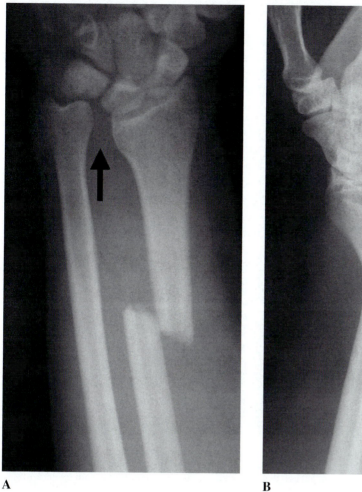

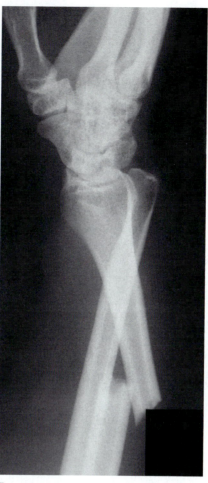

A   B

FIGURE 6-28.   Galeazzi fracture. *(A)* Anteroposterior radiograph shows the displaced fracture of the distal third of the radius. Note the widening of the distal radioulnar joint (arrow) indicating dislocation. *(B)* Lateral radiograph shows the angulated distal radius fracture and the offset of the distal radius and ulna.

the distal radius and capitate, almost always volarly. A change in shape of the lunate from rectangular to triangular on the AP radiograph indicates a lunate dislocation (Figure 6-35).

Carpal instability is due to ligament tears without frank carpal dislocation and consists of rotatory subluxation of the scaphoid, dorsal intercalated segmental instability (DISI), and volar intercalated segmental instability (VISI; see Chapter 11). An AP radiograph of rotatory subluxation of the scaphoid, also called *scapholunate dissociation*, shows a widened scapholunate distance (called the "Terry-Thomas" or "David Letterman" sign, named after the gap between the front teeth of these celebrities) and foreshortening of the scaphoid due to volar tilt of this bone. The tilted scaphoid also produces the "ring sign" as the x-ray beam passes tangentially along the long axis of the distal pole of the tilted scaphoid, forming a radiolucent oval with a thin sclerotic rim (Figure 6-36).

VISI and DISI refer to abnormal volar or dorsal tilting of the lunate due to tear of the lunotriquetral ligament and scapholunate ligament, respectively. DISI is more common. The diagnosis is made on the lateral radiograph: normally, the lunate sits like an

upright U on the distal radius, and a line drawn vertically through the center of the U should intersect a line drawn along the long axis of the scaphoid at an angle of 30° to 60° (Figure 6-37). In DISI, the lunate is tilted dorsally, and the resultant scapholunate angle is greater than 60°. In VISI, the lunate is tilted volarly, and the angle is less than 30°.

Hand

The most common metacarpal fracture is a fracture of the neck of the fifth metacarpal with volar angulation, called a *boxer's fracture* because the injury is due to a clenched fist striking something hard. A similar injury can occur in the fourth metacarpal (Figure 6-38).

Fractures of the first metacarpal occur at the base: a single fracture is called a *Bennet fracture* (Figure 6-39) and a comminuted fracture is a *Rolando fracture*. The fracture fragments stay with the first carpometacarpal joint, whereas the metacarpal shaft is displaced, but not dislocated, by the pull of the abductor and extensor tendons. A similar fracture can occur at the base

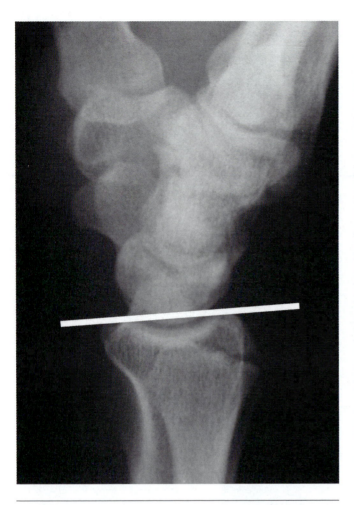

FIGURE 6-29. Lateral radiograph of a normal wrist shows the mild normal volar tilt of the distal articular surface of the radius (line). Incidentally noted is an old nonunited fracture of the ulnar styloid.

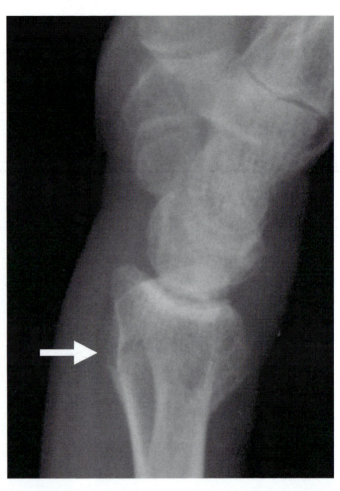

FIGURE 6-30. Colles fracture. Lateral radiograph shows the dorsally angulated distal articular surface. Fracture is indicated by the arrow.

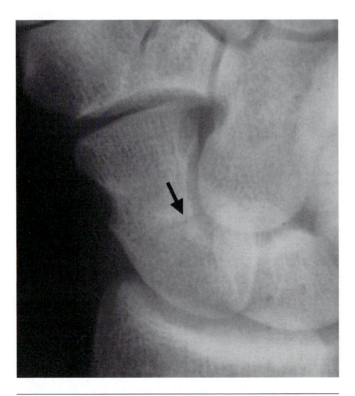

FIGURE 6-31. Anteroposterior radiograph of the wrist shows a thin radiolucent fracture through the waist of the scaphoid (arrow).

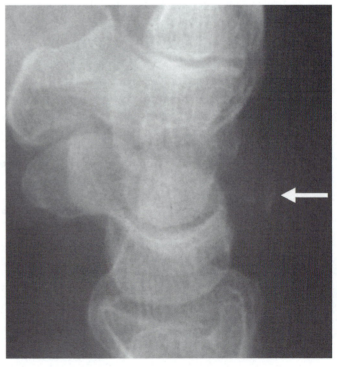

FIGURE 6-32. Lateral radiograph shows avulsion (arrow) of the dorsal aspect of the triquetrum.

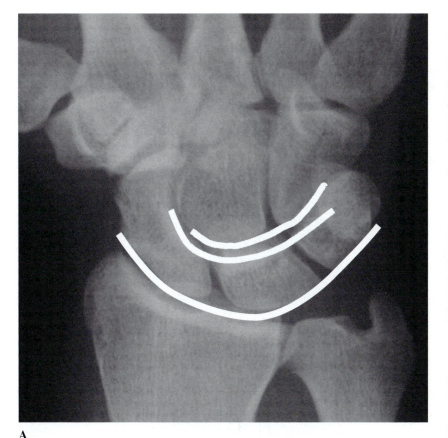

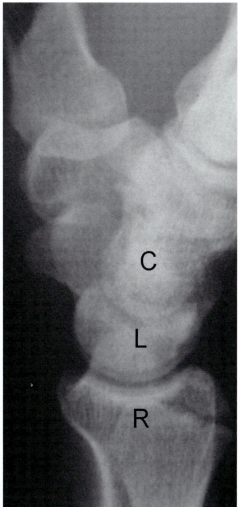

FIGURE 6-33. Normal wrist. *(A)* Anteroposterior radiograph shows the normal arcs of Gilula. *(B)* Lateral radiograph shows the normal colinear alignment of the distal radius, lunate, and capitate. This image shows the same patient as in Figure 6-29. C = capitate, L = lunate, R = radius.

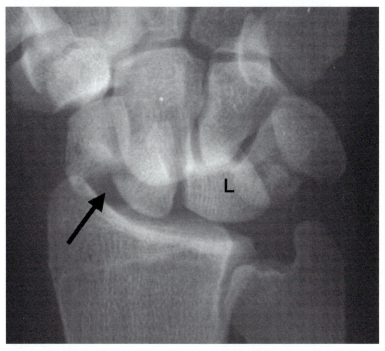

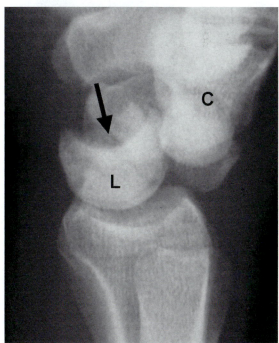

FIGURE 6-34. Transscaphoid perilunate fracture dislocation. *(A)* Anteroposterior radiograph shows overlap of the distal carpal row with the proximal carpal row. The lunate maintains its normal shape. There is a displaced fracture of the waist of the scaphoid (arrow), which typically accompanies a perilunate dislocation. *(B)* Lateral radiograph shows the dorsally dislocated capitate and hamate. Note the empty lunate fossa (arrow). C = capitate and hamate, L = lunate.

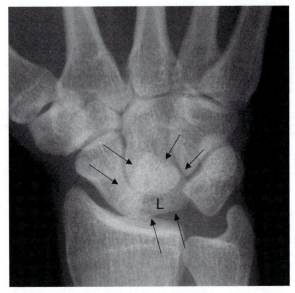

A

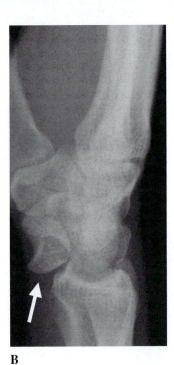

B

FIGURE 6-35.   Lunate dislocation. *(A)* Anteroposterior radiograph shows overlap of the distal and proximal carpal rows but note the triangular shape of the lunate (arrows), which indicates that it is the lunate which is dislocated and not the distal carpal row. *(B)* Corresponding lateral radiograph shows the volarly dislocated and rotated lunate (arrow). L = lunate.

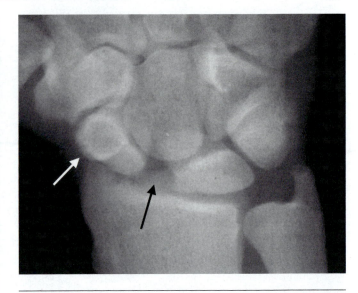

FIGURE 6-36.   Anteroposterior radiograph shows rotary subluxation of the scaphoid manifest as widening of the scapholunate distance (black arrow) and the ring sign (white arrow).

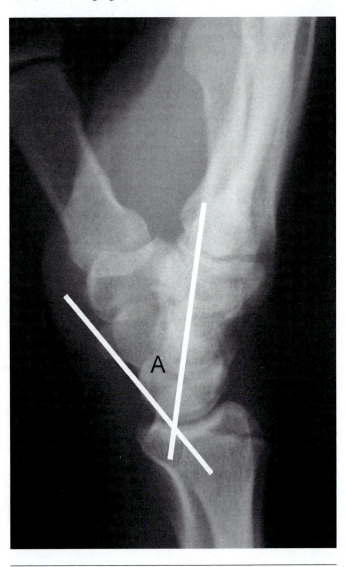

FIGURE 6-37.   Lateral radiograph shows the normal scapholunate angle. A = angle.

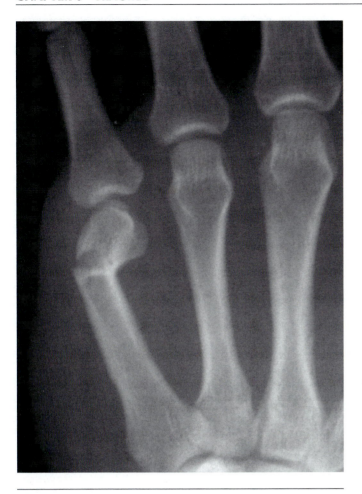

FIGURE 6-38. Anteroposterior radiograph of the hand shows the volarly angled boxer's fracture of the fifth metacarpal neck.

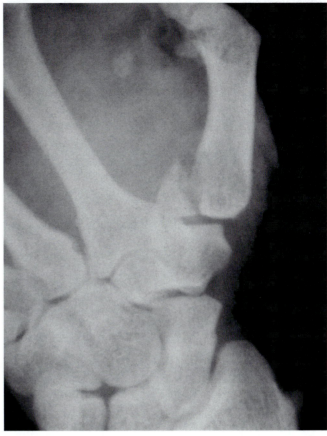

FIGURE 6-39. Anteroposterior radiograph of the hand shows a Bennet fracture.

of the fifth metacarpal but is less frequent and is termed a *baby Bennet fracture*.

A *gamekeeper's thumb* is an injury of the ulnar collateral ligament of the first metacarpophalangeal joint (see Chapter 11). The ligament may be ruptured or avulsed. If the latter, a bony fragment may be radiographically visible (Figure 6-40).

A common type of finger injury is a volar plate avulsion at the base of the middle phalanx, occurring secondary to forced hyperextension; lateral or off-lateral radiographs show a fracture fragment, which may be tiny, adjacent to the base of the phalanx. *Mallet finger* refers to an avulsion of the extensor tendon from the distal phalanx due to forced flexion. Finger dislocations are the most common dislocation of the hand and wrist and can occur in any direction, but dorsal dislocations are most common and most frequently occur at the interphalangeal joints rather than at the metacarpophalangeal joint.

Pelvis

Before the advent of classification systems for pelvic injury, descriptive terms were commonly used: *Malgaigne fracture* refers to the combination of a fracture or dislocation posterior to the acetabulum and a fracture or dislocation anterior to the acetabulum; *straddle fracture* refers to bilateral fractures of the superior and inferior pubic rami; *sprung pelvis* refers to dislocations of the sacroiliac joints bilaterally and the symphysis pubis. These terms may still be used but should be understood within a classification scheme.

Pelvic fractures may be categorized according to stability or mechanism of injury. The stability classification is based on the number of fractures or fracture "equivalents" (dislocation of the sacroiliac joints or the symphysis pubis). Examples of stable fractures are fracture of the iliac wing (*Duverney fracture*; Figure 6-41), avulsions (such as the sartorius muscle from the anterior superior iliac spine, the rectus femoris muscle from the anterior inferior spine, or the hamstrings from the ischial tuberosity; Figure 6-42), and single fractures of the sacrum or pubic rami, whereas Malgaigne, straddle, and sprung pelvis are examples of unstable injuries because of two or more fractures or equivalents around the pelvic ring.

The mechanism of injury classification separates injuries into anterior compression, lateral compression, and vertical shear, and all of these injuries are unstable. Lateral compression is the most common mechanism, with internal rotation of the affected hemipelvis and horizontally-oriented pubic rami fractures (Figure 6-43). An anterior compression vector results in vertically oriented pubic rami fractures (Figure 6-44) or a sprung pelvis (also called *the open book* pelvis) in which the symphysis pubis is diastatic and the sacroiliac joints are diastatic or fractured.

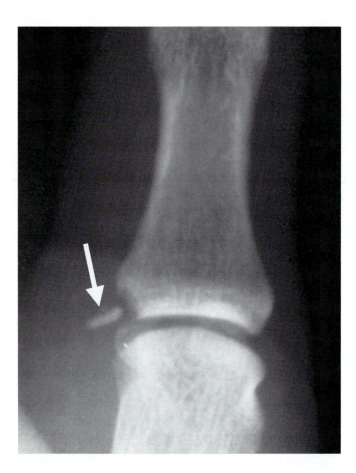

FIGURE 6-40. Anteroposterior radiograph of the thumb shows a small displaced and rotated avulsion fracture fragment (arrow) of the base of the first proximal phalanx, indicating avulsion of the ulnar collateral ligament.

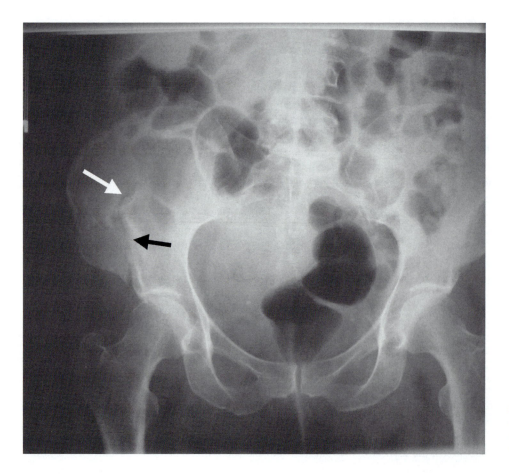

FIGURE 6-41. Anteroposterior radiograph of the pelvis shows a large Duverney fracture of the right iliac bone (arrows).

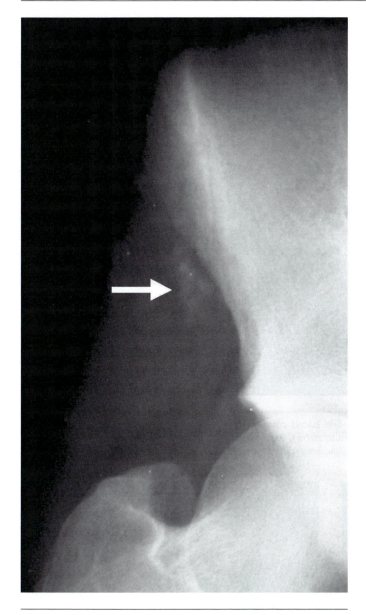

FIGURE 6-42. Anteroposterior radiograph of the right side of the pelvis shows faint periosteal new bone formation (arrow) at the site of a prior avulsion of the sartorius muscle from the anterior superior iliac spine.

Vertical shear injuries include superiorly displaced "straddle" fractures of the pubic rami and vertical offset of the hemipelvis (Figure 6-45). Because the term *Malgaigne* is nonspecific and merely refers to fracture or equivalents anterior and posterior to the acetabulum, all of these various unstable fractures are types of Malgaigne fractures.

Nonosseous complications of pelvic fractures are common and potentially life threatening, in particular vascular injury. The 10% mortality rate of pelvic fractures is directly related to vascular hemorrhage. Fractures of the medial aspects of the pubic rami can be associated with bladder and urethral tears.

Acetabular Fractures

There are six normal "lines" that can be identified around the acetabulum on a frontal radiograph, and disruption of any of them indicates an acetabular fracture (Figure 6-46). The iliopubic line represents the anterior column of the acetabulum, and the ilioischial line represents the quadrilateral plate, which is the medial wall and the thinnest portion of the acetabulum. The quadrilateral plate separates the anterior and posterior columns but is considered part of the posterior column. The pelvic "teardrop" is not an actual structure but rather a confluence of the ilioischial line medially and the anterior aspect of the acetabulum laterally.

Acetabular fractures should be described based on involvement of the anterior or the posterior column. The posterior column is more important because it is weight bearing. The modality of choice for evaluating acetabular fractures is CT (Figure 6-47). When assessing acetabular fractures, look for associated impaction or fracture of the femoral head and for any intraarticular bodies, in addition to column involvement.

Hip Fractures

Hip fractures are quite common and usually occur in osteoporotic patients. *Hip fracture* refers to fracture of the intraarticular portion of the proximal femur and may occur adjacent to the femoral head (subcapital), across the middle of the femoral neck (transcervical), at the base of the femoral neck (basicervical), or between the trochanters (intertrochanteric). The two most frequent locations are subcapital and intertrochanteric. These fractures occur at tremendous medical and social costs and have associated morbidity and mortality, particularly in elderly frail people who are medically "on the edge" and are pushed over by the debilitation of the fracture or the operative therapy.

Subcapital fractures have the worst prognosis medically and are described with the Garden classification. Type I fractures are valgus and incomplete. They may be subtle because the fracture line may not be radiographically visible. A clue is the change in direction of the normally vertically oriented compressive trabeculae of the neck (Figure 6-48). Garden type II fractures are complete but nondisplaced. Garden type III fractures are complete, with varus rotation of the femoral head. Garden type IV fractures are displaced but without rotation of the head (Figure 6-49). The usefulness of this classification is that it predicts the risk of avascular necrosis of the femoral head and thereby guides treatment: types I and II have a low risk of avascular necrosis and are treated with percutaneous pinning of the fracture, whereas types III and IV have a high risk of eventual avascular necrosis and are therefore treated with "prophylactic" hemiarthroplasty.

Intertrochanteric fractures have a better prognosis than subcapital fractures because the fracture is distal to the blood supply of the femoral head. The fracture is considered "2 parts" if there is a single fracture line and "3" or "4" parts if there are separate fractures of either or both trochanters, respectively (Figure 6-50).

If radiographs are normal in a patient with a clinically suspected hip fracture, MRI should be performed to look for occult

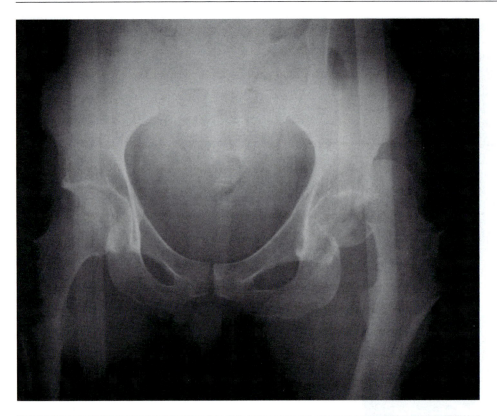

FIGURE 6-52.   Anteroposterior radiograph of a posterior dislocation of the left hip. Note that the femur is adducted and internally rotated.

seated rider is pushed out the back of the socket. A fall from a height can cause a similar injury. On the AP radiograph, the femur is adducted and internally rotated (Figure 6-52). Anterior dislocations are due to an abduction force with the femur in extension, and the head usually lies anteroinferior to the acetabulum. The femur is held in abduction and external rotation (Figure 6-53). Occasionally, the anteriorly dislocated head comes to lie within the obturator foramen, with frequent neurovascular injury. Hip dislocation also has a high risk of avascular necrosis (up to 50% of cases), which increases with increased delay to reduction.

An additional type of hip dislocation is termed *central*, although this is a misnomer because the injury is really an impaction of the femoral head into the acetabulum, resulting in fracture of the medial wall. In severe cases, the femoral head may be displaced medially to the acetabulum and into the pelvis.

Accompanying fractures of the acetabulum and femoral head may not be appreciated radiographically until the hip is reduced. Postreduction CT is useful for evaluating these injuries and to look for intraarticular fragments and the extent of acetabular involvement.

Midshaft and Distal Femur Fractures

Midshaft femur fractures usually require severe impact to occur and are associated with a large amount of periosteal callus

when healing. Distal femur fractures are usually seen in young adults and usually occur secondary to motor vehicle accidents. Commonly, these fractures involve the condyles in the Y and T patterns similar to those seen in the distal humerus, extending intercondylarly into the knee joint.

Knee

The most common fractures about the knee involve the patella and the tibial plateau. Patellar fractures can be stellate or horizontal. Stellate or comminuted fractures are usually due to a direct blow to the patella, such as occurs by falling on the knee or impacting the dashboard in a car accident. The horizontal patella fracture results from eccentric contraction of the quadriceps mechanism (see Chapter 13), which typically happens when someone stumbles (Figure 6-54). Quadriceps tension tends to displace the fragments.

A fracture of the medial rim of the patella is due to avulsion by the medial retinaculum, which occurs with lateral dislocation of the patella (Figure 6-55).

A pitfall in interpretation is the normal variant bipartite patella, in which there is a separate ossification center in the superolateral aspect of the patella that never unites to the rest of the patella. Clues to distinguish the bipartite patella are its characteristic location and its well-corticated edges, which the acute fracture does not have, and its lack of perfect fit into the patella, as opposed to fracture fragments.

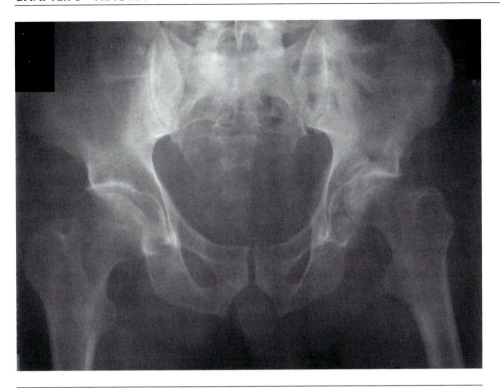

FIGURE 6-53. Anteroposterior radiograph of anterior dislocation of the left hip. The femur is externally rotated and abducted.

Tibial plateau fractures are due to impaction of the femoral condyles, usually with a valgus or, less often, a varus component, accounting for the more common occurrence of lateral than of medial fractures. The fracture may be a focal compression of the articular surface ("die-punch fracture"; Figure 6-56), a vertical

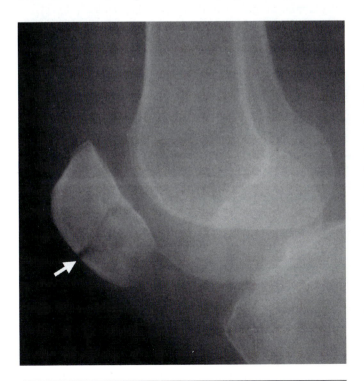

FIGURE 6-54. Lateral radiograph of the knee shows a nondisplaced horizontal fracture of the patella (arrow).

split or shear fracture, or a shallow oblique fracture that crosses under the tibial spines. The 6-type Schatzker classification is frequently used by orthopedic surgeons. Significant associated injuries are seen with plateau fractures and include medial collateral ligament tear, anterior cruciate ligament tear, and meniscal tears.

Most femoral condylar and tibial plateau fractures are radiographically visible, but some may be subtle or occult. If an effusion is present on the standard lateral radiograph without an obvious fracture, the technologist should perform a "cross-table lateral" view in which the patient is supine and the x-ray beam is horizontal; intraarticular fractures are accompanied by a lipohemarthrosis, which will appear on the cross-table view as a fat (lucent)–fluid (dense) level (Figure 6-57). CT is the method of choice for evaluating tibial plateau fractures to assess the amount of involvement of the articular surface, degree of displacement or inferior depression of the fracture fragments, and presence of intraarticular loose fragments, although some people advocate MRI to also assess meniscal injury.

Segond fracture of the anterolateral aspect of the tibia immediately distal to the plateau, avulsion of the anterior tibial spine, and chip fracture of the posteromedial aspect of the tibial plateau suggest anterior cruciate ligament (ACL) rupture and are discussed in Chapter 13. A fracture of the styloid of the fibular head is due to avulsion of the conjoined attachment of the biceps femoris tendon and fibular collateral ligament and is associated with ACL tear and posterolateral instability of the knee. Isolated proximal fibular fractures are often due to ankle injuries, where the force is transmitted proximally up the leg. Fractures of the fibular neck may injure the peroneal nerve.

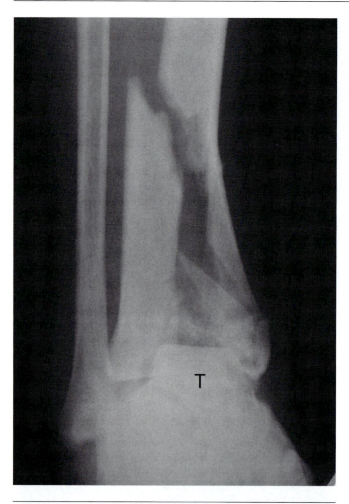

FIGURE 6-59. Anteroposterior radiograph shows the markedly comminuted pilon fracture of the distal tibia, due to impaction by the talus. T = talus.

tibial articular surface (the *plafond*; Figure 6-59). In children, a special type of Salter IV injury may occur, called a *triplane fracture*, which has a rotatory component of injury and is composed of a vertical fracture in the coronal plane through the metaphysis, a horizontal fracture through the physis, and a vertical fracture in the sagittal plane through the epiphysis (Figure 6-60). The *Tillaux fracture* is an avulsion of the anterolateral aspect of the tibial epiphysis, a Salter III injury (Figure 6-61).

Ankle

It is simple to classify ankle fractures by which malleolus is involved, but it is important to understand the mechanism of injury that produced the fracture. An inversion force pulls on the lateral ligament complex, thus rupturing it or causing a transverse fracture of the lateral malleolus, and causes compression of the talus against the medial malleolus, causing an oblique fracture of the medial malleolus. An eversion force does the opposite, with tear of the deltoid ligament or transverse fracture of the medial malleolus and oblique fracture of the lateral malleolus.

Lauge-Hansen, who performed experiments on cadaveric lower extremities, categorized ankle fractures based on the vector of injury (inversion or eversion) and the position of the foot (supination or pronation). He showed that there is a predictable pattern of fracture and ligament injury, but his classification has five types and many subtypes, making it cumbersome to use in daily practice. Instead, a more practical classification was described by Weber, which is based on the fibula fracture: Weber type A has a transverse fracture at or inferior to the level of the tibial plafond (Figure 6-62); Weber type B has an oblique fracture at the level of the joint space (Figure 6-63); and Weber

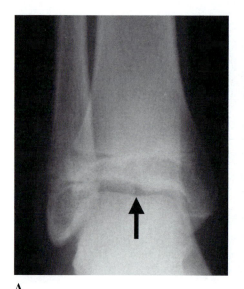

A

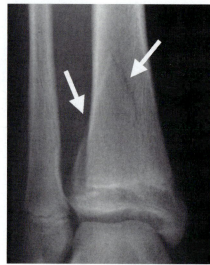

B

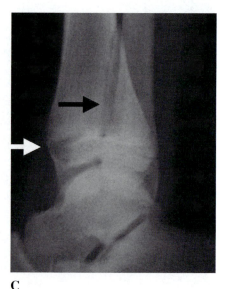

C

FIGURE 6-60. Triplane fracture. *(A)* Anteroposterior radiograph shows the sagittally oriented fracture of the tibial epiphysis (arrow). *(B)* Mortise view shows the coronally oriented fracture of the tibial metaphysis (arrows). *(C)* Lateral radiograph shows the coronally oriented fracture of the tibial metaphysis (black arrow) and the widened physis (white arrow) due to the horizontal fracture.

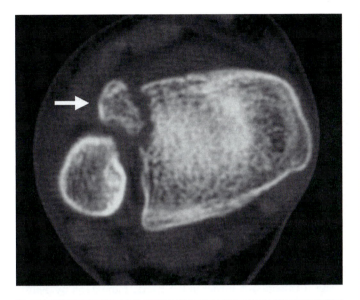

FIGURE 6-61. Axial computed tomographic image shows a displaced Tillaux fracture (arrow).

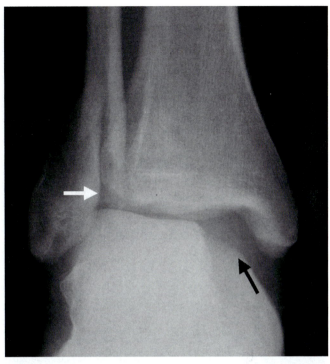

FIGURE 6-63. Anteroposterior radiograph of a Weber type B fracture shows the steep oblique fracture of the distal fibula (white arrow). Note that the distal aspect of the fibular fracture is at the level of the ankle joint and that the distal fibula and tibia remain overlapped, indicating sparing of the syndesmotic ligaments. Note also the widened mortise on the medial aspect of the ankle joint (black arrow), indicating rupture of the deltoid ligament.

type C has a fracture that is proximal to the ankle joint (Figure 6-64). Variations of Weber type C are *Dupuytren fracture*, in which the fibular fracture occurs in the distal third of the fibular shaft, and the *Maisonneuve fracture*, in which the fibular fracture is located in the proximal aspect of the fibular shaft. Regardless of how high up the fibular fracture is, the underlying cause is an ankle fracture in which the force has been transmitted proximally, rupturing the tibiofibular syndesmosis and interosseous membrane, and exiting through the fibular shaft (Figure 6-65).

The standard radiographic evaluation of the ankle includes an AP view, mortise view (15° internal rotation), and a lateral view. On the mortise view, the distal shafts of the fibula and tibia should overlap or touch, and the space (the *mortise*) formed around the talus by the medial malleolus, tibial plafond, and lateral malleolus should be uniform (Figure 6-66). Widening of the mortise can occur as a result of fracture of the malleoli or rupture of the lateral ligament complex or deltoid ligament or both (as a fracture equivalent). A fracture of the fibula proximal to the level of the plafond indicates rupture of the tibiofibular syndesmosis.

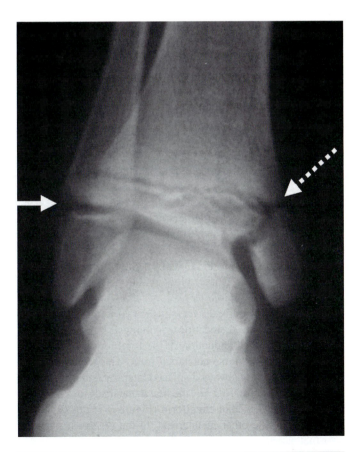

FIGURE 6-62. Anteroposterior radiograph in a child after an inversion injury shows a Weber type A fracture manifest as a horizontal widening of the fibular physis (solid arrow) and an oblique Salter type III fracture of the medial malleolus (dashed arrow).

Hindfoot

The hindfoot is composed of the talus and calcaneus and is subject to fracture and to dislocation.

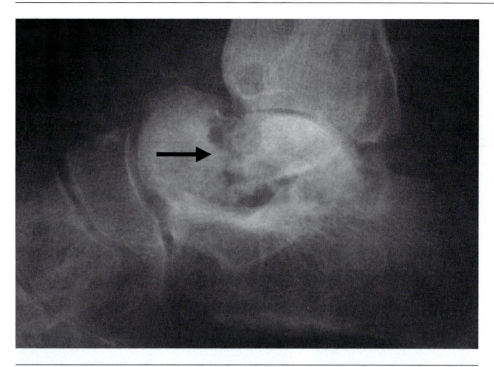

FIGURE 6-68. Lateral radiograph of the ankle shows an old fracture of the neck of the talus (arrow). Note that the body and dome of the talus are more dense than the surrounding bony structures, indicating that their blood supply has been disrupted and that avascular necrosis has occurred. This is a negative Hawkins sign.

medial cortex of the second metatarsal lines up with the medial cortex of the middle cuneiform, the medial cortex of the third metatarsal lines up with the medial cortex of the lateral cuneiform, and the bases of the fourth and fifth metatarsals sit in their respective shallow fossas on the distal articular surface of the cuboid (Figure 6-76). Any offset, no matter how subtle,

is abnormal. CT can be used to look for small fracture fragments and malalignment, and MRI is useful for evaluating damage to the ligaments that normally hold these bones together.

Metatarsal stress fractures are common, representing a fatigue-type injury, and most frequently involve the neck of the

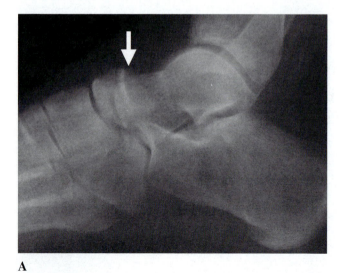

A

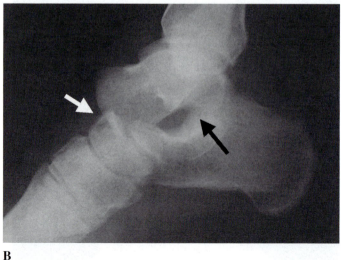

B

FIGURE 6-69. Subtalar dislocation. *(A)* Lateral radiograph shows a swivel talonavicular dislocation. Note the overlap of the head of the talus and navicular (arrow). The subtalar joint remains congruent. *(B)* Lateral radiograph of a different patient shows subtalar dislocation (black arrow) and talonavicular dislocation (white arrow).

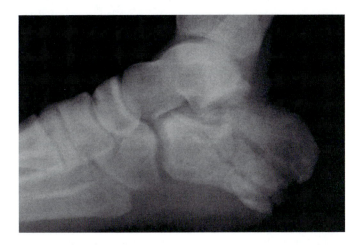

FIGURE 6-70.   Lateral radiograph of the calcaneus shows a tongue-type fracture.

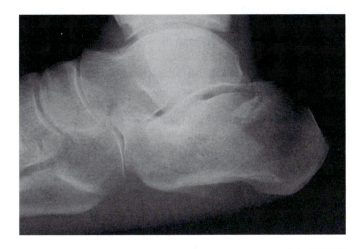

FIGURE 6-71.   Lateral radiograph shows a central depression type of fracture with loss of the Boehler angle.

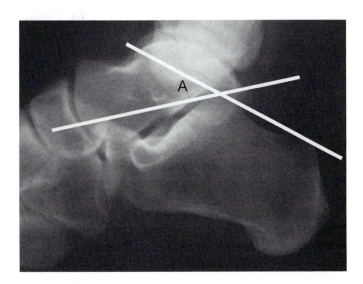

FIGURE 6-72.   Normal lateral radiograph shows a normal Boehler angle. A = angle.

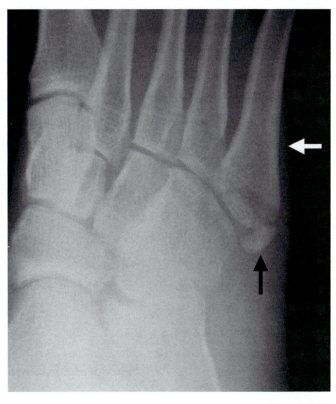

FIGURE 6-73.   Anteroposterior radiograph shows a comminuted avulsion fracture of the base of the fifth metatarsal (black arrow). A Jones fracture would occur more distally (white arrow).

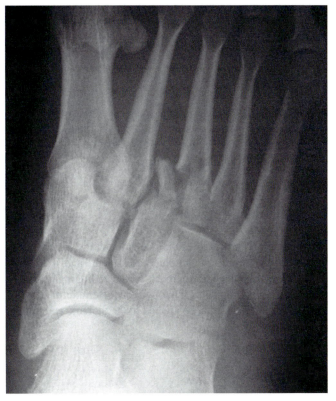

FIGURE 6-74.   Anteroposterior radiograph of the foot shows a homolateral Lisfranc fracture dislocation. Note that the first metatarsal remains aligned with the medial cuneiform.

TABLE 6-3

Extension Injuries

Signs
    Exaggerated lordosis
    Focal retrolisthesis >3 mm
    Teardrop fracture of C_2, avulsion fracture of anteroinferior aspect of
        other vertebrae
    Anterior disc space widening
    Prevertebral soft tissue swelling
Types
    Complex fractures of the facets
    Most hangman fractures
    Dens fractures
    Comminuted fracture of the posterior arch of C_1
    Avulsion of the anteroinferior aspect of the arch of C_1
    Extension teardrop injury

Unlike the thoracic and lumbar spine, axial loading is not a common vector in the cervical region. Compression fractures of the cervical vertebrae are rare but most often occur at C_1 and are called *Jefferson burst fractures*. These occur as the ring of C_1 is compressed between the occipital condyles of the skull and the lateral masses of C_2. The second most common site of cervical burst fracture is at C_7 (Table 6-4).

Lateral bending injuries are the least common type of mechanism of injury in the cervical spine and are rare. This type of injury encompasses fractures of the uncinate processes of the vertebrae, fractures of the lateral aspects of vertebral bodies, and fractures of transverse processes (Table 6-5).

Specific Sites of Injury

Rotatory malalignment of C_1 on C_2 is rare, and the nomenclature depends on the history and severity of rotation: rotatory *displacement* is transient, atraumatic, and mild; rotatory *fixation* is atraumatic and severe; rotatory *subluxation* is traumatic and mild; and rotatory *dislocation* is traumatic and severe. The atraumatic form usually occurs in children as a result of a viral pharyngitis and is self-limited. The traumatic form is usually due to a flexion-extension mechanism of injury. Patients typically complain of neck pain and may have torticollis, but neurologic impairment is absent unless the malalignment is severe. The malalignment can be assessed with open-mouth radiographs or with coronal and sagittal CT or MR images showing the offset of C_1 (Figure 6-83).

TABLE 6-4

Axial Loading Injuries

Burst fracture
    3 or 4 breaks in C_1
    Anterior and/or posterior displacement of vertebral body fragments
Vertebral body comminution
Anterior compression of the superior endplate
Disruption of the middle column

TABLE 6-5

Lateral Bending Injuries

Fracture of the transverse process
Fracture of the uncinate process
Lateral body fracture
Unilateral widening of the uncovertebral joint

C_1 fractures can occur anywhere in the bony ring (Table 6-6). Fractures of the anterior or posterior arch are the result of hyperextension (Figure 6-84). The Jefferson burst fracture is a 3- or 4-part fracture involving the anterior and posterior arches and is the result of axial load, as described above. Stability depends on the integrity of the transverse ligament; if the lateral masses of C_1 overhang C_2 by at least 7 mm, the ligament is disrupted and the fracture is unstable. Although radiographically severe, the Jefferson fracture usually is not associated with neurologic impairment, and 4-part fractures have a lower risk of impairment than do 3-part fractures.

Fractures of the dens may occur with flexion, extension, or rotational injuries. Type I fractures of the dens involve the tip and are due to an avulsion fracture of the alar ligament from the dens. This type is least common and is clinically insignificant except as a cause of pain. Type II fractures occur at the base of the dens and are unstable (Figure 6-85). Unfortunately, this is the most common type and is at risk for nonunion due to disruption of the blood supply to the dens. Type III fractures of the odontoid extend into the body of C_2 and are best appreciated on the lateral radiograph as disruption of the radiographic "ring" of the body of C_2 (Figure 6-86). They are stable and usually heal well (Table 6-7).

C_2 fractures (excluding the dens) involve the lateral masses or pedicles (see Table 6-7). Fractures of the lateral masses are due to an axial and lateral bending force. They are painful but stable injuries without neurologic sequelae. Bilateral fractures of the pedicles of C_2 are commonly called *hangman fractures*, but, although the mechanism of injury in judicial hanging is extension and distraction, the mechanism of injury of the more commonly encountered motor vehicle accident or fall is a mixture of hyperextension, hyperflexion, and compression. The associated soft tissue injury of a judicial hanging is also more severe, with complete disruption of the disc and ligaments between C_2 and C_3. A type I hangman fracture is nondisplaced and without angulation; a type II has angulation at the fracture site and displacement of the body of C_2; type IIa has fracture angulation but no vertebral displacement (Figure 6-87); type III is angled and displaced and has associated uni- or bilateral facet dislocation at

TABLE 6-6

Fractures of C_1

Jefferson burst
Hyperextension compression (comminuted fractures of the posterior arch without involvement of anterior arch)
Avulsion of the anterior atlantoaxial ligament from the inferior aspect of the anterior arch
Two thirds of C_1 fractures (especially Jefferson burst) are associated with C_2 fractures

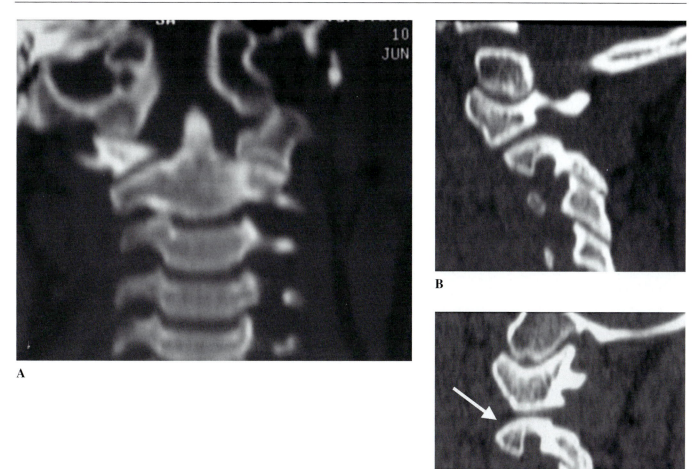

A

B

C

FIGURE 6-83. Rotatory displacement of C_1–C_2 in a child after an incident of strep throat. *(A)* Coronal reformatted computed tomographic image shows the mild rotation of the cervical spine. Note the asymmetric shape of the lateral masses of C_1, indicating that they are not in the same plane. *(B, C)* Sagittal reformatted computed tomographic images through the occipital condyles and lateral masses. Note the normal alignment in B and the offset at C_1 and C_2 in C (arrow).

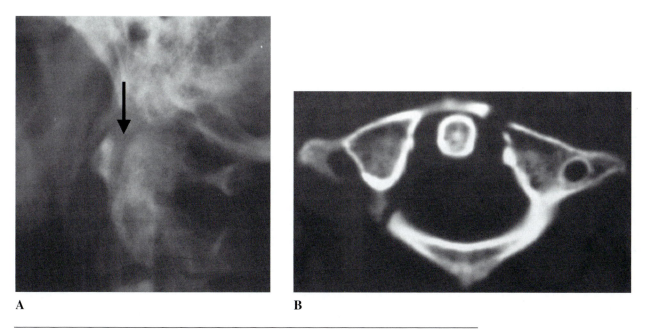

A   B

FIGURE 6-84. C_1 fracture. *(A)* Lateral radiograph shows widening of the pre-odontoid space (arrow). *(B)* Axial computed tomographic image shows fracture of the anterior and posterior arches.

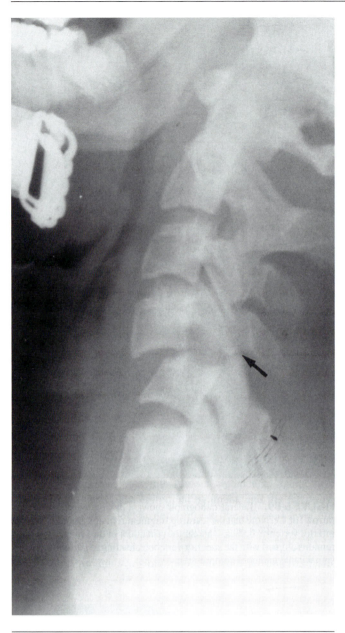

FIGURE 6-90.   Lateral radiograph shows perching of the facet joints bilaterally at C_4–C_5 (arrow).

THORACIC AND LUMBAR FRACTURES

Compression Fracture

Compression fracture is the most common type of fracture of the thoracic and lumbar spine and characteristically occurs between T_{10} and L_2. The severity of the anterior wedging or the endplate compression is variable. Traumatic anterior wedge compression fractures are the result of flexion injury with an associated axial load and are considered clinically significant if the compression is greater than 50% because of concomitant tear of the anterior longitudinal ligament. The degree of anterior wedging versus straight compression fracture will depend on which of these two injury vectors predominates.

Compression fractures are most commonly due to osteopenia or to focal disease within the vertebral bodies such as metastasis or myeloma. In such cases, the inciting trauma can be minimal such as mis-stepping off a curb or stair. Radiographs usually cannot discriminate between benign and malignant causes unless there is frank bony destruction to suggest tumor or the presence of the Kümmel phenomenon to suggest benignity. The *Kümmel phenomenon* is the development of a vacuum within a vertebral body due to collapse (see Chapter 2). When present, this vacuum excludes tumor as a cause of the fracture, but this phenomenon is rare. The MR evaluation of a radiographically evident compression fracture is a common clinical scenario in an attempt to determine underlying pathology.

Although it is not always easy to distinguish between pathologic and osteoporotic compressions, there are some general rules. In a pathologic fracture, the abnormal marrow signal affects the entire vertebral body and may extend into the pedicles, whereas in an osteoporotic compression, there tends to be some sparing of normal fatty marrow in the vertebral body and the pedicles are usually not involved. Osteoporotic compressions tend to show concave inward endplate compression with posterior prominence of the posterosuperior aspect of the vertebra (Figure 6-94), whereas pathologic compressions may show generalized outward bowing of the entire posterior cortex of the vertebra. A large paravertebral soft tissue mass or epidural component suggests pathologic fracture. Epidural hematoma can occur with an osteoporotic compression fracture but is usually small and infrequent. Diffusion-weighted MRI has been investigated for the differentiation of acute benign from pathologic compression fractures but is not able to reliably distinguish between them. Gradient echo images may be helpful for demonstrating frank trabecular destruction suggestive of pathologic fracture. If chronic osteoporotic compressions are present in other areas of the spine, manifest as loss of height but with normal fatty marrow signal, then the acute compression is most likely osteoporotic in origin. CT sometimes can be helpful for distinguishing benign from pathologic compression by showing frank bony destruction (in the case of malignancy) or mildly increased density of the benign compressed vertebra due to crowding of the osteoporotic trabeculae into a smaller space. If a distinction on MRI cannot be made, a follow-up scan in two to three months can be useful by showing resolution of the marrow edema, suggesting an osteoporotic compression, or showing no improvement, suggestive of pathologic injury. In some cases, a CT-guided biopsy is necessary to distinguish them. In cases of acute osteoporotic vertebral collapse or painful myelomatoid or metastatic disease, vertebroplasty or kyphoplasty can be performed as a therapeutic procedure (see Chapter 19).

Burst Fractures

The predominant vector of injury for burst fractures is axial compression, and burst fractures are a more severe form of compression fracture. The Dennis classification biomechanically

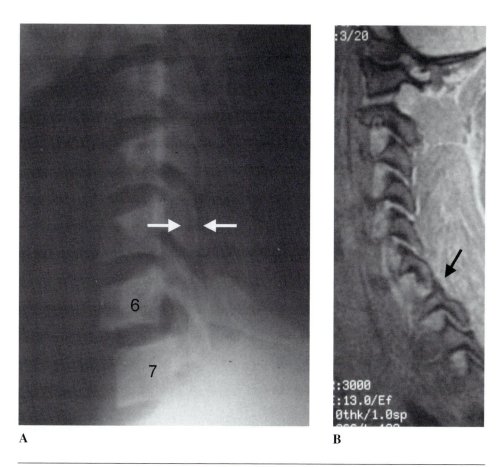

A   B

FIGURE 6-91. Unilateral locked facet. *(A)* Lateral radiograph shows mild anterior listhesis of C_6 and mild offset of the facet joints above this level due to rotation manifest as double lines (arrows) instead of being normally superimposed. *(B)* Corresponding sagittal fat-suppressed fast spin echo T_2-weighted image of the affected side shows the locked facet (arrow).

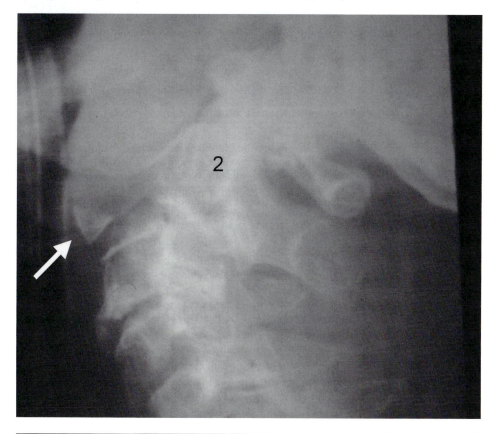

FIGURE 6-92. Lateral radiograph shows a hyperextension teardrop fracture of the inferior aspect of C_2 (arrow). Note the marked posterior displacement of the C_2 vertebra and head. $2 = C_2$ vertebra.

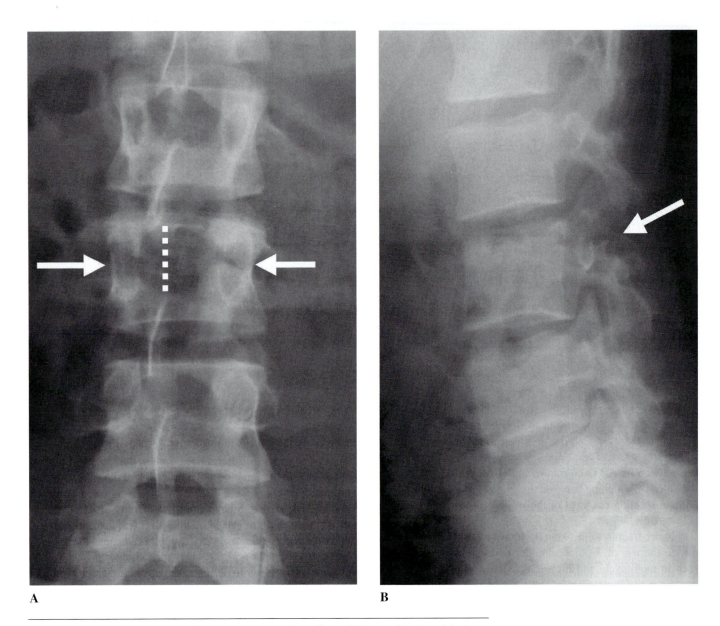

A   **B**

FIGURE 6-96.   Chance fracture of L₃. *(A)* Anteroposterior radiograph shows widening of the interspinous space (dashed line) and fractures of the pedicles (arrows). *(B)* Corresponding lateral radiograph shows the horizontal cleavage of the posterior elements (arrow) and the superior aspect of the vertebral body.

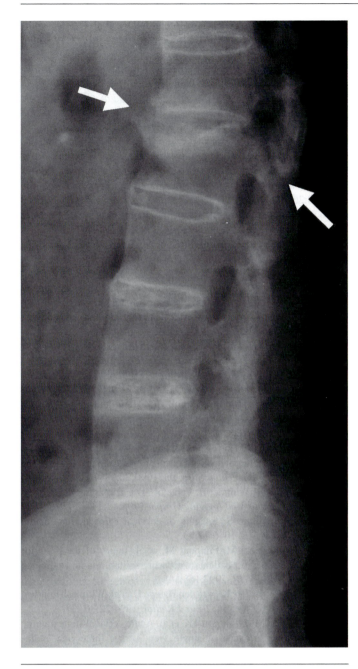

FIGURE 6-97. Fracture in ankylosing spondylitis. Lateral radiograph shows a fracture through the fused level between T$_{12}$ and L$_1$ (arrows). The fracture line extends through the posterior elements. Note the syndesmophytes and fusion of the posterior elements at other levels.

of the vertebral body. Offset of the spinous processes or increase in interspinous distances are other signs of instability.

SUGGESTED READINGS

Allen BL, Ferguson RL, Lehmann TR, et al. A mechanistic classification of closed indirect fractures and dislocations of the lower cervical spine. *Spine.* 1982;7:1–27.

Anderson LD, D'Alonzo RT. Fractures of the odontoid process of the axis. *J Bone Joint Surg Am.* 1974;56:1663–1674.

Anderson PA, Montesano PX. Morphology and treatment of the occipital condyle fractures. *Spine.* 1988;13:731–736.

Auletta AG, Conway WF, Hayes CW, Guisto DF, Gervin AS. Indications for radiography in patients with acute ankle injuries: role of the physical examination. *AJR.* 1991;157:789–801.

Barba CA, Taggert J, Morgan AS, et al. A new cervical spine clearance protocol using computed tomography. *J Trauma.* 2001;51:652–656.

Berne JD, Velmahos GC, El-Tawil Q, et al. Value of complete cervical helical computed tomographic scanning in identifying cervical spine injury in the unevaluable blunt trauma patient with multiple injuries: a prospective study. *J Trauma.* 1999;47:896–902.

Blackmore CC, Mann FA, Wilson AJ. Helical CT in the primary trauma evaluation of the cervical spine: an evidence-based approach. *Skeletal Radiol.* 2000;29:632–639.

Bogoch ER, Oullette G, Hastings DE. Intertrochanteric fractures of the femur in rheumatoid arthritis patients. *Clin Orthop.* 1993;294:181–186.

Brandser EA, El-Khoury GY. Thoracic and lumbar spine trauma. *Radiol Clin North Am.* 1997;35:533.

Bulas DI, Fitz CR, Johnson DL. Traumatic atlanto-occipital dislocation in children. *Radiology.* 1993;188:155–158.

Carr JB, Noto AM, Stevenson S. Volumetric three-dimensional computed tomography for acute calcaneus fractures: preliminary report. *J Orthop Trauma.* 1990;4:346–348.

Cattel HS, Filter DL. Pseudolaxation and other normal variations in the cervical spine in children. *J Bone Joint Surg Am.* 1965;47:1296–1309.

Cuenod CA, Laredo JD, Chevret S, et al. Acute vertebral collapse due to osteoporosis or malignancy: appearance on unenhanced and gadolinium-enhanced MR images. *Radiology.* 1996;198:515.

Daffner RH. Helical CT of the cervical spine for trauma patients: a time study. *AJR.* 2001;177:677–679.

Daffner RH, Deeb ZL, Goldberg AL, et al. The radiologic assessment of post-traumatic vertebral stability. *Skeletal Radiol.* 1990;19:103–108.

De Smet AA, Neff JR. Pubic and sacral insufficiency fractures: clinical course and radiological findings. *AJR.* 1985;145:601–606.

Denis F. The three column spine and its significance in the classification of acute thoracolumbar spinal injuries. *Spine.* 1983;8:817–831.

Deutsch AL, Mink JH, Waxman AD. Occult fractures of the proximal femur: MR imaging. *Radiology.* 1989;170:113–116.

Effendi B, Roy D, Cornish B, et al. Fractures of the ring of the axis. *J Bone Joint Surg Br.* 1981;63:319–327.

Ehara S, El-Khoury GY, Clark CR, et al. Radiologic evaluation of dens fracture: role of plain radiography and tomography. *Spine.* 1992;17:475–479.

El-Khoury GY, Kathol MH, Daniel WW, et al. Imaging of acute injuries of the cervical spine value of plain radiography, CT, and MR imaging. *AJR.* 1995;164:43.

El-Khoury GY, Whitten CG. Trauma to the upper thoracic spine: anatomy, biomechanics, and unique imaging features. *AJR.* 1993;160:95–102.

Garfin SR. Can burst fractures be predicted from plain radiographs? *J Bone Joint Surg Br.* 1992;74:147–150.

Gertzbein SD. Spine update: classification of thoracic and lumbar fractures. *Spine.* 1994;19:626–628.

Gilbert TJ, Cohen M. Imaging of acute injuries to the wrist and hand. *Radiol Clin North Am.* 1997;35:701.

Griffiths HJ, Olson PN, Everson LI, et al. Hyperextension strain of "whiplash" injuries to the cervical spine. *Skeletal Radiol.* 1995;24:263.

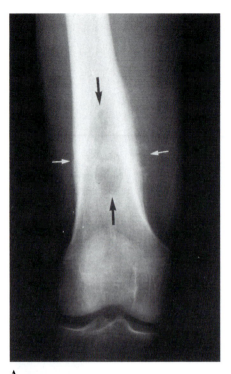
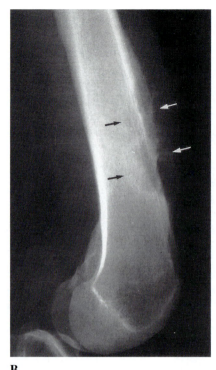
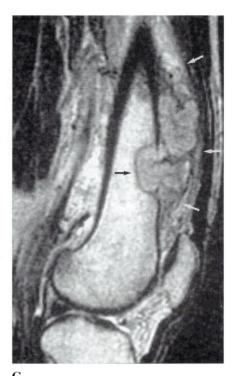

A   B   C

FIGURE 7-4. Bacillary angiomatosis. *(A)* Anteroposterior and *(B)* lateral radiographs of the distal femur shows a lobulated lytic lesion (black arrows) with disorganized periosteal reaction (white arrows). *(C)* Contrast-enhanced T$_1$-weighted magnetic resonance image demonstrates the intraosseous (black arrow) and prominent extraosseous lobulated soft tissue component (white arrows). The mass enhances heterogeneously with contrast. Extraosseous soft tissue extension is common with bacillary angiomatosis. *(Courtesy of Dr. Rolando Singson.)*

Lymphomatous involvement of muscle has been reported to occur in 8.8% of AIDS patients with non-Hodgkin lymphoma and occasionally has been reported as the initial manifestation of AIDS. In these instances, patients present with soft tissue swelling or a mass with or without tenderness. The differential diagnosis of lymphomatous involvement of muscle includes pyomyositis and thrombophlebitis, both of which can be clinically difficult to differentiate. MRI helps to distinguish muscle lymphoma from pyomyositis by demonstrating infiltration of the overlying subcutaneous tissue, which typically does not occur with pyomyositis. Thrombophlebitis can be evaluated by sonographic Doppler studies. Although MRI and ultrasound can confirm and define the presence of a soft tissue mass, they may not be able to distinguish infection from neoplasm.

Musculoskeletal neoplasms reported in children with HIV include Ewing sarcoma and leiomyosarcoma, with leiomyosarcoma occurring with disproportionately greater frequency than found in the general population.

SERONEGATIVE SPONDYLOARTHROPATHY ASSOCIATED WITH HIV

Reiter syndrome, in addition to other types of seronegative spondyloarthropathy, is generally believed to be the most common arthritic disorder to affect HIV$^+$ individuals, with

reports showing a greater prevalence of Reiter syndrome in the HIV$^+$ population than would be expected by coincidence. Arthritis of inflammatory bowel disease and ankylosing spondylitis are not associated with HIV. Although Reiter syndrome occurs in HIV$^+$ homosexuals and intravenous drug abusers, it is more commonly encountered in the former. Genital tract infection and diarrheal illness occurring before the onset of Reiter syndrome in some patients have implicated an infectious etiology, but this association remains unproven.

Most of the clinical features of HIV$^+$ patients with Reiter syndrome are the same as those encountered in the HIV$^-$ population, namely oligoarthritis mainly involving the lower extremities, painful enthesopathy, tendonitis, conjunctivitis, keratodermia blennorrhagicum, and circinate balanitis. An exception, however, is the lower incidence of sacroiliitis and spondylitis and the absence of radiographic findings in the spine and pelvis even in those few HIV$^+$ patients who do have clinical evidence of sacroiliitis and spondylitis.

Psoriasis and psoriatic arthritis also have been reported to occur with greater frequency in the HIV$^+$ population, but this is controversial. As is the case of HIV$^+$ patients with Reiter syndrome, oligoarthritis of the lower extremities predominates and sacroiliac involvement occurs less frequently than it does in HIV$^-$ individuals, and HIV$^+$ patients have absent radiographic and scintigraphic findings even in the presence of symptoms. Enthesopathy of the heel and foot and sausage digits of the feet are common.

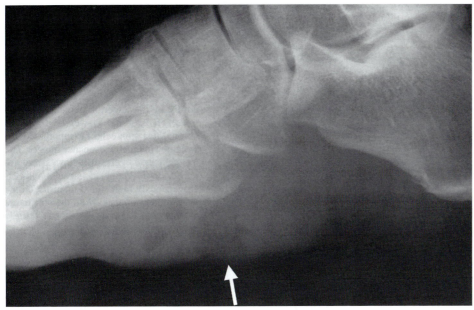

A

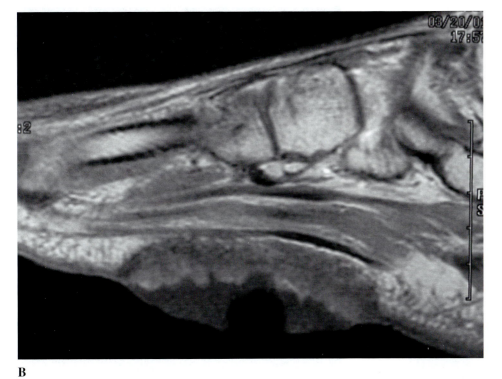

B

FIGURE 7-5. Kaposi sarcoma. *(A)* Lateral radiograph of the foot shows a large plantar soft tissue mass with heterogeneous density due to a large ulcer (arrow). *(B)* Sagittal T$_1$-weighted image after intravenous contrast shows the ulcerated, large, soft tissue mass. There is no bony involvement. *(Courtesy of Dr. Rolando Singson.)*

Undifferentiated spondyloarthropathy, also termed *incomplete Reiter syndrome*, is the name used for those HIV-infected individuals who demonstrate some of the features of Reiter syndrome and psoriatic arthritis (oligoarthritis and enthesopathy) but lack other clinical manifestations such as urethritis and conjunctivitis. Sacroiliac and spinal involvement also are characteristically unusual in undifferentiated spondyloarthritis.

The presence of Reiter syndrome, psoriatic arthritis, or undifferentiated spondyloarthropathy in an HIV$^+$ patient indicates a poor prognosis. The severity of these disorders is greater in the HIV$^+$ population than in the general population, and treatment is problematic because conventional therapy for these disorders consists of immunosuppressive agents.

Radiographic findings of these three arthropathies are similar and include erosive arthritis of the feet, calcaneal osteophytes, thickening of the plantar fascia, periostitis, and sausage toes. In the less frequently affected upper extremities, erosive arthritis of the distal interphalangeal joints of the hand with fluffy periostitis, enthesopathy of the greater tuberosity of the humerus associated with rotator cuff tendinitis, and epicondylitis of the elbow have been reported. Atlantoaxial subluxation and juxtaarticular osteoporosis of the hands and feet with subluxation of the metatarsal and phalangeal joints, features associated with rheumatoid arthritis (RA) and not with seronegative spondyloarthropathy, also have been reported, although these radiologic findings appear to be the exception rather than the rule.

RHEUMATOID ARTHRITIS AND AIDS

In contrast to seronegative spondyloarthropathy, the prevalence of RA in HIV$^+$ individuals is lower than that found in the general population. Early investigators believed that HIV was responsible for clinical remission of RA, whereas others went so far as to claim that these two diseases are mutually exclusive. The lower levels of the T-helper lymphocyte cell, CD4, found in HIV$^+$ patients was thought to be responsible for this phenomenon because the CD4 lymphocyte has been implicated in the pathogenesis of RA, but reports of coexisting RA and AIDS have disproved this theory. Thus, the role of CD4 lymphocytes in RA is unclear.

The radiologic findings described in the hands of HIV$^+$ patients with RA are no different from those seen in patients without HIV and include periarticular osteoporosis, soft tissue

CHAPTER 8

MISCELLANEOUS DISEASES

TERRY L. LEVIN / THEODORE T. MILLER

The scope of this book is not meant to cover every abnormal condition of bone; therefore, in this chapter we restrict ourselves to some commonly encountered diseases and other diseases that are not common but may be important differential diagnostic considerations.

PAGET DISEASE

Osteitis deformans, described by Sir James Paget in the 1870s and which now bears his name, is a fascinating disease. Its etiology is unknown but is probably viral, and it has a predilection for people of European, in particular Welsh, descent. Any bone in the body may be affected, although most commonly it involves the skull, spine, pelvis and sacrum, femur, and humerus. Histologically, the hallmark is a mosaic pattern of primitive woven bone.

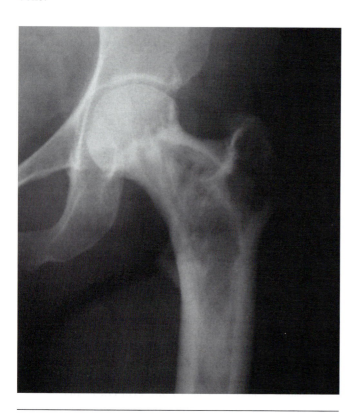

FIGURE 8-1. Anteroposterior radiograph of the hip shows mixed lytic and sclerotic Paget disease. It affects the greater trochanter as an end-of-bone equivalent in this case.

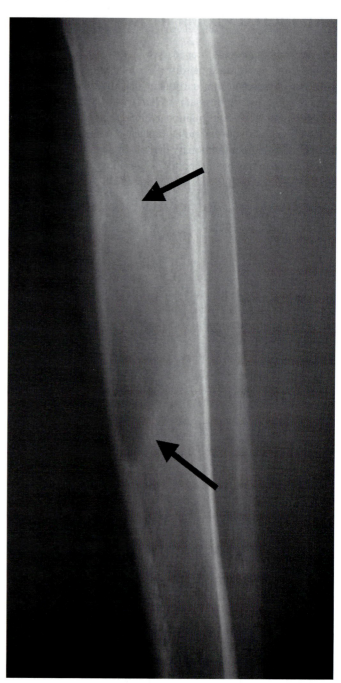

FIGURE 8-2. Lateral radiograph of the tibia shows lytic Paget disease in the midshaft of the bone. Note the "blade of grass" appearance of the ends of the lesion (arrows).

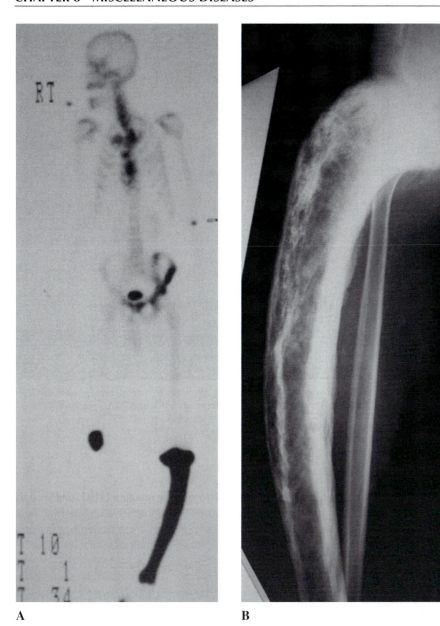

A   B

FIGURE 8-3.   Paget disease. *(A)* Anterior whole body bone scan shows marked diffuse uptake in the tibia, with enlargement and bowing. The patient also has Pagetic involvement of the contralateral patella, the ilium, cervical thoracic spine, and sternum. *(B)* Corresponding lateral radiograph of the affected tibia shows the coarsened appearance and anterior bowing. *(Courtesy of Dr. Frieda Feldman.)*

The disease has three phases: an active, lytic phase that appears radiographically as lucency; a mixed lytic and sclerotic phase; and a quiescent sclerotic phase. Paget's original term denotes the typical features of the disease: in the active phase, the affected bone is hyperemic and seemingly inflamed (hence the term *osteitis*); in the sclerotic phase, the affected bone eventually deforms due to enlargement. The marked hyperemia of the bones may cause high-output cardiac failure.

The disease is polyostotic in approximately two-thirds of cases, and different sites in the same person may show different phases. Moreover, an affected site does not have to progress from one phase to the next. The disease is usually asymptomatic and found incidentally on radiographs or other imaging examinations done for some other reason. If symptomatic, the usual

complaint is aching pain, although sometimes the enlargement or deformity of the bone may be noticed by the patient, such as the person whose hat size increases. The serum alkaline phosphatase and urinary hydroxyproline levels are elevated in the lytic and mixed phases and usually normal in the quiescent sclerotic phase. Men are affected slightly more commonly than are women, and the disease is usually not present until middle or old age.

Involvement of a long bone is always an "end-of-bone" process, but one must remember that apophyses, such as the greater and lesser trochanters of the femur and tibial tubercle, are end-of-bone equivalents as are flat bones such as those of the pelvis and skull (Figure 8-1). The major exception to the end-of-bone rule is the tibia, in which Paget disease may be

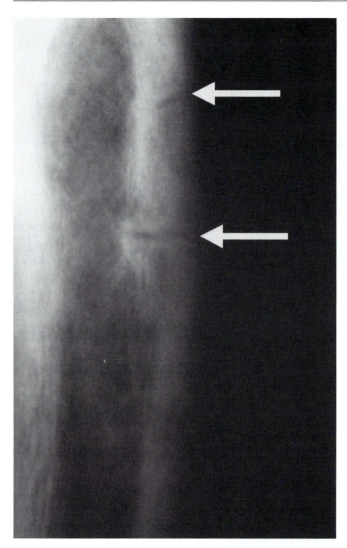

FIGURE 8-8. Anteroposterior radiograph of the proximal femur shows Looser lines perpendicular to the outer cortex of the bone (arrows).

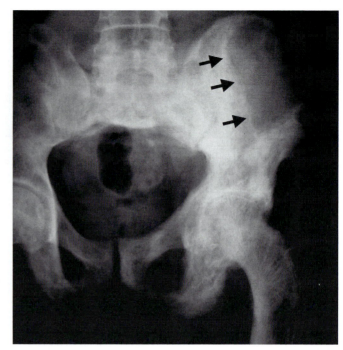

A

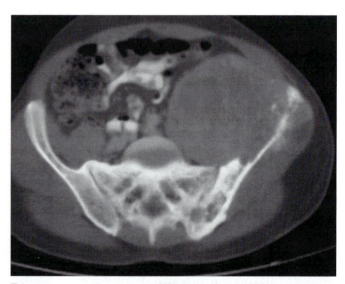

B

FIGURE 8-9. Malignant degeneration of Paget disease. *(A)* Anteroposterior radiograph shows Paget disease of the pelvis and left femur, with a large lucent area in the left ilium (arrows). *(B)* Corresponding axial computed tomographic scan shows a large heterogeneous soft tissue mass with destruction of the underlying bone.

On MRI, the affected vertebra may have a heterogeneous "zebra-stripe" appearance of low and high signal intensity (Figure 8-7).

Complications of Paget disease are: (*a*) deformity of the long bone due to bowing, eg, in the proximal femur, bowing manifests as varus deformity of the femoral neck; (*b*) pathologic fracture, where the fracture may be complete, or may be an incomplete, insufficiency type that appears as short, radiolucent Looser lines perpendicular to the convex (outer) surface of the bowed bone (Figure 8-8). Looser zones of osteomalacia occur on the concave, or inner surface, of the bone; (*c*) basilar invagination of the skull and resultant hydrocephalus; (*d*) deafness due to otosclerosis and enlargement of the temporal bone and ossicles of

the inner ear; (*e*) degenerative arthritis due to joint incongruence resulting from the enlarged bone; and (*f*) tumor. Pagetic bone is at risk for the development of giant cell tumors, particularly of the jaw, and at risk of malignant degeneration into osteosarcoma (most commonly), chondrosarcoma, and fibrosarcoma. Malignant degeneration occurs in fewer than 1% of cases, and the radiographic features are bone destruction and soft tissue mass, without periosteal reaction (Figure 8-9).

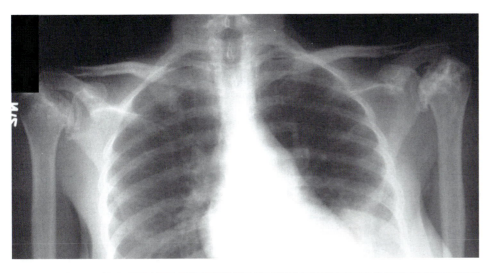

FIGURE 8-10. Anteroposterior radiograph of the chest shows osteonecrosis and collapse of the humeral heads bilaterally in this patient with sickle cell disease.

SICKLE CELL DISEASE

The bony manifestations of sickle cell disease typically are related to osteonecrosis and infection (Figure 8-10). The bones may have a chalky or mildly dense appearance due to infarct. A particular feature of osteonecrosis in sickle cell patients is infarction of the center of the vertebral body leading to a characteristic H-shape collapse of the endplates (Figure 8-11). Osteonecrosis of the phalanges causes patchy medullary sclerosis and periosteal reaction, called *sickle dactylitis* or *hand-foot syndrome*, in which the patient complains of finger pain and

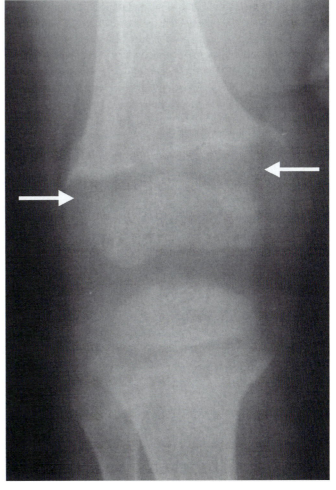

FIGURE 8-12. Anteroposterior radiograph of the knee shows widening of the physis of the distal femur (arrows) and fraying and irregularity of the metaphysis.

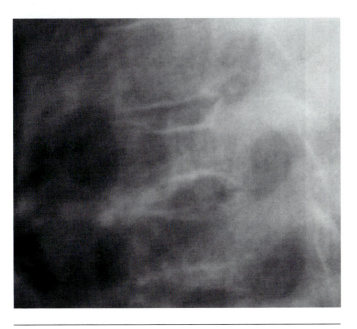

FIGURE 8-11. Lateral radiograph shows the H-shape deformity of the osteonecrotic vertebral body.

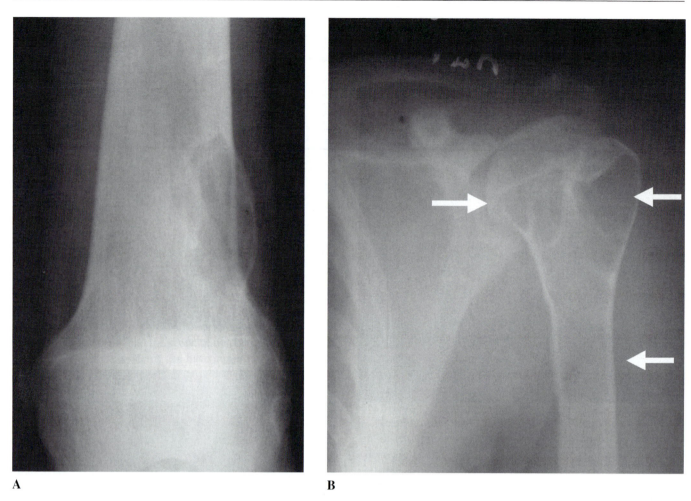

A   B

FIGURE 8-15.   Brown tumors in two patients. *(A)* Anteroposterior radiograph of the distal femur shows an eccentrically located, mildly expansile lesion with well-defined margins. *(B)* Anteroposterior radiograph of the shoulder shows brown tumors in the humeral head and proximal shaft (arrows). *(B courtesy of Dr. James Naidich.)*

Patients on renal dialysis also are at risk for secondary complications such as spontaneous rupture of tendons and an increased susceptibility to osteomyelitis. They also are at increased risk for amyloid deposition because the cuprophane membrane of the hemodialysis unit does not allow β_2-microglobulin to be filtered out of the blood. Amyloid deposition also can occur in other diseases such as multiple myeloma, rheumatoid arthritis, and inflammatory bowel disease. Amyloid can be deposited in the soft tissues and, when it occurs around the shoulders, gives the patient the appearance of wearing football shoulder pads. On MRI, amyloid has a low signal intensity on all pulse sequences. In the bones, it can have a lytic and a lace-like trabecular appearance. Deposition in the joints is called *amyloid arthropathy* and commonly occurs in the spine, hips, and wrists. The typical appearance of amyloid is well-circumscribed erosion without joint space narrowing (see Chapter 3). The differential diagnosis of erosion without joint space narrowing is amyloidosis, pigmented villonodular synovitis, tuberculosis, and primary synovial

chondromatosis. In the spine, amyloid deposition can cause endplate erosion, mimicking infectious spondylodiscitis (see Chapter 1).

RED MARROW HYPERPLASIA

Residual red marrow, or mild hyperplasia, is commonly found incidentally on MR images of the hip, knee, and shoulder and should not be mistaken for a malignant infiltrative disorder. At birth, red marrow normally occupies the entire shaft and metaphysis of the bone and the flat bones; during childhood and the teenage years, the red marrow in long bones regresses, beginning in the center of the shaft and moving toward the proximal and distal ends. Once regression has occurred, marrow has a fatty signal intensity on all pulse sequences, representing yellow marrow. Even the pelvis and vertebral bodies, which remain the main source of hematopoiesis in the adult, display yellow

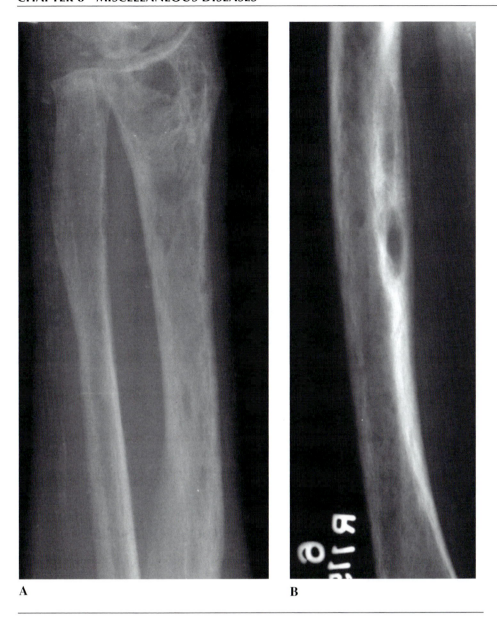

A   B

FIGURE 8-16. Osteitis fibrosa cystica in two patients. Anteroposterior radiographs of the *(A)* fore-arm and *(B)* the femur show a patchy, moth-eaten appearance due to a combination of bone resorption and focal brown tumors in the medullary canal and cortex. *(Courtesy of Dr. James Naidich.)*

marrow signal intensity. Sometimes red marrow persists in the proximal humeral shaft, the proximal femoral shaft, and the distal femoral shaft and appears on MRI as patchy intermediate signal intensity on T_1-weighted sequences, which becomes mildly high signal intensity on fat-suppressed T_2-weighted images (Figure 8-19). This should not be misinterpreted as an infiltrative marrow disorder such as myeloma or lymphoma; those processes tend to be lower signal intensity on T_1-weighted images and higher signal intensity on T_2-weighted images and have a more "solid" appearance. Moreover, red marrow does not affect the femoral head, humeral head, or femoral condyles, whereas a true infiltrative tumor would not spare these ends of bones. Causes of residual red marrow in the adult are smoking, chronic

disease, anemia, endurance sports, and obesity. The red marrow expansion of sickle cell anemia, thalassemia, and erythrocyte-stimulating drugs such as erythropoietin may involve the ends of the bones.

SCLEROSING DYSPLASIAS

The sclerosing dysplasias are a group of developmental abnormalities of cortical bone. They are benign and have typical appearances. A bone island (enostosis) is an ectopic focus of cortical bone in the medullary canal of flat or long bones. It is typically round or oval and may have a finely spiculated

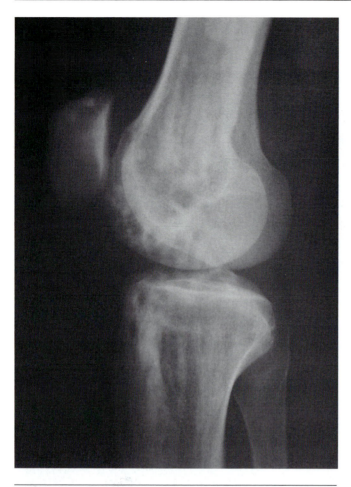

FIGURE 8-21.   Osteopathia striata. Lateral radiograph of the knee shows the intramedullary cortical striations in the distal femur and proximal tibia.

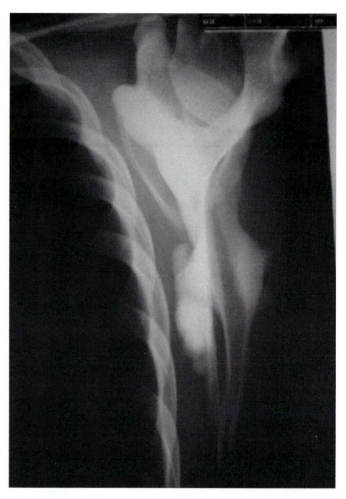

FIGURE 8-22.   Y-scapular view of the shoulder shows the thick undulating hyperostosis of melorheostosis. *(Courtesy of Dr. Frieda Feldman.)*

force, dentinogenesis imperfecta (small, deformed teeth with a gray opalescent appearance), and blue sclerae. Multiple fractures may cause the affected long bone to "telescope" into itself, causing a dwarfing deformity (Figure 8-25). OI can be classified into two types, the severe congenita form and the more mild tarda form, or into four types. Type 1 is the most common and corresponds to the tarda form. It is autosomal dominant. Fractures become apparent in older children or young adults but usually without bowing of the bones or dwarfing due to the fractures. It is subtyped into A or B, depending on the absence or presence of dentinogenesis imperfecta, respectively. The sclerae are blue, and patients may be deaf due to otosclerosis. Type 2 can be autosomal recessive or dominant or due to spontaneous mutation, but it is the lethal form of the disease and corresponds to the congenital type. Fractures occur in utero, and the babies are stillborn or die shortly after birth. The ribs are thin and ribbon-like, and the sclerae are blue. Type 3 is rare and may be fatal in infancy. It is usually autosomal dominant and less often recessive. Affected individuals have markedly fragile bones, fractures of which cause the most severe dwarfing deformities of any type, and kyphoscoliosis. Dentinogenesis imperfecta and wormian bones ("extra" bones in the sutures of the skull) may

be present, but the sclerae become normal by adolescence. Type 4 is autosomal dominant and has variable presentations that may be mild or severe. Sclerae are normal.

Thus, although abuse and OI can have fractures of various ages, the typical appearance of the gracile, bowed, and deformed bones of OI should be an immediate distinguishing feature. Moreover, the fractures of abuse tend to involve the metaphysis, whereas fractures of OI affect the shaft. The distinction between them may be difficult in milder forms of OI, but the clinical features, such as family history, blue sclerae, wormian bones of the skull, and dentinogenesis imperfecta, help to distinguish it from abuse.

PYCNODYSOSTOSIS

Pycnodysostosis is an autosomal recessive condition characterized by short stature and increased density of the entire skeleton. It is usually diagnosed by the age of 5 years. The characteristic radiographic findings include osteosclerosis, mandibular hypoplasia and an increased mandibular angle, frontal and occipital bossing, and patency of the anterior fontanelle into

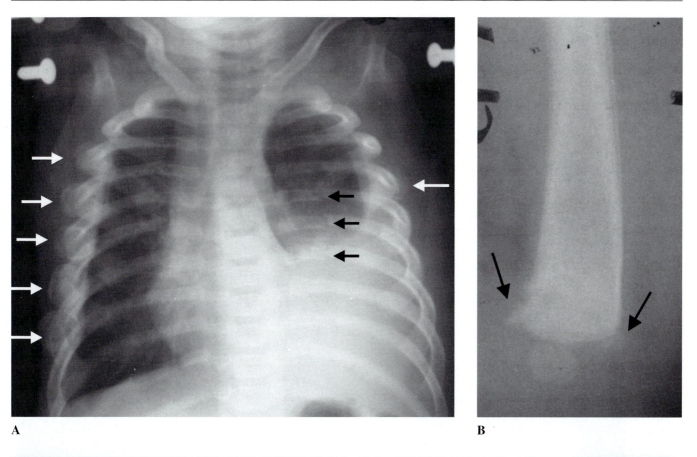

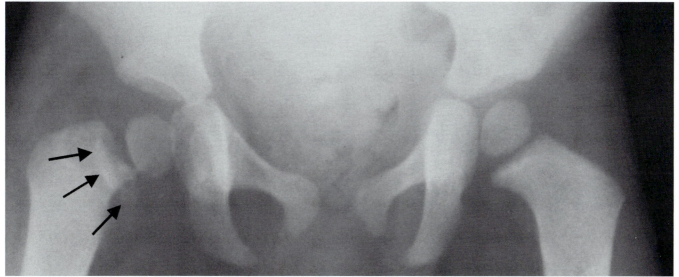

FIGURE 8-23.   Child abuse in three children. *(A)* Anteroposterior radiograph of the chest shows acute fractures in the posterior aspects of the left ribs (black arrows), abundant callus of healed fractures of the right and left ribs (white arrows), and an old fracture of the right clavicle. The opacity in the left hemithorax is a hemothorax due to the trauma. *(B)* Coned radiograph of the distal femur shows corner fractures of the metaphyses (arrows). Note the periosteal reaction along the femoral shaft. *(C)* Anteroposterior radiograph shows a bucket-type fracture of the right metaphysis (arrows). Note the contralateral normal metaphysis for comparison. *(A and B courtesy of Dr. Henry Pritzker.)*

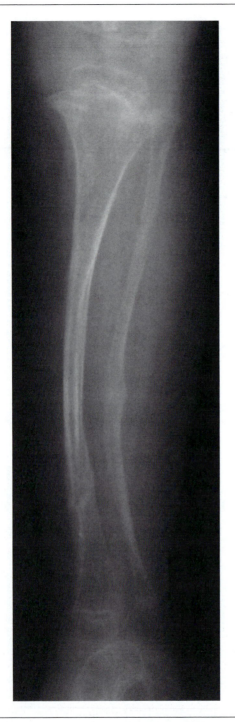

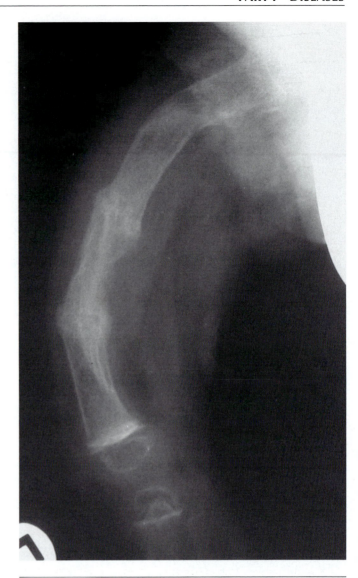

FIGURE 8-25. Lateral radiograph of the femur in osteogenesis imperfecta shows generalized osteopenia with multiple fractures and resultant bowing and foreshortening.

FIGURE 8-24. Anteroposterior radiograph of a child with osteogenesis imperfecta shows the gracile and osteopenic bones and mild bowing deformity. There are old fractures of the tibia and fibula.

adulthood. Wormian bones may be present, and there may be resorption of the distal ends of the clavicles. The distal phalanges may be hypoplastic, and the fingernails are often abnormal (Figure 8-26). Despite the osteosclerosis, these patients are not anemic, unlike patients with osteopetrosis. In addition, neural foraminal overgrowth with cranial nerve compression does not occur.

OSTEOPETROSIS

There are two forms of osteopetrosis and both are characterized by generalized osteosclerosis. The first form, osteopetrosis congenita, is an autosomal recessive condition that appears within the first few months of age. Infants present with failure to thrive, anemia, thrombocytopenia, and hypocalcemia. Sepsis may rarely occur. Hyperostosis in the skull may lead to encroachment on neural foramina, resulting in blindness or deafness. The second form of osteopetrosis is osteopetrosis tarda. This is inherited in an autosomal dominant pattern and presents in childhood, adolescence, or adulthood. Patients present with bone pain and fractures and may have cranial nerve abnormalities due to hyperostotic encroachment. Anemia is present.

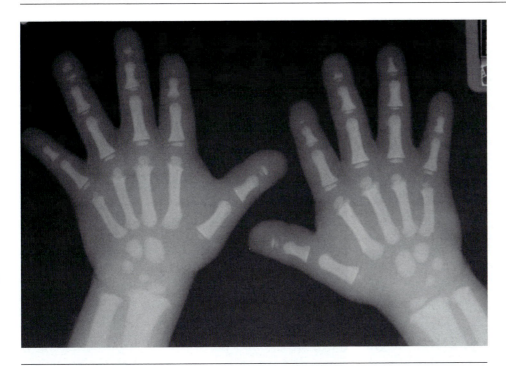

FIGURE 8-26. Anteroposterior radiograph of the hands in pycnodysostosis shows hypoplasia of the distal phalanges and generalized density of the bones.

The pathogenesis of both forms of osteopetrosis is failure of absorption of primary spongiosa during enchondral bone formation. Increased bone density results from persistence of primary spongiosa, and lack of bone remodeling results in under-tubulation of bone, giving an "Erlenmeyer flask" configuration to the metaphyseal portions of long bones, in particular the femur (Figure 8-27).

Radiographically, the bones are dense. All portions of the bones, including epiphyses, metaphyses, and diaphyses, are uniformly affected, and there is resultant lack of distinction between cortex and medulla (Figure 8-28). A bone-within-bone appearance, or alternating radiopaque and radiolucent lines, may be present. These lines may be particularly prominent in the iliac crests (Figure 8-29). In the spine, sclerosis at the endplates of the vertebrae mimics the rugger jersey spine of renal osteodystrophy (Figure 8-30).

PERIOSTITIDES

In children, periosteal new bone formation can be divided into that occurring before age 6 months and that occurring after age 6 months (Table 8-2).

Before Age 6 Months

In the infant, periosteal new bone formation may be normal or physiologic. This occurs in at least one-third of all full-term infants after age 1 month. It is usually seen in the femurs, humeri, and tibias and is characterized by a thin line of periosteal new bone that parallels the cortex of the diaphysis. This is eventually incorporated into the bone and is not seen after age 6 months.

Prostaglandin E_1, a vasodilator used in newborns with cyanotic congenital heart disease to keep the ductus open, can cause periosteal new bone formation in the ribs and long bones.

Malignancy, such as neonatal leukemia, is an unusual cause of periosteal new bone in an infant younger than 6 months.

Caffey disease (infantile cortical hyperostosis) is a rare condition of unknown etiology but may be viral. The condition affects males and females with equal frequency and is characterized by soft tissue swelling and cortical thickening. Clinically, the child is often irritable, and the affected area is tender. The sedimentation rate is usually elevated as is the serum alkaline phosphatase. Anemia also may be present. The mandible and ribs are most frequently affected, but other bones such as the clavicle, scapula, and long bones (in particular the ulna) and the hands and feet may be (Figure 8-31). Usually, multiple sites are affected; less commonly, a single site is affected. The periosteal new bone is generally thick and occurs in the diaphyses, with sparing of the metaphyses and epiphyses. The disease is self-limited, and no therapy is generally necessary.

A cause of neonatal osteomyelitis is syphilis. Syphilis tends to affect the metaphyses and diaphyses of long bones, and multiple bones are often affected. Trophic changes may develop in the metaphyses, leading to a lucent metaphyseal zone. Metaphyseal destruction may occur and is called *Wimberger's sign* when it occurs in the medial aspect of the proximal tibia. Additional features of syphilis include diaphysitis and periostitis (Figure 8-32).

PART II

DISEASES BY REGION

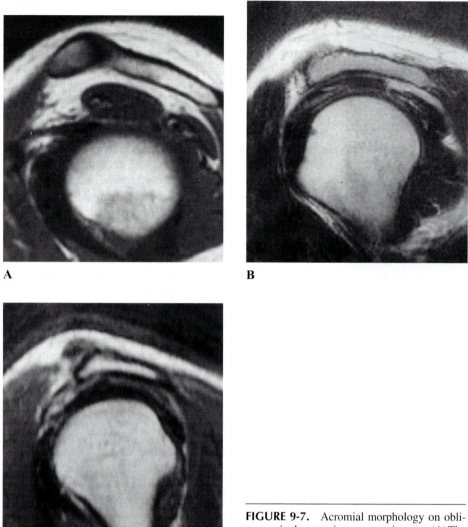

A

B

C

FIGURE 9-7. Acromial morphology on oblique sagittal magnetic resonance images. *(A)* The type I acromion is flat. *(B)* The type II acromion is curved. *(C)* The type III acromion is hooked.

Subscapularis tendon tear or fracture of the lesser tuberosity may be associated with injuries to the glenohumeral ligaments and/or medial displacement of the tendon of the long head of the biceps. The teres minor tendon is typically spared even in the setting of massive rotator cuff tear.

Rotator cuff tears may be full or partial thickness: full-thickness tears allow communication between the bursal and articular spaces, whereas partial tears do not. A full-thickness tear may be a focal process or a complete rupture of the tendon, whereas a partial tear may involve the articular or bursal side or be entirely interstitial (ie, entirely within the substance of the tendon). Complete cuff tears may be quantitatively described based on the size of the defect in the coronal plane: small tears are smaller than 1 cm, medium tears are 1 to 3 cm, large tears are 3 to 5 cm, and massive tears are larger than 5 cm in maximal dimension. The amount of retraction of the tendon should be reported by using quantitative measurement or by describing the anatomic location of the retracted tendon edge, such as to the level of the top of the humeral head or to the level of the glenoid.

Imaging

CONVENTIONAL RADIOGRAPHY. A typical radiographic shoulder series includes AP projections with the humerus in internal and external rotations. The glenohumeral joint space can be "opened up" by using an AP oblique Grashey view in which the x-ray beam is angled tangential to the anterior and posterior rims of the glenoid. Axillary or Stryker notch views delineate the glenohumeral articulation in the transverse plane and are helpful in the evaluation of glenohumeral alignment (Figure 9-12). The transscapular or "Y" view demonstrates acromial morphology and acromioclavicular arthropathy in the oblique sagittal plane, which is helpful for evaluating the osseous boundaries of the supraspinatus outlet. This view also demonstrates the relation of the humeral head to the glenoid.

Chronic rotator cuff tear is manifest as narrowing of the distance between the undersurface of the acromion and superior aspect of the humeral head due to upward migration of the humeral head, which is drawn cephalad by the deltoid muscle. This may be readily appreciated on conventional AP radiographs.

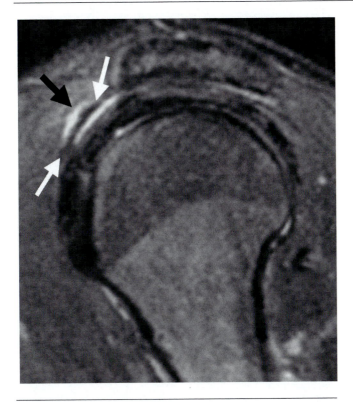

FIGURE 9-8. Oblique sagittal fat-suppressed T$_2$-weighted image shows high signal intensity edema (black arrow) surrounding the cora-coacromial ligament (white arrows).

Associated degenerative changes, including osteophyte formation (especially at the inferior aspect of the humeral articular surface), sclerosis and degenerative pseudocyst formation at the greater tuberosity, and faceting and sclerosis of the undersurface of the acromion may be seen on conventional radiographs, and such degenerative change occurring as a result of chronic cuff tear is called *secondary cuff arthropathy*. Occasionally, an "active abduction view," performed while weight bearing in the AP oblique projection, may demonstrate narrowing of the subacromial space, which is not evident on non–weight-bearing AP radiographs; this suggests an acute or subacute rotator cuff tear.

CONVENTIONAL ARTHROGRAPHY. Conventional arthrography is used most frequently to determine the integrity of the rotator cuff in those patients for whom MRI is contraindicated. Postinjection postexercise radiographs are required to adequately coat the joint surfaces and force the contrast through any potential defect in the rotator cuff. Full-thickness cuff tears allow free communication of contrast between the articular and bursal sides of the torn tendon. Contrast may also extend into the acromioclavicular joint, an appearance called the *geyser phenomenon* due to an associated tear of the acromioclavicular joint capsule (Figure 9-13). Partial tears of the articular surface of the cuff may be demonstrated as insinuation of contrast into the substance of the tendon without communication into the subdeltoid bursa (Figure 9-14). Visualization of bursal surface partial tears

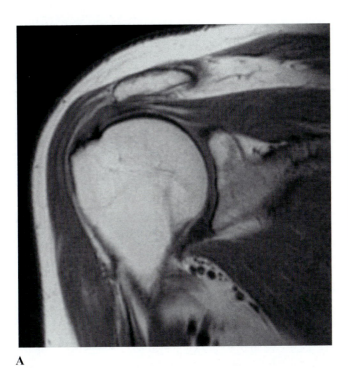

A

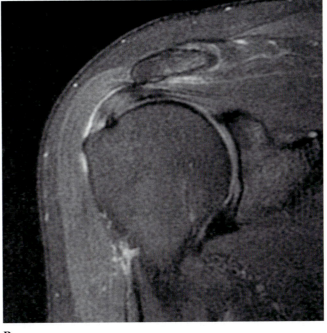

B

FIGURE 9-9. Supraspinatus tendinosis. *(A)* Oblique coronal T$_1$-weighted image shows intermediate signal intensity throughout a thickened supraspinatus tendon. *(B)* Corresponding oblique coronal fat-suppressed fast spin echo T$_2$-weighted image shows the heterogeneous high signal intensity throughout the tendon, particularly at its insertion, but not as bright as the fluid signal in the overlying subdeltoid bursa.

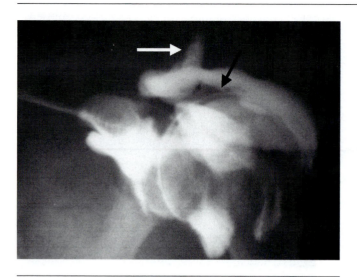

FIGURE 9-13. Arthrographic image after injection into the glenohumeral joint shows contrast outlining the torn and retracted supraspinatus tendon (black arrow), with flow into the overlying subacromial-subdeltoid bursa and into the acromioclavicular joint (white arrow), forming the geyser phenomenon.

indicated sensitivity and specificity greater than 90% for detection of rotator cuff tear. Results are better for full-thickness than for partial-thickness tears and for massive or large tears than for small tears.

Sonographic criteria for full-thickness rotator cuff tears include nonvisualization of the tendon (Figure 9-15), a focal hypoechoic gap in the tendon, loss of normal convex curvature of the overlying subdeltoid bursa with sagging of the peribursal fat

stripe into the defect, and clear visualization of hyaline cartilage at the humeral head ("naked cartilage sign"). Partial-thickness tear may appear as a focal well-defined hypoechoic region that does not involve the entire thickness of the tendon (Figure 9-16). Even though sonography cannot evaluate the deep aspect of the acromioclavicular joint and thus cannot evaluate indentation of the supraspinatus, it can dynamically assess the supraspinatus and overlying bursa during arm abduction by demonstrating entrapment of these soft tissue structures between the acromion and greater tuberosity in the case of impingement.

MAGNETIC RESONANCE IMAGING. MRI is the imaging standard for evaluation of shoulder abnormalities. It allows evaluation of the entire shoulder region, including the glenohumeral joint, the supraspinatus outlet, and the bony structures themselves. Its larger field of view and unobstructed visualization of soft tissue structures that are blocked sonographically allow definition of the extent and location of partial- and full-thickness cuff tears and evaluation of tendon retraction and associated muscle atrophy.

Oblique coronal and oblique sagittal planes are the most useful for detection of rotator cuff tear, with greater accuracy for full-thickness than for partial-thickness defects. Tears may be evaluated with conventional spin echo sequences, fast spin echo sequences with or without fat suppression, or gradient echo sequences. Criteria for full-thickness tear are discontinuity of the tendon, usually with high signal intensity fluid in the gap on T_2-weighted images, and nonvisualization of the tendon due to retraction (see Fig. 9-15). The geyser sign also may be seen (Figure 9-17). Chronic ruptures usually do not have associated

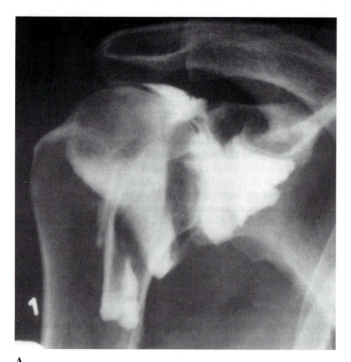

A

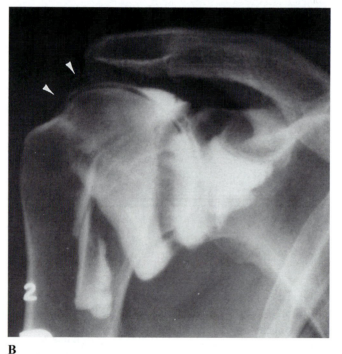

B

FIGURE 9-14. Partial tear of the supraspinatus tendon. *(A)* Initial arthrographic image after injection into the glenohumeral joint shows no evidence of insinuation of contrast into the tendon or through it. *(B)* Repeat image after mild exercise of the joint shows a thin stripe of contrast (arrowheads) entering the substance of the supraspinatus tendon, indicating articular surface partial tear.

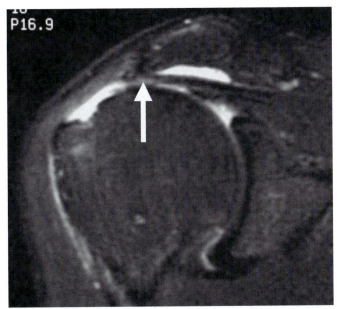

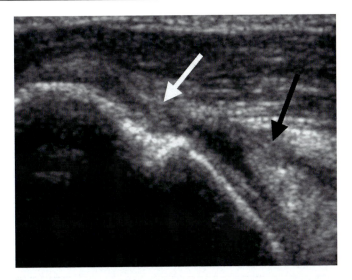

B

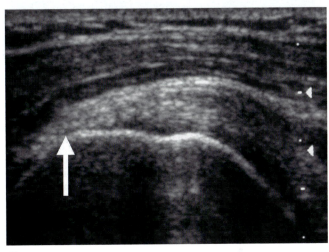

C

FIGURE 9-15.   Full-thickness tear of the supraspinatus tendon. *(A)* Oblique coronal fat-suppressed T_2-weighted image shows the torn supraspinatus tendon (arrow) that has retracted to the "12 o'clock position," with high signal intensity fluid filling the tendon gap. *(B)* Corresponding longitudinal sonogram shows the retracted tendon edge (black arrow). The peribursal fat is sagging into the defect (white arrow). *(C)* Longitudinal sonogram of the patient's contralateral normal shoulder shows an intact supraspinatus tendon attaching to the greater tuberosity (arrow). *(Continued)*

A

joint fluid to outline the gap. In those instances, secondary signs of rupture, such as retraction of the torn tendon edge, elevation of the humeral head, and fatty atrophy of the muscle, may be helpful (Figure 9-18).

Partial tears appear as localized high signal intensity on T_2-weighted images with an associated tendinous contour defect involving the bursal or articular side (see Fig. 9-16). Occasionally, partial tears may remain entirely intrasubstance, thus limiting distinction from tendinosis.

On conventional MR images, it may be difficult or impossible to differentiate the abnormal signal intensity of a partial tear from that of tendinosis and hard to distinguish a large partial-thickness tear from a full-thickness injury. The presence of a joint effusion may aid in these distinctions by outlining or filling the tear. In the absence of native joint fluid, MR arthrography using dilute gadolinium contrast or normal saline may help to distinguish these abnormalities. Although commonly used for MR arthrography, intraarticular gadolinium contrast is not approved by the US Food and Drug Administration.

SURGICAL REPAIR AND POSTOPERATIVE IMAGING.   Surgical repair of the rotator cuff tear varies according to the surgeon's pref-

erence and depends on the extent of the tear, degree of tendon retraction, and associated fatty atrophy of the muscle. Small tears may be addressed by "side-to-side" suturing, whereas larger tears require reattachment to the bone. Reattachment requires creation of an osseous defect at the lateral aspect of the greater tuberosity. The tendon is reattached to a bed of bleeding cancellous bone by means of a variety of nonabsorbable or absorbable sutures and anchors. Larger tears may be augmented with rotator cuff or Achilles tendon allograft or by incorporation of the adjacent subscapularis or long head of biceps tendon. Partial tears may be treated conservatively, débrided, or repaired.

As arthroscopic and open rotator cuff repairs become more common, so does imaging of the postsurgical shoulder. MRI may be degraded by staples, suture anchors, and nonmetallic suture, which limit the quality and diagnostic value of the study. This limitation may be especially prominent in tendon-to-humerus repairs in which a surgical trough is created at the superolateral aspect of the humeral head. Sonography is an excellent method to evaluate for rerupture of the postoperative cuff if MRI is technically suboptimal or nondiagnostic. Conventional arthrography and MR arthrography may be misleading because most surgical repairs of cuff rupture are not "water tight," and contrast

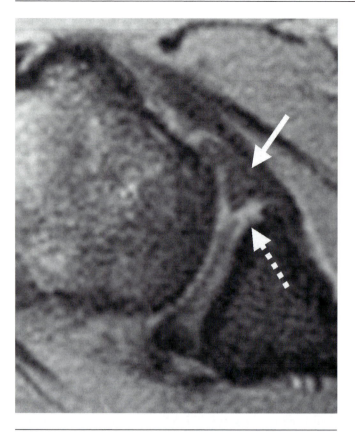

FIGURE 9-25. Axial gradient echo magnetic resonance image shows a torn and detached anterior labrum (solid arrow), which has taken a piece of articular cartilage with it, manifest as irregularity of the anterior edge of the cartilage (dashed arrow), forming a glenolabral articular disruption lesion.

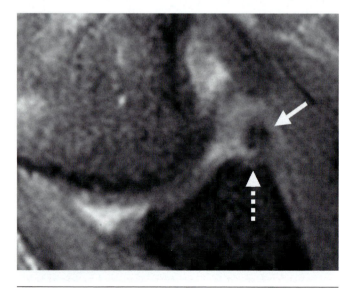

FIGURE 9-26. Axial gradient echo T_2-weighted image shows a detached tear of the inferior aspect of the anterior labrum (solid arrow), which has taken a piece of the bony glenoid with it, manifest by the small defect in the anterior aspect of the glenoid (dashed arrow), constituting a Bankart fracture.

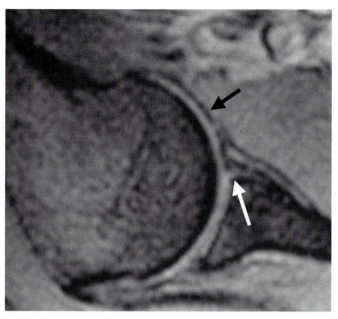

FIGURE 9-27. Anterior labral tear. In the abducted externally rotated position, the stretched inferior glenohumeral ligament (black arrow) pulls on the labrum, outlining the tear (white arrow).

lesion and fracture are the result of anterior dislocation of the humeral head. If the capsulolabral injury is not identified on routine axial images but clinical suspicion is high because the shoulder is unstable, additional imaging can be performed with the patient's humerus in the abducted externally rotated (ABER) position. This position is achieved by having the patient place the hand on the back of the head, thus stretching the anterior band of the inferior glenohumeral ligament and stressing the attachment of the inferior aspect of the anterior labrum (Figure 9-27).

A Hill-Sachs impaction fracture of the posterolateral superior aspect of the humeral head is also a result of anterior dislocation and can be a clue to injury of the anterior labroligamentous complex. One must be careful to distinguish a true Hill-Sachs deformity, occurring above the level of the coracoid process, from the normal posterolateral contour indentation of the anatomic neck of the humerus at a level caudal to the coracoid (Figure 9-28).

The Perthes lesion is a variant of the Bankart lesion in which the scapular periosteum is stripped medially from the glenoid neck but is not torn, and the anterior labrum, although also torn, remains in its normal location (Figure 9-29). Over time, the labrum may fibrose in reasonable anatomic alignment, but the periosteal anchors for the capsule and capsular ligaments remain incompetent, and the patient therefore may have persistent anterior instability.

The anterior labroligamentous periosteal sleeve avulsion (ALPSA) lesion is avulsion of the anterior labrum with its capsular and periosteal attachment from the glenoid. Unlike the Perthes lesion in which the anterior labrum remains in its normal location, the anterior labrum and capsular periosteum are displaced medially and inferiorly as an intact sleeve. This is also called a *medialized Bankart lesion*. Due to the loss of the capsular attachment, the inferior glenohumeral ligament may no longer function, resulting in recurrent dislocations of the

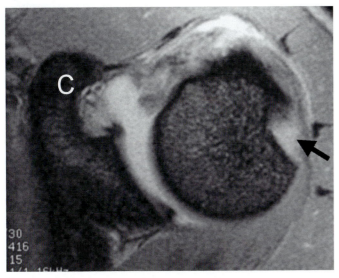

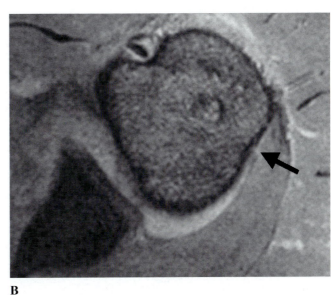

A   B

FIGURE 9-28.   Hill-Sachs Lesion. *(A)* Axial gradient echo image shows the defect in the humeral head (arrow). Note that the image is at the level of the coracoid process. *(B)* Axial gradient echo image in this same patient more inferiorly shows the normal flattening of the posterior aspect of the humeral head (arrow), which should not be mistaken for a Hill-Sachs defect. Note that this image is below the level of the coracoid. C = coracoid process.

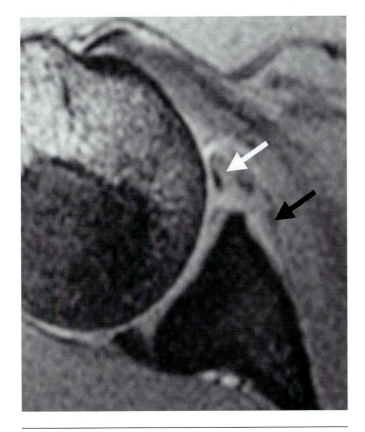

FIGURE 9-29.   Perthes lesion. Axial gradient echo image shows the torn anterior labrum (white arrow) and the stripped periosteum (black arrow) with a small amount of high signal intensity edema or hemorrhage intervening between the capsule and the bony glenoid.

glenohumeral joint. Fractures of the anterior lip of the glenoid also may be present.

A *posterior* or *reverse Bankart lesion* refers to injury of the posterior labrum and may be seen after posterior dislocation (Figure 9-30). The Bennett lesion is a bony spur at the posterior glenoid due to avulsion of the posterior band of the inferior glenohumeral ligament and is associated with posterior labral and rotator cuff injury. An impaction fracture at the anterosuperior aspect of the humeral head in the region of the lesser tuberosity may be referred to as a *reverse Hill-Sachs deformity* or a *trough sign* and is indicative of the posterior dislocation but may also be seen in bidirectional instability with a posterior component.

The capsuloligamentous complex also may be injured at its humeral attachment instead of at the labral attachment. Humeral avulsion of the (inferior) glenohumeral ligament (HAGL) describes an avulsion of the inferior glenohumeral ligament from the humerus. The ligamentous disruption is sufficient to cause anterior instability. Associated labral tear may or may not be present. The injury can be appreciated on axial and oblique coronal MR images as detachment of the inferior glenohumeral ligament from the bone, forming the *J sign* on the oblique coronal images (Figure 9-31). Bony humeral avulsion of the (inferior) glenohumeral ligament (BHAGL) describes an avulsion of the inferior glenohumeral ligament with a fragment of bone from the humerus. This is simply a humeral avulsion of the inferior glenohumeral ligament with an additional piece of bone torn off the humerus in addition to the inferior glenohumeral attachment. A posterior humeral avulsion of the (inferior) glenohumeral ligament (PHAGL) lesion also has been described

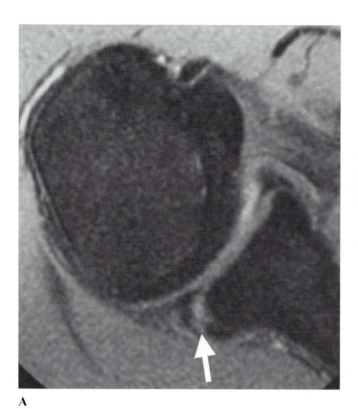

A

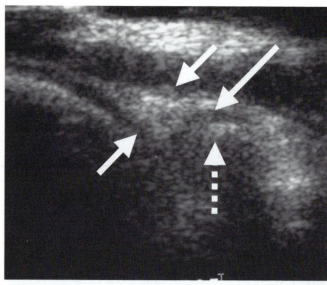

B

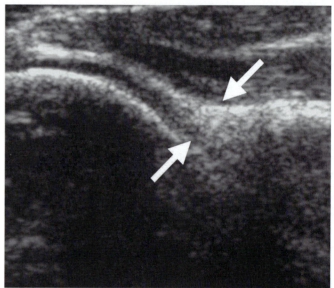

C

FIGURE 9-30. Posterior labral tear. *(A)* Axial gradient echo image shows the tear through the base of the posterior labrum (arrow). *(B)* Corresponding transverse sonographic image in this same patient shows the echogenic triangular posterior labrum (small arrows) separated from the underlying bony cortex of the glenoid (dashed arrow) by the hypoechoic fluid of the tear (large arrow). *(C)* Transverse sonogram through the patient's contralateral normal shoulder shows the hyperechoic posterior labrum (arrows) inserting directly into the glenoid without an intervening hypoechoic tear.

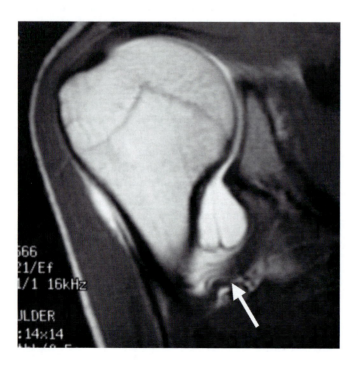

FIGURE 9-31. Humeral avulsion of the (inferior) glenohumeral ligament lesion. Oblique coronal T_1-weighted magnetic resonance arthrographic image shows the torn inferior glenohumeral ligament (arrow) detached from the humeral shaft, forming the J sign. *(Courtesy of Dr. Rolando Singson).*

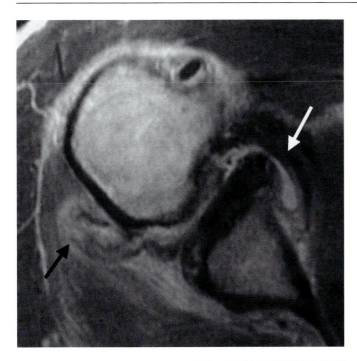

FIGURE 9-32. Axial fast spin echo proton density image shows the torn posterior band of the inferior glenohumeral ligament (black arrow). Note that the anterior band is intact (white arrow).

recently, in which the posterior band of the inferior glenohumeral ligament is avulsed from its humeral attachment (Figure 9-32).

One should keep in mind that, although unidirectional instability is a posttraumatic event, most cases of dislocation do not, in fact, progress to instability. When instability ensues, it is typically in the direction of the original dislocation, most commonly anterior, and is termed *traumatic unidirectional instability with a Bankart lesion requiring surgical intervention* (TUBS). Unidirectional posterior instability can occur after posterior dislocation and may be accompanied by a reverse Bankart lesion, but it is less common than anterior instability, reflecting the more rarely occurring posterior dislocation. Traumatic unidirectional instability with a Bankart lesion requiring surgical intervention should be distinguished from nontraumatic multidirectional instability, called *atraumatic multidirectional and bilateral instability that is often treated with rehabilitation or surgically by inferior capsule and rotator cuff interval capsulorrhaphy* (AMRI). This type of instability is usually due to physiologic ligamentous laxity or glenoid hypoplasia, and the patient may be able to voluntarily dislocate.

ADHESIVE CAPSULITIS

Adhesive capsulitis is a self-limited condition in which the glenohumeral capsule is thickened and contracted. The etiology can be idiopathic or traumatic. Clinically, the patient complains of pain and has severely reduced range of motion. Joint capsule thickness exceeding 4 mm at the axillary recess has been suggested as the criterion for the MR diagnosis of adhesive capsulitis. Arthrography demonstrates a markedly shrunken capsule,

and the joint will only accept a few milliliters of contrast instead of the normal 12 to 15 mL. Iatrogenic rupture of the joint capsule by overdistention with saline or contrast (the *Brisman procedure*) can be therapeutic.

BICEPS INJURIES

The tendon of the long head of the biceps is another potential site of injury and pain. Bicipital tendinosis has two separate etiologies. The most common is injury of the biceps tendon as part of the impingement syndrome or coexistent with disruption of the rotator cuff tendons. The second and more rare etiology is stenosis at the bicipital groove, usually due to periostitis, which may result in subsequent biceps tendon rupture. On MRI, biceps tendinosis is manifest as abnormal high signal intensity on T_2-weighted sequences within the normally low signal intensity tendon, the tendon may be thickened, and fluid may surround the tendon. Tendon thickening, anechoic surrounding fluid, and possibly focal areas of altered echotexture may be seen sonographically, and hyperemia may be demonstrated when using power Doppler (Figure 9-33). Sonography also can guide needle placement into the tendon sheath for corticosteroid injection therapy. Although fluid surrounding an otherwise normal-appearing biceps tendon is considered evidence of tenosynovitis, the biceps tendon sheath normally communicates with the glenohumeral joint, and fluid from a joint effusion may track into the tendon sheath; therefore, one should not diagnose tenosynovitis unless the amount of fluid surrounding the biceps tendon is much larger than the amount of fluid in the glenohumeral joint.

Rupture of the subscapularis tendon or partial tear of its deep surface will disrupt the transverse humeral ligament, which normally helps hold the extracapsular portion of the long head of the biceps tendon within the bicipital groove. Such injury of the subscapularis may allow the biceps tendon to dislocate medially out of the groove. These two injuries almost always go together, so recognition of one should prompt suspicion of and search for the other. The appearance is well shown on axial MR images and transverse sonographic images as an empty bicipital groove, with the biceps present in the anterior aspect of the glenohumeral joint and an abnormal-appearing subscapularis tendon (Figure 9-34).

Inflammation of the rotator cuff interval also can cause anterior shoulder pain. The rotator cuff interval is the space between the supraspinatus and subscapularis tendons, through which run the coracohumeral and superior glenohumeral ligaments and the tendon of the long head of the biceps on its way to attach to the supraglenoid tubercle.

Inflammation of the rotator cuff interval is visualized on oblique sagittal fat-suppressed T_2-weighted sequences as high signal intensity within the interval and may represent sprain of the ligaments (Figure 9-35).

ENTRAPMENT NEUROPATHIES

The most common entrapment syndromes at the shoulder involve the suprascapular nerve and the axillary nerve.

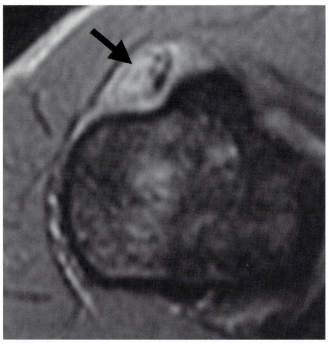

A

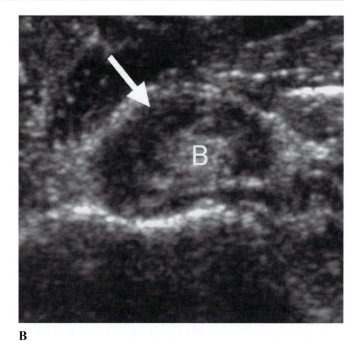

B

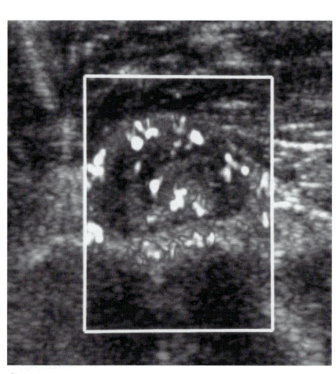

C

FIGURE 9-33.   Biceps tendinosis and tenosynovitis. *(A)* Axial gradient echo T$_2$-weighted image shows heterogeneously high signal intensity within the markedly thickened biceps tendon (arrow), with mild surrounding high signal intensity fluid or synovial thickening. *(B)* Corresponding transverse sonographic image shows the heterogeneous biceps and the hypoechoic synovial thickening or fluid (arrow). *(C)* Corresponding power Doppler image at this same level shows the marked hyperemia within the tendon and in the surrounding thickened tendon sheath. B = biceps.

The suprascapular nerve travels through the suprascapular notch and spinoglenoid notch and is vulnerable to compression by ganglion cysts and perilabral cysts, scapular fractures, glenohumeral dislocation, and suprascapular varices. Perilabral cysts or ganglia of the notches are the most common causes of compression and are readily identified as fluid signal intensity masses on MRI. Perilabral cysts are almost always caused by an underlying labral tear, and the presence of such cysts should heighten one's suspicion of labral tear. Acute compression of the nerve causes denervation edema of the innervated muscle,

seen as high signal intensity in the muscle on fat-suppressed T$_2$-weighted images (Figure 9-36), whereas chronic compression eventually causes fatty atrophy, seen as streaky high signal intensity fat in the muscle on T$_1$-weighted images and decreased muscle mass. Compression of the suprascapular nerve in the suprascapular notch affects the supraspinatus and infraspinatus muscles, whereas compression in the spinoglenoid notch may cause isolated involvement of the infraspinatus muscle. Symptoms of gradually increasing pain and weakness due to the compressive neuropathy may mask underlying shoulder instability

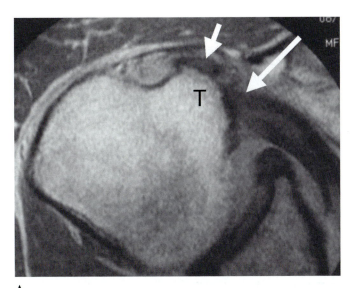

A

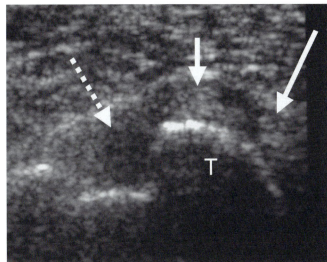

B

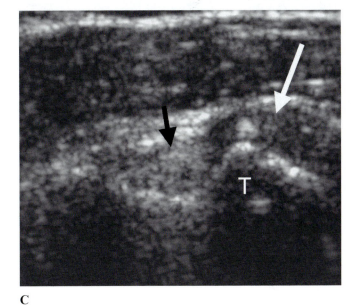

C

FIGURE 9-34. Dislocated biceps tendon. *(A)* Axial proton density image shows the torn and retracted subscapularis tendon (large arrow). The biceps tendon (small arrow) has dislocated medially and is perched over the lesser tuberosity. Notice that the biceps groove itself now appears empty. *(B)* Corresponding transverse sonographic image shows the empty bicipital groove (dashed arrow). The echogenic biceps tendon (small arrow) is perched on the lesser tuberosity, and the retracted end of the subscapularis is also visualized (large arrow). *(C)* Transverse sonogram of the patient's contralateral normal side shows the echogenic biceps tendon (black arrow) located normally within the groove and the subscapularis (white arrow) attaching to the lesser tuberosity. T = lesser tuberosity.

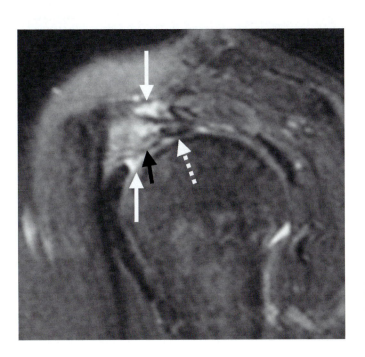

FIGURE 9-35. Oblique sagittal fat-suppressed T$_2$-weighted image shows high signal intensity (solid white arrows) in the rotator cuff interval, with thickening of the coracohumeral ligament (black arrow) indicating a sprain. Biceps tendon is also visible (dashed white arrow).

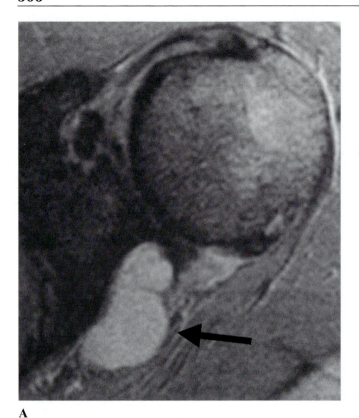

A

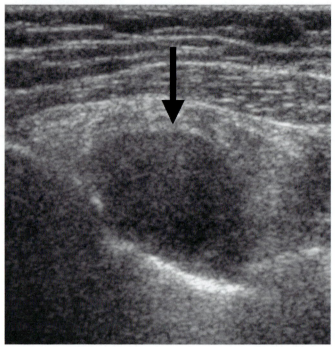

B

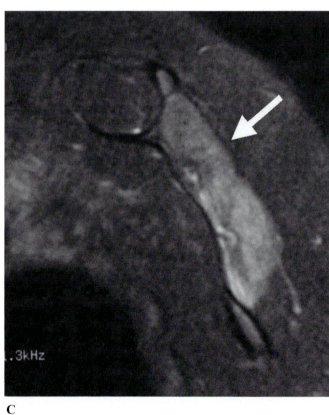

C

FIGURE 9-36. Acute denervation edema of the infraspinatus tendon due to a posterior cyst. *(A)* Axial gradient echo T_2-weighted image shows a large cyst (arrow) in the spinoglenoid notch. *(B)* Corresponding ultrasound image shows the large hypoechoic cyst (arrow) with the subjacent echogenic scapular cortex. *(C)* Oblique sagittal fat-suppressed T_2-weighted image shows the infraspinatus muscle (arrow), with internal high signal intensity edema.

related to the original labral injury. In the case of ganglia or perilabral cysts, palliation of the entrapment neuropathy may be accomplished by sonographically guided aspiration of the cystic mass.

Acute brachial neuritis (*Parsonage-Turner syndrome*) is acute denervation edema of the supraspinatus, infraspinatus, and, occasionally, deltoid muscles. The cause is unknown but is thought to be viral or postinfectious. The onset of severe shoulder pain is sudden, unlike that of a compressive neuropathy, but the process is self-limited.

The axillary nerve innervates the deltoid and teres minor muscles and is most often injured as a result of anterior dislocation of the humeral head and fractures of the surgical neck and proximal shaft of the humerus. This nerve also may become entrapped by

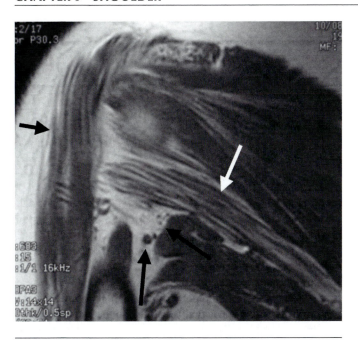

FIGURE 9-37. Oblique coronal T_1-weighted image shows streaky high signal intensity fatty atrophy of the teres minor muscle (white arrow) and the deltoid muscle (small black arrow), indicating quadrilateral space syndrome. The quadrilateral space itself in this patient is normal (large black arrows); in most cases; no discrete cause is identified.

small fibrous bands, a chronic and nontraumatic process, within the quadrilateral space of the shoulder. This space is formed by the medial cortex of the surgical neck of the humerus, the long head of triceps, and the teres major and teres minor muscles; the axillary nerve and posterior humeral circumflex artery course through this space. The diagnosis of chronic *quadrilateral space syndrome* may be made with MRI, which demonstrates fatty atrophy of the deltoid and/or teres minor muscles (Figure 9-37).

Subclavian arteriography demonstrates occlusion of the posterior humeral circumflex artery during abduction and external rotation of the arm, which resolves when the arm is adducted.

SUGGESTED READINGS

Atay OA, Aydingoz U, Doral MN, Leblebigioglu G. Anterior labroligamentous periosteal sleeve avulsion lesion at the superior glenoid labrum. *Knee Surg Sports Traumatol Arthrosc.* 2002;10:122–125.

Balich SM, Sheley RC, Brown TR, Sauser DD, Quinn SF. MR imaging of the rotator cuff tendon: interobserver agreement and analysis of interobserver errors. *Radiology.* 1997;204:191–194.

Chung CB, Dwek JR, Sorenson SM, Resnick DL. Posterior band humeral avulsion of the inferior glenohumeral ligament (PHAGL): magnetic resonance arthrogram (MRA) imaging findings and clinical correlation in 10 patients. *Radiology.* 2002;225(P):422.

Connell DA, Potter HG. Magnetic resonance evaluation of the labral capsular ligamentous complex: a pictorial review. *Australas Radiol.* 1999;43:419–426.

Kreitner KF, Botchen K, Rude J, Bittinger F, Krummenauer F, Thelen M. Superior labrum and labral bicipital complex: MR imaging with pathologic-anatomic and histologic correlation. *AJR.* 1998;170:599–605.

Rafii M, Minkoff J. Advanced arthrography of the shoulder with CT and MR imaging. *Radiol Clin North Am.* 1998;36:609–633.

Seibold CJ, Mallisee TA, Erickson SJ, Boynton MD, Raasch WG, Timins ME. Rotator cuff: evaluation with US and MR imaging. *Radiographics.* 1999;19:685–705.

Tirman PFJ, Steinbach LS, Belzer JP, Bost PW. A practical approach to imaging of the shoulder with emphasis on MR imaging. *Orthop Clin North Am.* 1997;28:483–515.

Uri DS. MR imaging of shoulder impingement and rotator cuff disease. *Radiol Clin North Am.* 1997;35:77–96.

Wischer TK, Bredella MA, Genant HK, Stoller DW, Bost FW, Tirman PF. Perthes lesion (a variant of the Bankart lesion): MR imaging and MR arthrographic findings with surgical correlation. *AJR.* 2002;178:233–237.

CHAPTER 10

ELBOW

THEODORE T. MILLER

The elbow is a joint not imaged frequently unless one is involved in a practice that has a large sports medicine referral base. The injuries are typically those of sports and overuse, such as epicondylitis from tennis and golf, ulnar collateral ligament injury from pitching a baseball, and injury to the triceps and biceps typically from weight lifting.

ANATOMY

The elbow joint is composed of three bones, the humerus, ulna, and radius, and three articulations, the ulnohumeral articulation, the radiocapitellar articulation, and the radioulnar articulation. The hinge-like motion of flexion and extension occurs at the ulnohumeral articulation, and supination and pronation occurs at the radioulnar joint, as the head of the radius rotates in the sigmoid notch of the lateral side of the ulna. The radial head is held within the sigmoid notch by the anular ligament. The flat radial head articulates with the hemispherical capitellum of the humerus, permitting supination and pronation and flexion and extension.

The radial collateral ligament (RCL) further stabilizes the radial head at the radiocapitellar joint by coursing from the lateral side of the capitellum and blending with the anular ligament (Figure 10-1). Posterior to the RCL is a thin band of tissue called the *lateral ulnar collateral ligament* (LUCL), which arises slightly posterior to the RCL on the lateral aspect of the capitellum, and courses posteroinferiorly, behind the radial neck, to insert on a small tubercle on the lateral side of the ulna (see Fig. 10-1). The LUCL acts as a sling to support the radial head and prevent posterolateral instability.

The medial side of the elbow is stabilized by the ulnar collateral ligament (UCL), which is composed of anterior, posterior, and transverse bands. Of these three structures, the anterior band is functionally most important for maintaining stability against valgus stress of the elbow, is therefore the band of clinical concern, and is routinely seen on magnetic resonance imaging (MRI; see Fig. 10-1). It is composed of anterior and posterior bundles, but these are not distinguishable from each other on imaging. The anterior band originates on the undersurface of the medial epicondyle and extends across the ulnohumeral joint to insert on the sublime tubercle of the coronoid process of the ulna. The proximal attachment is shaped somewhat like a fan, and the middle and distal aspects typically are thin.

There are four tendons about the elbow that are of clinical importance: the common extensor tendon laterally, the com-

mon flexor tendon medially, the biceps tendon anteriorly, and the triceps tendon posteriorly. The common extensor tendon originates from the lateral aspect of the lateral epicondyle (see Fig. 10-1) and is composed of contributions by the extensor carpi radialis brevis, the extensor digitorum communis, the extensor carpi radialis longus, and the extensor digiti minimi. These four structures share a common origin, and neither imaging nor anatomic dissection can actually distinguish the individual bundles. The common flexor tendon arises from the medial aspect of the medial epicondyle and is composed of contributions from the pronator teres, flexor carpi radialis and flexor carpi ulnaris, palmaris longus, and flexor digitorum sublimis, but these individual components also cannot be distinguished from each other. The common flexor tendon lies superficially to the medial collateral ligament and is shorter and broader than the common extensor tendon (see Fig. 10-1).

The distal musculotendinous junction of the biceps is located in the distal arm, and the distal biceps tendon crosses the elbow joint to insert on the radial tubercle of the proximal radius. It is a rounded or cord-like structure in its proximal aspect, which flattens out into a more band-like structure near its attachment on the tubercle. The chief functions of the biceps are to flex and supinate the forearm, but other muscles, such as the brachialis and supinator muscles, also contribute to these actions. The triceps tendon posteriorly is a short broad structure that inserts onto the olecranon process of the ulna. Its function is extension of the elbow.

LIGAMENT INJURY

The UCL is the primary restraint against valgus stress of the elbow and is consequently injured in overuse activities that put stress on this ligament, such as throwing a baseball. Chronic stress can cause radiographically visible heterotopic ossification along the course of this ligament or small traction osteophyte formation at its insertion on the coronoid (Figure 10-2). More acute injury, such as sprain or rupture, is best visualized with MRI or sonography. The UCL is usually well seen on coronal MR images of the elbow in full extension. Injuries are best demonstrated with fat-suppressed T_2-weighted sequences. Mild or moderate sprain appears as soft tissue edema surrounding the ligament and the ligament may have intrasubstance high signal intensity, and rupture is manifest as nonvisualization of the "blown-out" ligament with marked soft tissue edema in the expected location (Figure 10-3) or as focal discontinuity of the ligament with high

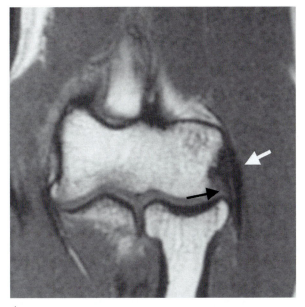

A

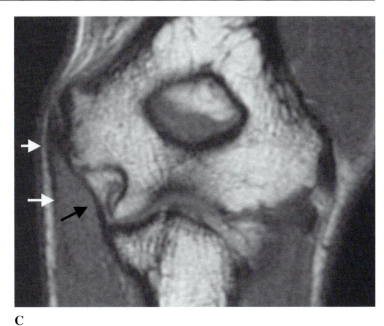

C

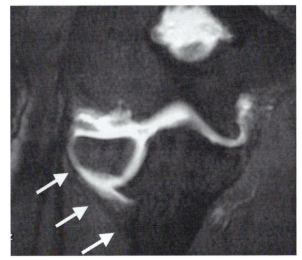

B

FIGURE 10-1. Normal anatomy. *(A)* Coronal T₁-weighted image shows the common extensor tendon (white arrow) and the underlying radial collateral ligament (black arrow). *(B)* Coronal fat-suppressed T₁-weighted magnetic resonance arthrogram shows the lateral ulnar collateral ligament (white arrows) acting as a sling posterior to the neck of the radius and inserting on the ulnar. *(C)* Coronal T₁-weighted magnetic resonance image shows the common flexor tendon (white arrows) and the ulnar collateral ligament (black arrow).

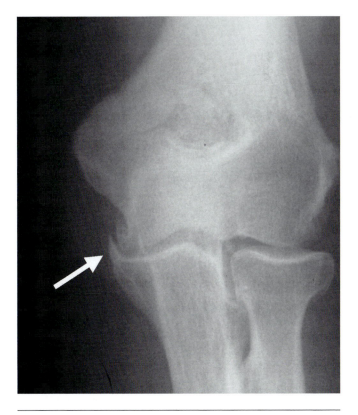

FIGURE 10-2. Anteroposterior radiograph shows a large traction spur arising from the coronoid process of the ulna at the attachment of the ulnar collateral ligament (arrow).

signal intensity fluid in the gap. Sonographically, it is best assessed in the longitudinal plane with the transducer placed across the medial side of the elbow and normally appears as a hyperechoic structure. Similar to the MRI appearance, sprain appears as hypoechoic edema around the ligament with swelling of and decreased echogenicity of the ligament, and rupture is manifest as focal discontinuity or nonvisualization with complex echogenicity due to hemorrhage and edema. An advantage of sonography over MRI is the ability to dynamically stress this ligament in order to look for widening of the ulnohumeral joint space as a clue to functional incompetence. Comparison should be made with the patient's normal contralateral elbow, since mild widening of the joint space of the throwing arm may not necessarily indicate functional incompetence of this ligament.

There is a type of partial tear of the UCL that occurs on the deep surface of the ligament at its ulnar attachment and is

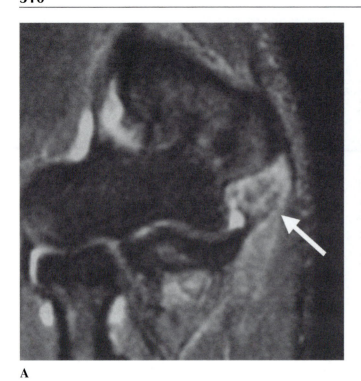

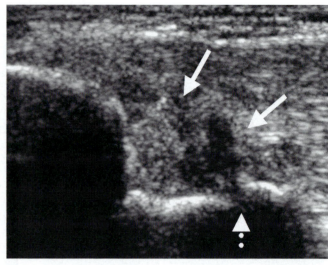

B

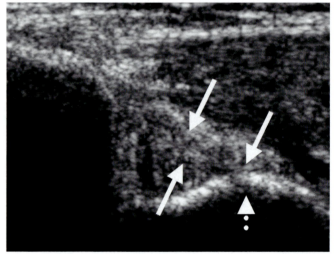

C

FIGURE 10-3. Rupture of the ulnar collateral ligament. *(A)* Coronal fat-suppressed fast spin echo T$_2$-weighted image shows the "blown-out" medial collateral ligament with surrounding high signal intensity edema (arrow). *(B)* Longitudinal sonogram shows the poorly defined and blown-out ligament (white arrows). The joint space is outlined by the dotted arrow. *(C)* Longitudinal sonogram of the patient's contralateral normal elbow shows a well-defined echogenic ligament (white arrows). The joint space is demarcated by the dotted arrow.

best assessed with MR arthrography or computed tomographic arthrography. The contrast insinuates itself between the distal aspect of the ligament and its ulnar attachment, forming the "T sign."

Little leaguer's elbow is a spectrum of injury in skeletally immature patients, ranging from avulsion of the UCL from the medial epicondyle to widening of the physis of the medial epicondyle (a Salter I injury) due to the chronic pull of the UCL and common flexor tendon. Avulsion of the UCL may take a piece of the bony epicondyle with it and will be radiographically visible. A widened physis is usually detectable radiographically, especially in comparison with the contralateral elbow.

The RCL and the LUCL are less commonly injured than the UCL. The RCL is deep to the common extensor tendon and sometimes can be difficult to distinguish from this larger overlying structure to which it is closely apposed. The RCL can be injured by the same chronic overuse that produces lateral epicondylitis, so it is important not to overlook this ligament when evaluating the common extensor tendon. The LUCL is

best assessed on coronal MR images using thin slice thicknesses (≤ 3 mm thick). This ligament is usually injured as a result of dislocation of the radial head, and rupture of this ligament can be a cause of recurrent posterolateral instability of the radial head. The MRI appearance of injury of the RCL and the LUCL is similar to that of UCL injury.

TENDON INJURY

Epicondylitis is an overuse injury of the common extensor tendon at its attachment to the lateral epicondyle or of the common flexor tendon on the medial epicondyle. Although *epicondylitis* implies inflammation, the term is a misnomer because histologic studies of involved tendons show no acute inflammatory cells. Rather, overuse leads to mucinous or angiofibroblastic degeneration of the common tendon, which may progress to partial tearing or complete rupture. Lateral epicondylitis, also called *tennis elbow*, is more common and usually involves the extensor

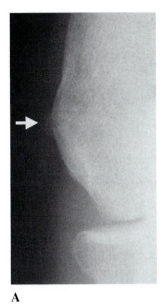

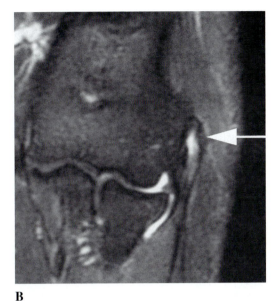

A   **B**

FIGURE 10-4. Lateral epicondylitis. *(A)* Coned view of the lateral epicondyle shows a small chronic focus of calcification in the region of the tendinous insertion. *(B)* Coronal fat-suppressed T$_2$-weighted fast spin echo sequence shows the outwardly bowed common extensor tendon (white arrow) with high signal edema and/or mucinous change deep to it. *(C)* Longitudinal sonogram of the same patient shows the outwardly bowed common extensor tendon (black arrows) with subjacent hypoechoic edema. The small focus of calcification is visible (white arrow). *(D)* Longitudinal sonogram of the patient's contralateral asymptomatic elbow shows the normal thin common extensor tendon (black arrows) inserting onto the lateral epicondyle; a small echogenic focus of calcification is also present in this elbow (white arrow). LE = lateral epicondyle, R = radial head.

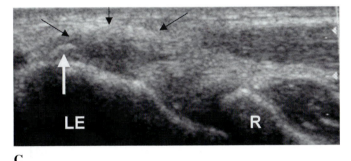

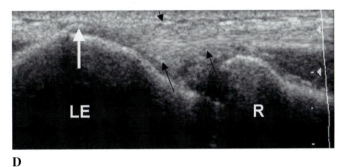

C   **D**

carpi radialis brevis component. Medial epicondylitis is referred to as *golfer's elbow*. Clinically, lateral epicondylitis is manifest by point tenderness over the lateral epicondyle and pain with forced dorsiflexion of the wrist.

The imaging appearance is the same, regardless of whether the medial or lateral side is affected. Radiographs occasionally show small foci of calcification adjacent to the epicondyle. The tendon should be assessed in the coronal and axial planes on MRI and in the longitudinal and transverse planes on sonographic imaging. MRI is more sensitive and specific than sonography, but sonographic evaluation can be performed much more rapidly. On MRI, the injured tendon can appear thickened or thinned, may have abnormal high signal intensity within it or between it and the underlying epicondyle on T$_2$-weighted images, and may be bowed outward. An analogous appearance can be seen sonographically with hypoechoic regions corresponding to the areas of high signal intensity on MRI (Figure 10-4).

Unlike chronic overuse, which leads to epicondylitis, the distal tendon of the biceps is typically injured in a single traumatic episode that the patient can often recall. The mechanism of injury is usually eccentric contraction of the muscle occurring by a sudden flexion jerk during which the patient tries to quickly lift something that is too heavy to be lifted or by the patient falling and grabbing on to something and trying to pull up while the arm is actually being extended. The classic clinical appearance of distal biceps rupture is pain and a palpable defect in the ante-

cubital fossa with a bulge in the mid aspect of the arm due to the torn and retracted biceps muscle. The bulging retracted muscle has been termed the *Popeye sign*, after the cartoon character's bulging biceps. Clinically, supination of the forearm and flexion of the elbow are weakened due to the ruptured biceps but not completely absent due to the preservation of these functions by the supinator and brachialis muscles, respectively. Not all patients present with the classic Popeye sign because it is possible for the distal biceps tendon to rupture but not retract if the biceps aponeurosis remains intact. The biceps aponeurosis (aka, *lacertus fibrosus*) is a sheet of fascial tissue that connects the distal biceps tendon to the common flexor mass on the medial aspect of the forearm. It is difficult to clinically distinguish a partial tear of the distal biceps tendon, which may be treated conservatively, from a non-retracted ruptured tendon, which needs surgical repair. For this reason, imaging can be helpful.

The distal biceps tendon can be evaluated with MRI and sonography. A ruptured tendon is discontinuous, with a balled-up end that may or may not be retracted. It is important to measure the degree of retraction from the radial tuberosity, so that the orthopedic surgeon knows where to find the torn retracted end during surgical repair. Sagittal MR images and longitudinal sonographic images are best for evaluating the degree of retraction. Edema and hemorrhage typically fill the tendon gap, seen as high signal intensity on T$_2$-weighted MR sequences and heterogeneous hypoechogenicity on sonography (Figure 10-5).

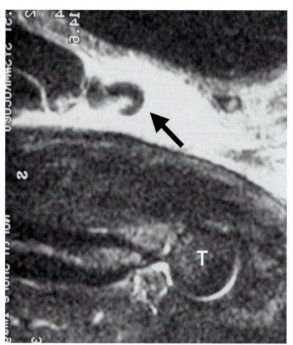

A

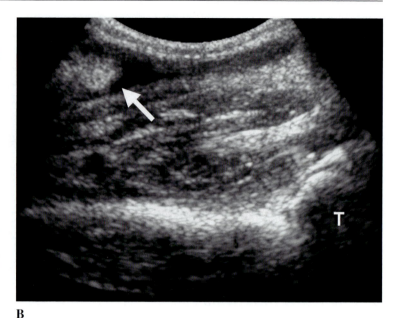

B

FIGURE 10-5. Ruptured and retracted distal tendon of the biceps. *(A)* Sagittal fat-suppressed fast spin-echo T_2-weighted sequence shows the torn and retracted tendon that has balled up on itself (black arrow), with high signal intensity edema and hemorrhage in the gap. The tendon has retracted proximally to the level of the distal humeral shaft. *(B)* Longitudinal sonogram performed with a curved array transducer to increase the field of view shows the torn and retracted distal tendon (white arrow), with hypoechoic edema and hemorrhage in the gap. The tendon retraction relative to the trochlea is well seen. T = trochlea.

Partial tearing can be visualized as thickening or thinning of the distal tendon with internal heterogeneous signal intensity or echogenicity (Figure 10-6). Sonographically, visualization in the longitudinal and transverse planes can be optimized by maximally supinating the patient's forearm and by comparison with the presumably normal contralateral elbow.

Injuries of the distal triceps tendon are rare. Partial tears are manifest as thinning or thickening of the tendon, and the patient, usually a weight lifter, complains of pain during arm extension such as with bench press or overhead pressing. In the case of complete rupture, the patient may have inability to extend the arm, and there may be a palpable defect at the insertion on the olecranon. Lateral radiographs may show soft tissue swelling and, occasionally, a small avulsed fragment of bone separated from the tip of the olecranon process. MRI may show discontinuity of the distal triceps tendon with high signal intensity edema and hemorrhage on T_2-weighted images in and around the tendon. Similarly, sonography shows discontinuity and disruption of the normal striated fibrillar appearance of the tendon. Longitudinal sonographic scanning during passive flexion and extension of the patient's elbow can help to distinguish a large partial tear of the tendon from a ruptured but non-retracted tendon, similar to the evaluation of quadriceps tendon tears of the knee (Figure 10-7). This distinction has implications for management because a partial tear can be treated conservatively, whereas a ruptured tendon needs to be repaired surgically.

OSTEOCHONDRITIS DISSECANS

Osteochondritis dissecans of the elbow is similar to that of the knee and the ankle. In fact, the elbow is the third most common site of osteochondritis dissecans in the body, and, within the elbow, the capitellum is most commonly affected. The injury can be due to microfracture from repetitive impaction of the radial head against the capitellum, such as occurs in baseball pitchers with valgus stress of the elbow, or can be due to a single traumatic incident. As in the ankle and knee, the injury may be chondral or osteochondral, and the fragment may be stable or unstable. The radiographic and MRI appearances are similar to those in the femoral condyles of the knee and the talus (see Chapter 2). Sonography also has been used to evaluate foci of osteochondritis dissecans anteriorly located in the capitellum and shows irregularity of the cortical surface, but cannot determine whether the fragment is stable or unstable (Figure 10-8).

INTRAARTICULAR LOOSE BODIES

Intraarticular loose bodies can be cartilaginous, osseous, or osteochondral. To be seen on radiographs, the fragment must be large enough and ossified or calcified. The loose bodies will collect in the recesses of the joint such as the olecranon fossa, coronoid fossa, and radial neck recess. Computed tomography

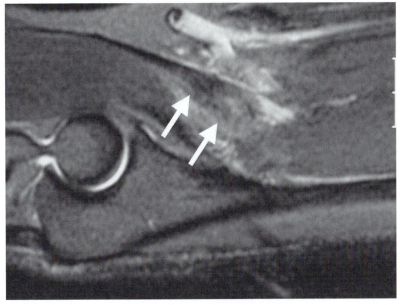

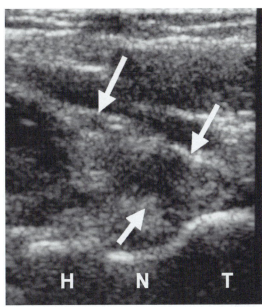

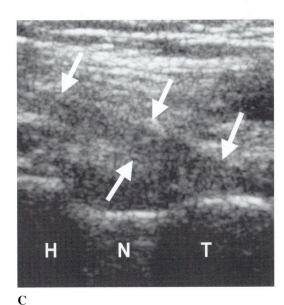

FIGURE 10-6. Partial tear of the distal tendon without retraction. *(A)* Sagittal fat-suppressed fast spin-echo T$_2$-weighted sequence shows thickening and heterogeneous signal within the distal biceps tendon (white arrows) at its insertion on the radial tuberosity. The tuberosity itself is out of the plane of this image. *(B)* Longitudinal sonogram shows the thickened and abnormally heterogeneously echogenic distal tendon (white arrows) inserting on the radial tuberosity. The radial head and radial neck are visualized. *(C)* Longitudinal sonogram of the patient's contralateral normal side shows a uniformly thick and hypoechoic tendon inserting on the radial tuberosity. H = radial head, N = radial neck, T = radial tuberosity.

is more sensitive than plain radiographs for the detection of small mineralized loose bodies because of its tomographic nature. Some investigators have advocated computed tomography arthrography using the single or double contrast technique; in the single contrast technique, the non-mineralized loose body will be seen as a radiolucent defect within the pool of contrast; with a double contrast technique, the loose body will be outlined by a thin rim of contrast in the air-filled radiolucent joint cavity. On MRI, an ossified loose body should have the same signal characteristics as marrow, whereas a calcified loose body will have low signal intensity on all pulse sequences (Figure 10-9). The non-mineralized loose body can be difficult to see unless a joint effusion is present. Similarly, ossified and calcified loose bodies are visualized sonographically by their echogenic surface

and posterior acoustic shadowing (Figure 10-10). As with MRI, non-mineralized loose bodies can be difficult to see sonographically without the presence of a joint effusion to distend the joint capsule.

ULNAR NERVE

At the level of the elbow, the ulnar nerve is posterior to the medial condyle. It is surrounded by fat and enclosed within the cubital tunnel by the overlying retinaculum (*ligament of Osborne*; Figure 10-11). Just distal to the medial condyle, it divides into superficial sensory and deep motor branches within the flexor carpi ulnaris muscle. On MRI and sonography, the nerve has

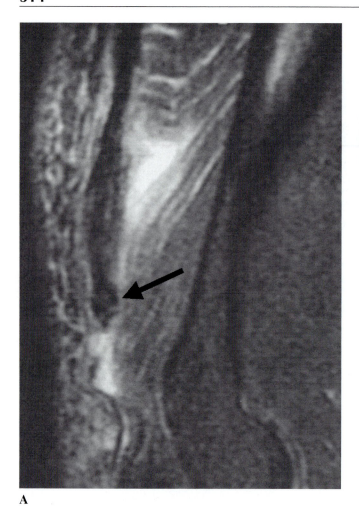

A

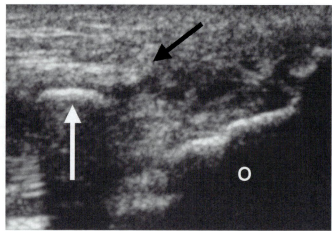

B

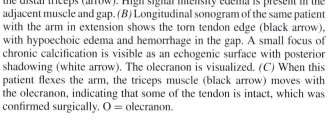

C

FIGURE 10-7. Triceps tendon tear. *(A)* Sagittal fat-suppressed fast spin-echo T$_2$-weighted sequence shows a torn and retracted edge of the distal triceps (arrow). High signal intensity edema is present in the adjacent muscle and gap. *(B)* Longitudinal sonogram of the same patient with the arm in extension shows the torn tendon edge (black arrow), with hypoechoic edema and hemorrhage in the gap. A small focus of chronic calcification is visible as an echogenic surface with posterior shadowing (white arrow). The olecranon is visualized. *(C)* When this patient flexes the arm, the triceps muscle (black arrow) moves with the olecranon, indicating that some of the tendon is intact, which was confirmed surgically. O = olecranon.

a uniform thickness, and on axial T$_2$-weighted MR images, the normal nerve may have high signal intensity. Sonography shows a fibrillar appearance due to the interfaces of the individual nerve fascicles.

Acute ulnar neuritis may not show any structural abnormality initially but eventually may be manifest as mild swelling of the nerve. Cubital tunnel syndrome is a more chronic form of ulnar neuritis due to compression of the ulnar nerve between the medial condyle and the overlying retinaculum. The cause of compression is usually osteophytes or cortical deformity from previous fractures. Chronic compression of the nerve within the cubital tunnel will cause focal nerve atrophy at the level of compression and proximal swelling of the nerve (Figure 10-12).

The ulnar nerve is also subject to anterior dislocation, in which it snaps anteriorly over the medial epicondyle during flexion. It is usually associated with similar snapping of the medial head of the triceps, which actually pushes the ulnar nerve out of its normal position. MRI can demonstrate the dislocation in static imaging performed in flexion and extension, whereas sonography can demonstrate the phenomenon in real time while the patient flexes and extends the elbow (Figure 10-13).

BURSITIS

Olecranon bursitis results from chronic irritation to the bursa that overlies the olecranon process, such as from chronic

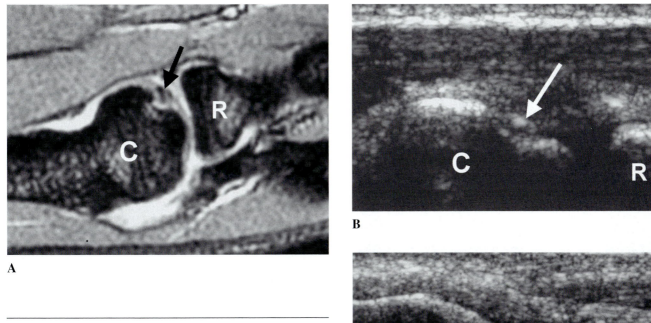

FIGURE 10-8. Osteochondritis dissecans of the capitellum. *(A)* Sagittal gradient echo T_2-weighted sequence shows a small detached loose fragment (black arrow) in the donor pit of the anterior aspect of the capitellum. *(B)* Corresponding longitudinal sonogram in the same patient shows the osteochondral fragment (white arrow) in the underlying donor pit of the capitellum. *(C)* Longitudinal sonogram of the patient's contralateral normal elbow shows a smooth contour of the anterior aspect of the capitellum. C = capitellum, R = radial head.

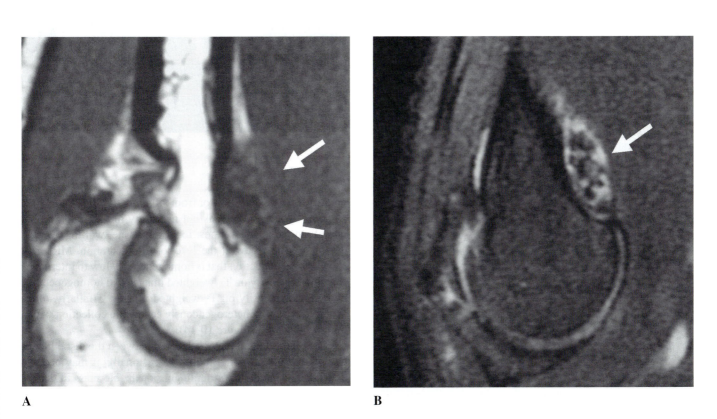

FIGURE 10-9. Intraarticular loose bodies. *(A)* Sagittal T_1-weighted sequence shows low signal intensity loose bodies in the coronoid fossa of the humerus (white arrows). *(B)* Corresponding sagittal fat-suppressed fast spin-echo T_2-weighted image shows the low signal loose bodies (white arrow) surrounding by a small amount of high signal intensity joint fluid.

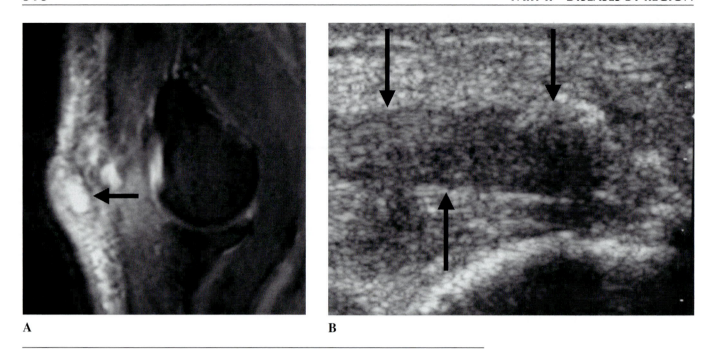

A   B

FIGURE 10-14.   Olecranon bursitis. *(A)* Sagittal fat-suppressed fast spin-echo T_2-weighted sequence shows focal high signal intensity representing the inflamed bursa (arrow) with surrounding soft tissue edema. *(B)* Corresponding longitudinal sonogram shows the heterogeneously echogenic bursa (arrows).

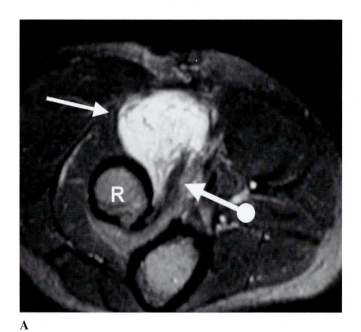

A

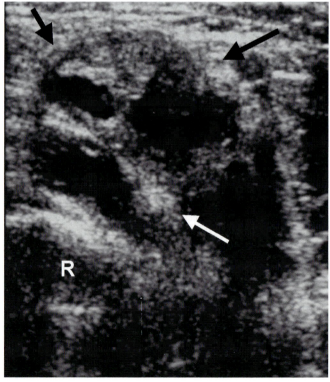

FIGURE 10-15.   Bicipitoradial bursitis. *(A)* Axial fat-suppressed fast spin echo T_2-weighted sequence shows a heterogeneously appearing, distended bursa (straight arrow) between the distal tendon of the biceps (round-tail arrow) and the radius. *(B)* Corresponding transverse sonogram shows the distended and heterogeneous bursa (black arrows) surrounding the distal biceps tendon (white arrow). R = radius.

B

SUGGESTED READINGS

Chiou HJ, Chou YH, Cheng SP, et al. Cubital tunnel syndrome diagnosis by high-resolution ultrasonography. *J Ultrasound Med.* 1998;17:643–648.

Connell D, Burke F, Coombes P, et al. Sonographic examination of lateral epicondylitis. *AJR.* 2001;176:777–782.

Falchook FS, Zlatkin MB, Erbacher GE, Moulton JS, Bisset GS, Murphy BJ. Rupture of the distal biceps tendon: evaluation with MR imaging. *Radiology.* 1994;190:659–663.

Martin CE, Schweitzer ME. MR imaging of the epicondylitis. *Skeletal Radiol.* 1998;27:133–138.

Miller TT, Adler RS. Sonography of tears of the distal biceps tendon. *AJR.* 2000;175:108–116.

Mulligan, SA, Schwartz ML, Broussard, MF, Andrews JR. Heterotopic calcification and tears of the ulnar collateral ligament: radiographic and MR imaging findings. *AJR.* 2000;175:1099–1102.

Rosenberg ZS, Beltran J, Cheung YY, Yun Ro S, Green SM, Lenzo SR. The elbow: MR features of nerve disorders. *Radiology.* 1993; 188:235–240.

Sasaki J, Masatoshi T, Toshihko O, Kashiwa H. Ultrasonography assessment of the ulnar collateral ligament and medial elbow laxity in college baseball players. *J Bone Joint Surg Am.* 2002;84A:525–531.

Skaf AY, Boutin RD, Dantas RWM, et al. Bicipitoradial bursitis: MR imaging findings in eight patients and anatomic data from contrast material opacification of bursae followed by routine radiography and MR imaging in cadavers. *Radiology.* 1999;212:111–116.

Timmerman LA, Schwartz ML, Andrews JR. Preoperative evaluation of the ulnar collateral ligament by magnetic resonance imaging and computed tomography arthrography. *Am J Sports Med.* 1994;22:26–32.

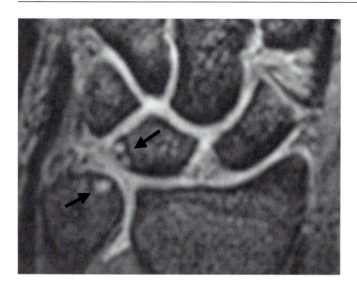

FIGURE 11-5. Coronal gradient echo T_2-weighted image shows positive ulnar variance with subchondral fibrocystic change on the apposing surfaces of the distal ulna and ulnar side of the lunate (arrows). The triangular fibrocartilage is degenerated and torn.

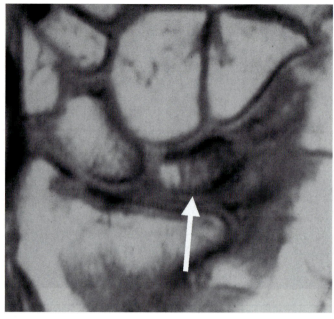

FIGURE 11-6. Coronal T_1-weighted magnetic resonance image shows low signal intensity in the lunate (arrow) but with some sparing of normal fatty marrow signal intensity. This is the appearance of stage I Kienböck disease.

the most commonly perforated. Membranous perforations can be painful, but do not lead to instability and are therefore biomechanically unimportant. The dorsal and ulnar aspects are thought to be more important biomechanically, but these are, unfortunately, the more difficult portions of the ligaments to evaluate reliably. As with evaluation of the TFC, MRI is the modality of choice, and assessment of ligament integrity is aided by the presence of fluid in the radiocarpal and midcarpal joints on coronal images. The SL and LT ligaments are located along the proximal aspects of the bones. As a consequence, fluid or contrast in the radiocarpal joint normally should not extend into the intercarpal intervals and the midcarpal joint, whereas fluid in the midcarpal joint will extend into the intercarpal intervals but normally should not extend proximally past these bones into the radiocarpal joint (Figure 11-7). Coronal T2W MRI and arthrography best evaluate the membranous portion of these ligaments; tears are manifest as fluid extension between the bones (Figures 11-8 and 11-9) or nonvisualization of the ligament (Figure 11-10). However, the LT ligament sometimes is not visualized on MRI, even if it is anatomically present and normal, because it is a thin ligament; the presence of high signal intensity fluid is used as a secondary sign for injury in such cases. Another potential

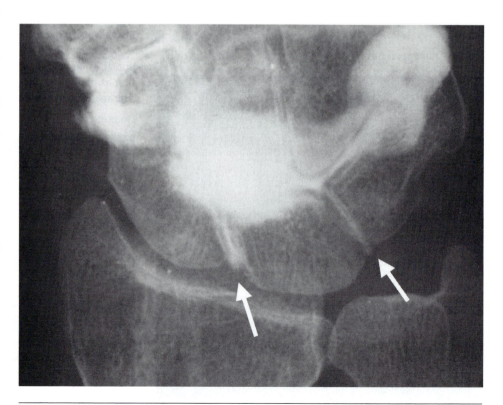

FIGURE 11-7. Anteroposterior radiograph after direct injection of contrast into the midcarpal joint shows contrast in the intercarpal intervals between the scaphoid and lunate and between the lunate and triquetral bones (arrows). The proximal flow of contrast is blocked from entering the radiocarpal joint by the intact intercarpal ligaments.

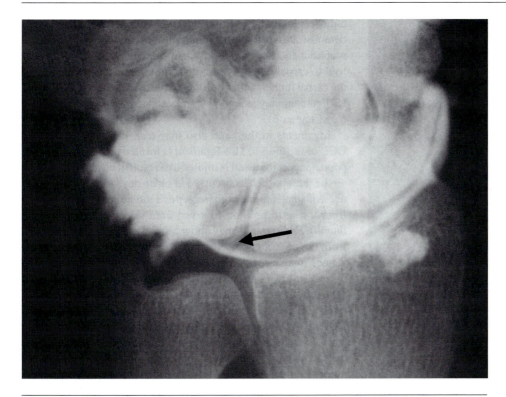

FIGURE 11-8.   Anteroposterior view of the wrist after injection into the midcarpal joint shows flow of contrast through a torn lunotriquetral ligament (arrow) into the radiocarpal joint.

pitfall of interpretation of coronal T2WI is high signal intensity of the articular cartilage of the bones, which undercuts the ligament attachment and may mimic a tear. Axial MR images and transverse sonographic scanning may be more helpful than coronal MR images for the evaluation of the dorsal and volar aspects of these ligaments (Figure 11-11).

Failure of fluid to enter the intercarpal interval is a sign of chronic ligament tear with scarring. Also, the presence of osteophytes and focal articular disease are signs of chronic ligament dysfunction, as are focal offset of two adjacent carpal bones and lack of the normal articular parallelism.

The extrinsic ligaments of the wrist, in particular the volar set, also are important for carpal stability and can be assessed with sagittal or thin-section coronal MR images.

Tears of the intrinsic ligaments may lead to "dissociative" instability, such as rotatory subluxation of the scaphoid and dorsal intercalated segmental instability in the case of SL ligament tears. A wrist with SL advanced collapse (SLAC) also may occur in patients with an SL ligament tear, in which there is proximal migration of the capitate between the splayed scaphoid and lunate. This leads to focal arthritis at the capitoscaphoid and capitolunate joints, with eventual arthritis at the

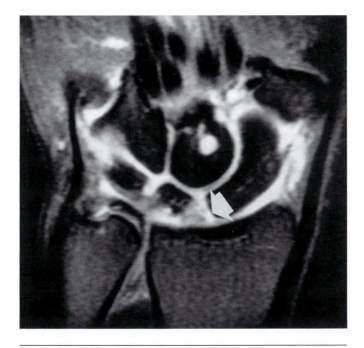

FIGURE 11-9.   Fat-suppressed T_1-weighted coronal magnetic resonance image after intravenous injection of gadolinium contrast shows high signal intensity contrast (arrow) extending through a tear of the radial side of the scapholunate ligament.

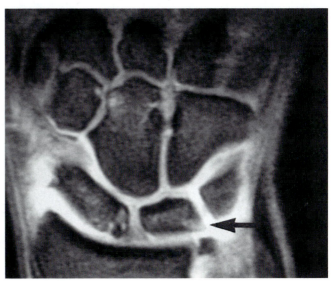

FIGURE 11-10.   Coronal fat-suppressed T_1-weighted image after intravenous injection of gadolinium contrast shows nonvisualization of the lunotriquetral ligament with contrast flowing freely across the lunotriquetral interval (arrow).

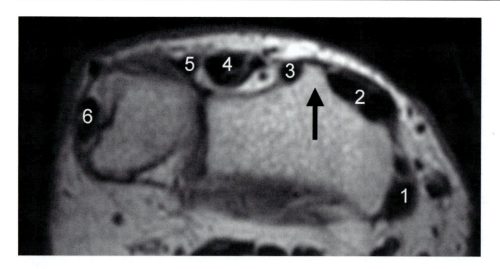

FIGURE 11-23.   Normal axial T_1-weighted magnetic resonance image shows the 6 extensor tendon compartments (1 to 6). Lister tubercle (arrow) is the small bony protuberance on the dorsal aspect of the distal radius that separates compartments 2 and 3 and acts as an attachment for some of the extrinsic dorsal ligaments of the wrist.

fractures, but the imaging modality of choice is MRI. Bone scan may show increased tracer uptake in the scaphoid but cannot distinguish bone bruise from fracture, an important distinction because a fracture requires casting and a bone bruise does not. CT can miss some subtle fractures and cannot demonstrate bone bruise as the cause of the pain. Moreover, many patients with clinically suspected scaphoid fracture actually have soft tissue injuries, such as ligament and TFC tears, which will be missed on bone scan and CT. A modified screening MR protocol can be performed, consisting of coronal T1WI and fat suppressed T2WI only. If the marrow is normal, there is no bony injury. Abnormal marrow signal intensity on T1WI and fat-suppressed T2WI

represents a true fracture, whereas marrow edema seen only on fat-suppressed T2WI represents a bone bruise. A discrete fracture line may not be visible within the marrow edema of T1WI and T2WI, but cortical disruption or stepoff may be present (Figure 11-27).

Avascular necrosis (AVN) of the proximal pole of the scaphoid occurs in approximately 60% of scaphoid fractures, and displaced fractures have a higher risk of AVN than nondisplaced fractures (see Chapter 2). The demonstration of AVN is clinically important because it suggests that the fracture will not heal, even if operated upon. Low signal intensity within the proximal pole on all pulse sequences is the best MR sign of posttraumatic AVN, but it is not completely reliable. Some investigators have advocated the use of intravenous contrast to look for enhancement of the proximal pole, indicating an intact vascular supply. Normal marrow signal intensity in the proximal pole at the time of the initial injury is unreliable to exclude AVN because AVN may take a few months to appear. Posttraumatic cysts can occur in the proximal pole but have better defined margins than does AVN. Marrow edema in the distal pole is usually secondary to reactive changes at the site of the fracture.

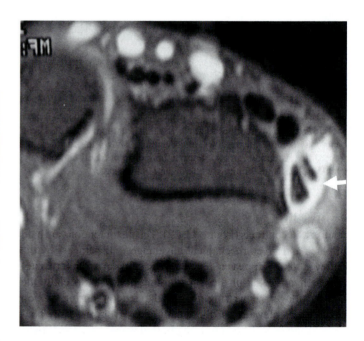

FIGURE 11-24.   Axial T_1-weighted magnetic resonance image in a patient with a de Quervain tenosynovitis shows enlargement of the first extensor compartment tendons, with low signal intensity fibrosis replacing the overlying subcutaneous fat (arrow).

FIGURE 11-25.   Fat-suppressed T_1-weighted axial magnetic resonance image after intravenous administration of gadolinium shows thickening and enhancement of the synovium (arrow) surrounding the first extensor compartment in this patient with de Quervain stenosing tenosynovitis.

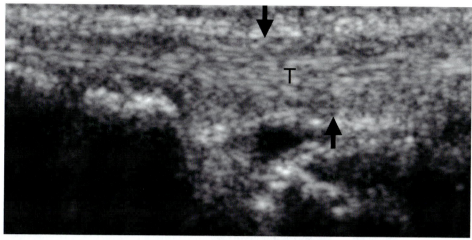

A

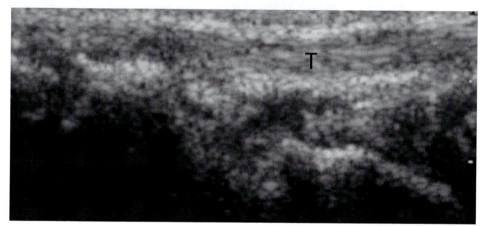

B

FIGURE 11-26. Sonography of de Quervain tenosynovitis. *(A)* Longitudinal sonogram of the affected side shows the thickened tendon, with thickening of the overlying tendon sheath (arrows). *(B)* Sonography of the same patient's normal contralateral wrist shows a normal appearance of the tendon. T = tendon.

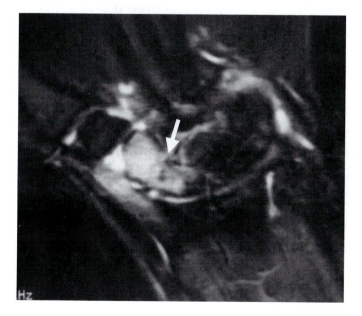

FIGURE 11-27. Coronal fat-suppressed T_2-weighted magnetic resonance image shows a fracture through the waist of the scaphoid. Although the fracture line is not well visualized, there is disruption and stepoff of the cortical surfaces (arrow). Note also the marked high signal intensity marrow edema within the fractured scaphoid and the surrounding high signal intensity soft tissue edema.

Scaphoid fractures have a relatively high incidence of nonunion, only partly related to the risk of AVN. Scaphoid nonunions may be fibrous, cartilaginous, or synovial (pseudoarthrosis).

A fibrous nonunion demonstrates low signal on T1WI and T2WI. Because this appearance is similar to the MR appearance of some united fractures, this appearance can be definitively defined as nonunion only when motion is present on physical examination. Motion is indirectly visible by MRI as high signal about the fracture on T2WI. Cartilaginous nonunion shows signal similar to that of cartilage and may demonstrate motion-related edema about the fracture line. If fluid-like signal intensity is present in the fracture gap after 6 months, the diagnosis of pseudoarthrosis or synovial nonunion should be suggested (Figure 11-28). Pseudoarthrosis is the only nonunion that is almost always surgically treated. The high signal intensity of the pseudoarthrosis should be differentiated from the periosseous edema of healing by using heavily T2WI: the granulation tissue of normal fracture healing will fade on these images with long echo times.

CT often is employed to evaluate healing of a scaphoid fracture by looking for trabecular or cortical bridging of the fracture site. Even after the surgical placement of a screw across the fracture, the images provide useful information (Figure 11-29).

CHAPTER 12

HIP

TERRY L. LEVIN / THEODORE T. MILLER

Abnormalities of the hip affect the entire age range of life, with different abnormalities affecting different ages. With the exception of developmental dysplasia, these abnormalities typically present due to pain. Depending on the patient's age, the cause of symptoms can be intra- or extraarticular.

INTRAARTICULAR CAUSES

Infant

Developmental dysplasia of the hip (DDH) refers to a shallow acetabulum and resultant subluxation or dislocation of the femoral head. It occurs in between 1.5 and 10 per 1000 live births. It is more common in infants who are white, female, born by breech delivery, and first born. The left hip is much more commonly affected, but the condition is bilateral in 5 to 20% of cases. Bilaterality may be associated with other conditions such as arthrogryposis and torticollis. The etiology of DDH is likely multifactorial. There is a component of ligament laxity that is induced by circulating maternal hormones, although other factors are clearly involved.

Before the advent of sonography, anteroposterior (AP) radiographs were used to evaluate suspected DDH, but because the epiphysis is radiolucent until the age of approximately 6 months, its location had to be inferred; the acetabulum was divided into quadrants by drawing Hilgenreiner's line (a horizontal line through the triradiate cartilage) and Perkin's line (a line perpendicular to Hilgenreiner's line, drawn along the lateral margin of the acetabular roof), and a normal epiphysis is located in the lower inner quadrant (Figure 12-1). Confirmation of normal position can be made with Shenton's line, a curved line connecting the medial margin of the femoral metaphysis and the superior margin of the obturator foramen. The acetabular angle (the slope of the acetabular roof relative to the horizontal) also can be measured on AP radiographs and normally should be less than 30°.

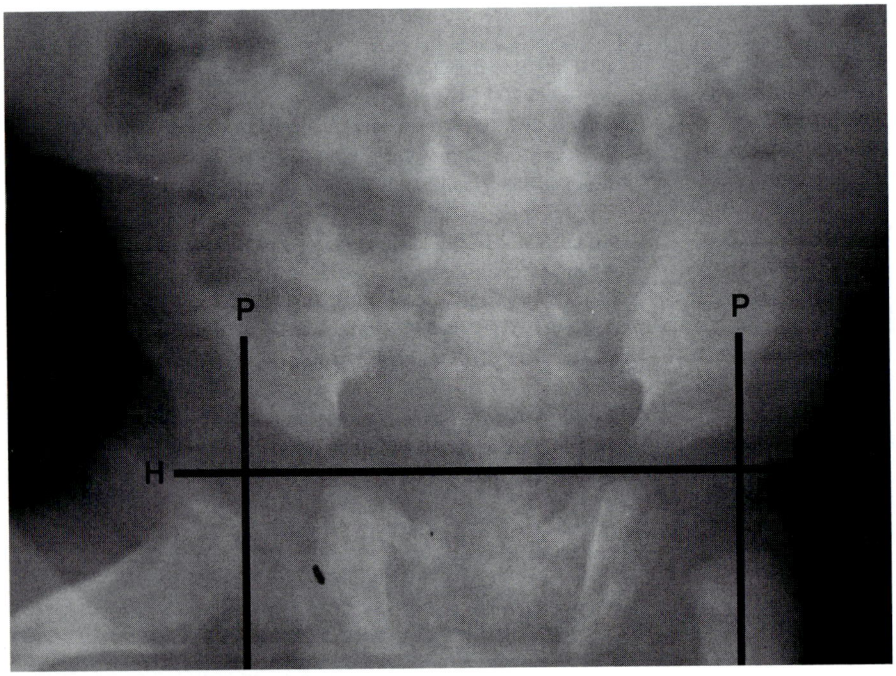

Real-time ultrasound (US) has become the modality of choice in assessing infants with suspected DDH for several reasons: (*a*) the cartilaginous femoral head can be directly visualized on US; (*b*) sonography is a dynamic examination in which the hip can be flexed, extended, and stressed under direct US visualization; (*c*) the bony acetabulum can be measured by using the Graf alpha angle (normal is greater than 60°); and (*d*) the appearance and position of the fibrocartilaginous labrum may be determined, and interposition of the labrum between the femoral head and acetabulum may be diagnosed (Figure 12-2).

Complications of untreated DDH include the development of a pseudoacetabulum, delayed and abnormal ossification of the femoral head, labral tear, and eventual premature degenerative arthritis.

FIGURE 12-1. Anteroposterior view of a neonatal pelvis shows the horizontal Hilgenreiner's line and the vertical Perkin's line. The femoral metastases should be pointing to the lower inner quadrant for the expected location of the unossified epiphysis. In this image these lines are obliqued in order to be horizontal and perpendicular to the pelvis, which is obliqued in this case. H = Hilgenreiner's line, P = Perkin's line.

Child

In a child, intraarticular causes of hip pain include septic arthritis (see

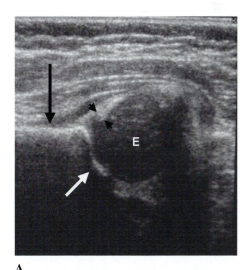

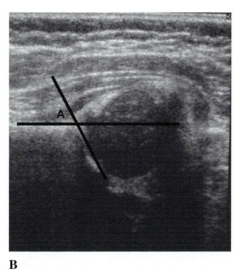

A   B

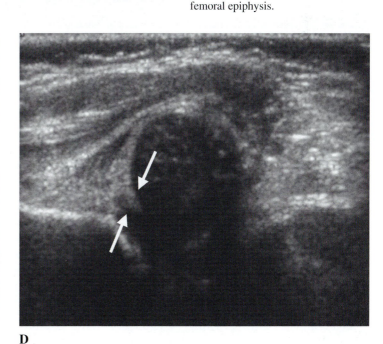

C   D

FIGURE 12-2. Hip dysplasia. *(A)* Coronal flexed view of a normal hip shows a normal iliac bone (large black arrow) and normal acetabulum (white arrow). The hypoechoic cartilaginous epiphysis (E) is well seated in the acetabulum. Note the echogenic triangular labrum (small black arrow). *(B)* Coronal flexed view of a normal hip shows the intersection of the iliac line and acetabular line, forming the Graf A angle. *(C)* Corresponding coronal flexed view of the patient's contralateral symptomatic side shows a shallow acetabulum (white arrow) and a laterally dislocated femoral epiphysis (E). Echogenic fibrofatty (F) material is present between the head and the acetabulum, and the acetabular labrum is dysmorphic (black arrow). *(D)* Coronal flexed view of a different patient with dysplasia shows a similar shallow acetabulum and displaced femoral head. The labrum (arrows) has become interposed between the acetabulum and the femoral epiphysis.

Chapter 1), transient viral synovitis, Perthes disease, and slipped capital femoral epiphysis (SCFE). Transient synovitis of the hip, a nonspecific inflammatory reaction of the synovium, occurs in children between ages 5 and 10 years. A history of an antecedent viral infection may be obtained, but this is not always the case. Clinically, the child presents with hip pain and limitation of motion, in particular hip extension. Plain radiographs are often unhelpful. Hip US demonstrates the presence of a joint effusion, and joint aspiration yields sterile fluid (Figure 12-3). These children generally are treated with rest or nonsteroidal antiinflammatory agents, leading to eventual resolution of symptoms.

The differential diagnosis includes Perthes disease and septic arthritis.

Perthes disease is idiopathic osteonecrosis of the femoral head, which typically occurs between ages 4 and 8 years (see Chapter 2). SCFE is a Salter I injury of unknown etiology, affecting the proximal femoral physis. It occurs approximately 3 times more commonly in boys than in girls and occurs around the time of the pubertal growth spurt, which is usually slightly earlier in girls than in boys. There is a higher incidence of SCFE in overweight children and in children with delayed skeletal maturation. SCFE may present at unusual ages in children with

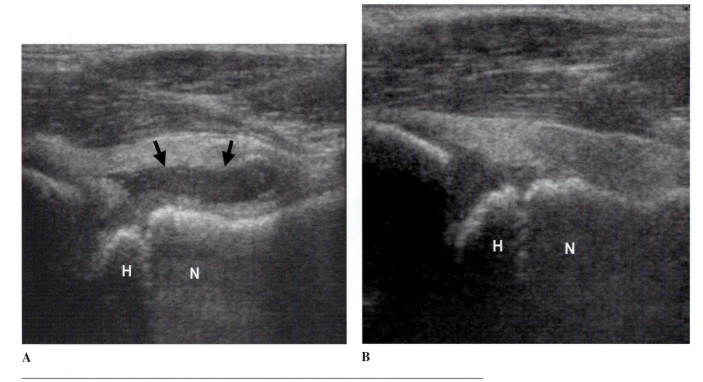

A   B

FIGURE 12-3.   Transient synovitis of the hip. *(A)* Longitudinal sonogram of the symptomatic side shows a hypoechoic joint effusion (arrows). Note the outline of the femoral neck and the early ossification of the femoral head. *(B)* Corresponding image of the patient's contralateral normal side shows the absence of the joint effusion. H = femoral head, N = femoral neck.

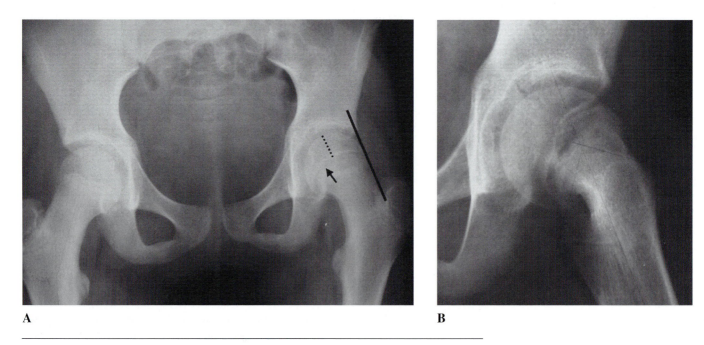

A   B

FIGURE 12-4.   Slipped capital femoral epiphysis. *(A)* Anteroposterior radiograph of the pelvis with left-side slipped capital femoral epiphysis shows widening of the physis (arrow), decreased height of the epiphysis (dashed line), and failure of a line drawn along the lateral cortex of the femoral neck to intersect the head. Compare with the contralateral normal hip. *(B)* Frog lateral view shows the posteromedial slip, with the appearance of ice cream sliding off the cone.

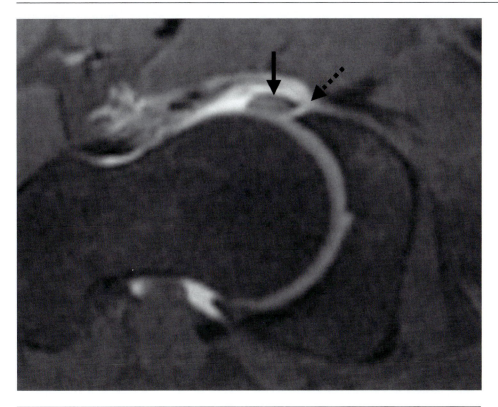

FIGURE 12-5. Oblique axial fat-suppressed T_1-weighted magnetic resonance arthrographic image shows detachment of the anterior aspect of the acetabular labrum (arrow), with high signal intensity contrast (dashed arrow) interposed between the labrum and the acetabulum.

Adult

In an adult, causes of intraarticular hip pain such as arthritis, fracture, infection, and osteonecrosis have been covered in their respective chapters. Another cause of hip pain in teenagers and adults is tear of the acetabular labrum. The acetabulum is shaped like an upside down U and has a fibrocartilaginous labrum along the bony rim, similar to that of the shoulder. As with the shoulder, the acetabular labrum can tear, typically due to repetitive microtrauma that occurs with pivoting and twisting during athletic activity, but acute trauma such as hip dislocation, degenerative arthritis, and DDH also can be causes. Symptoms of labral tear include pain, a clicking or clunking sensation, locking, or giving way.

MRI, in particular MR arthrography, is the procedure of choice for evaluating the acetabular labrum. In cross section, the labrum appears as a low signal intensity triangle. The joint capsule typically inserts on the acetabulum at the base of the anterior and posterior labrum and superiorly on the acetabulum a few millimeters above the base of the superior labrum; thus, fluid in the distended joint fills the perilabral sulcus and surrounds the labrum. The criteria for tear are similar to those for tears of the meniscus and glenoid labrum, namely an abnormal signal that reaches the articular surface, frank labral detachment, and intraarticular contrast material entering the substance of the labrum (Figure 12-5). Tears occur most commonly in the anterior labrum. As with the glenoid labrum of the shoulder, there is normal anatomic variation such as small size or even absence. There is also some controversy as to whether there is a sublabral foramen in the anterosuperior aspect of the acetabular labrum; however, if it exists, it is shallow. Therefore, marked undercutting of the base of the labrum, even if the periphery remains attached, should be considered a tear. Occasionally, paralabral cysts arise due to the underlying labral tear, just as in the shoulder and knee, and have the typical MR appearance of a fluid-filled cyst. On sonography, these cysts can be identified and sonography can guide percutaneous aspiration (Figure 12-6). The cysts tend to be associated with posterior labral tears. One should also look for defects in the articular cartilage of the acetabulum and femoral head when evaluating the labrum because labral tears are often accompanied by articular cartilage injury.

A commonly encountered finding on radiographs and MRI of the hip is the synovial herniation pit (also called *Pitt's pits* after the person who first described them). It usually occurs in the anterior and superior aspects of the femoral neck and is due

hypothyroidism, rickets, or renal osteodystrophy and in children receiving growth hormone. The condition more commonly affects the left hip and may be bilateral in 25% of cases. Clinically, children with SCFE typically present with hip pain and limp, although the presenting symptom occasionally is knee pain.

The femoral capital epiphysis slips medially and posteriorly. Radiographic findings on AP and frog leg lateral views of the hips include widening of the physis, apparent decreased height of the capital epiphysis, poor definition of the trabeculae in the metaphysis immediately adjacent to the physis, and failure of a line drawn along the lateral margin of the femoral neck to intersect the femoral head (Figure 12-4). Magnetic resonance imaging (MRI) in cases of painful hip with normal radiographs (called a *pre-slip*) may demonstrate edema in the physis and metaphysis. In cases of chronic SCFE, remodeling of the femoral neck may occur, with rounded buttressing of the lateral aspect.

Complications of SCFE include avascular necrosis (AVN) and chondrolysis. AVN occurs in 10% of SCFE cases, with a greater incidence in those with a more severe degree of slip. AVN also may occur as a result of the treatment of SCFE, which is percutaneous pinning of the affected hip. Chondrolysis is rare, and its etiology is unclear but may be related to an ischemic event. Radiographically, there is marked and rapid narrowing of the hip joint space, with osteoporosis and subchondral erosive changes, accompanied by severe hip pain and limitation of motion.

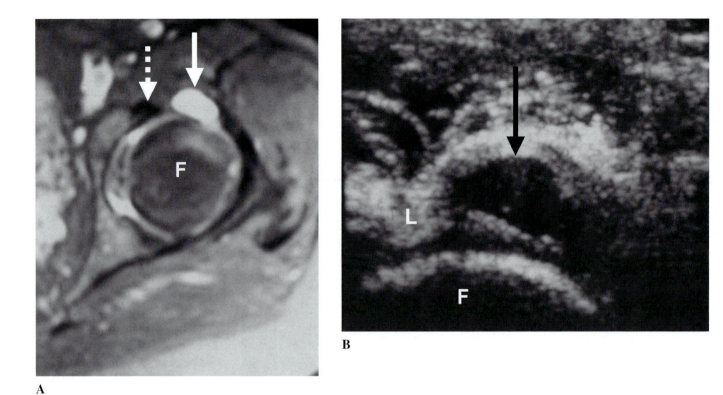

FIGURE 12-6. Perilabral cyst. *(A)* Axial fat-suppressed fast spin echo T_2-weighted magnetic resonance image shows a cystic-appearing structure (solid arrow) anterior to the femoral head and adjacent to the acetabular labrum (dashed arrow). *(B)* Corresponding transverse sonogram shows the anechoic cyst (arrow) anterior to the femoral head. F = femoral head, L = labrum.

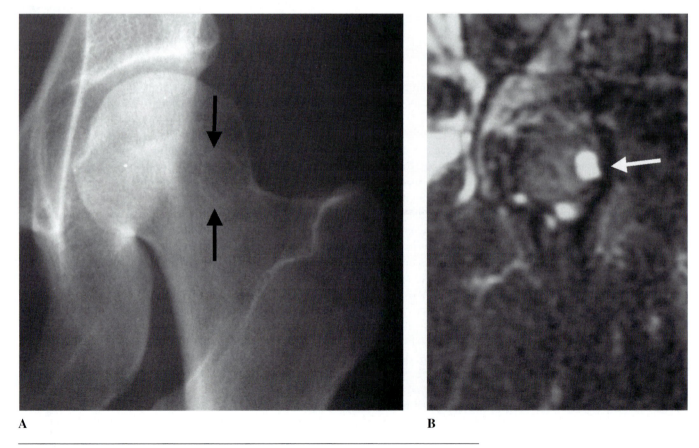

FIGURE 12-7. Synovial herniation pit. *(A)* Anteroposterior radiograph shows an oval lucency with a thin sclerotic rim (arrows). *(B)* Corresponding fat-suppressed fast spin echo T_2-weighted image show the fluid appearing pit (arrow) in the anterosuperior aspect of the femoral head. Small foci of high signal intensity joint fluid are present at the inferior aspect of the head.

to invagination of the overlying joint capsule into the femoral neck. They are almost always incidental and asymptomatic findings, although in some people they may be a secondary sign of femero-acetabular impingement. If large, the overlying cortex may fracture, thus causing pain. Radiographically, they appear as a thin sclerotic circle or oval and on MRI have the signal characteristics of fluid (Figure 12-7). Bone scan may show increased uptake, even in asymptomatic pits.

Not uncommonly, radiographically subtle arthritis may present with articular hip pain in adults. This is especially true for subtle traumatic or degenerative cartilage defects. Subchondral edema is often seen on MRI with these symptomatic defects. Because of the subtlety of these defects, lidocaine should be added to all direct MR arthrograms. The importance of the lidocaine is to differentiate intra- from extraarticular etiologies of pain;

if the symptoms do not improve after the arthrogram, then the cause may be outside the joint.

EXTRAARTICULAR CAUSES

Hip pain can come from surrounding tendons and bursae and can be referred to the hip region from degenerative disc disease of the lumbar spine and from degenerative arthritis of the knee.

The tendons of the gluteus medius and minimus muscles insert along the lateral aspect of the greater trochanter. These tendons are subject to degenerative tendinosis and to partial tearing and symptomatic calcific tendinitis. On MRI, there is typically high signal intensity edema on T_2-weighted imaging in and around these tendons, which occasionally may track into

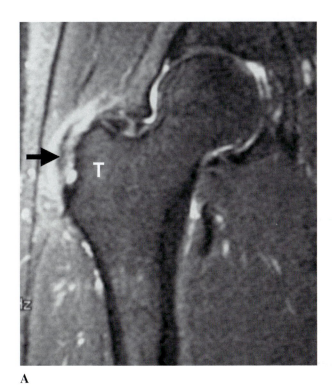

A

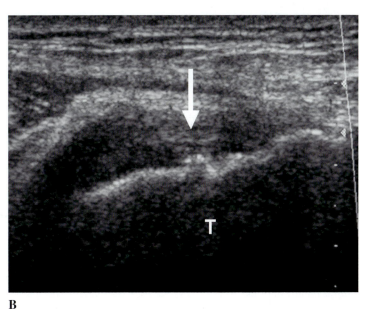

B

C

FIGURE 12-8. Gluteal tendinitis. *(A)* Coronal fat-suppressed fast spin echo T_2-weighted magnetic resonance image shows high signal intensity edema in and around the gluteal tendons (arrow) as they insert on the greater trochanter. *(B)* Corresponding longitudinal sonogram in the same patient shows the hypoechogenic edema surrounding the tendon (arrow). *(C)* Corresponding longitudinal sonogram of the patient's contralateral asymptomatic side shows the normal-appearing attachment (arrow). T = greater trochanter.

Pelsser V, Cardinal E, Hobden R, Aubin B, Lafortune M. Extraarticular snapping hip: sonographic findings. *AJR*. 2001;176:67–73.

Petersilge CA. Chronic adult hip pain: MR arthrography of the hip. *Radiographics*. 2000;20:S43–S52.

Petersilge CA. MR arthrography for evaluation of the acetabular labrum. *Skeletal Radiol*. 2001;30:423–430.

Pitt MJ, Graham AR, Shipman JH, Birkby W. Herniation pit of the femoral neck. *AJR*. 1982;138:1115–1121.

Schnarkowski P, Steinbach LS, Tirman PFJ, Peterfy CG, Genant HK. Magnetic resonance imaging of labral cysts of the hip. *Skeletal Radiol*. 1996;25:733–737.

Sopov V, Fuchs D, Bar-Meir E, Gorenberg M, Groshar D. Clinical spectrum of asymptomatic femoral neck abnormal uptake on bone scintigraphy. *J Nucl Med*. 2002;43:484–486.

Umans H, Liebling MS, Moy L, Haramati N. Slipped capital femoral epiphysis: a physeal lesion diagnosed by MRI, with radiographic and CT correlation. *Skeletal Radiol*. 1998;27:139–144.

Vaccaro JP, Sauser DD, Beals RK. Iliopsoas Bursa imaging: efficacy in depicting abnormal iliopsoas tendon motion in patients with internal snapping hip syndrome. *Radiology*. 1995;197:853–856.

Wunderbaldinger P, Bremer C, Matuszewski L, Marten K, Turetschek K, Rand T. Efficient radiological assessment of the internal snapping hip syndrome. *Eur Radiol*. 2001;11:1743–1747.

CHAPTER 13

KNEE

THEODORE T. MILLER

In most practice settings, the knee is the most commonly imaged joint, and the second most commonly imaged body part after the lumbar spine.

ANATOMY

The osseous anatomy of the knee is inherently unstable, consisting of the rounded femoral condyles resting on the flat tibial plateau. Stability is created by the presence of medial and lateral menisci, which deepen the surfaces of the plateau and increase contact area, and by numerous ligaments and tendons that act to control anterior and posterior subluxation of the tibia, rotatory subluxation, and varus and valgus angulation.

The menisci are crescentic wedges of fibrocartilage whose purposes are to deepen the surface of the tibial plateau, thus providing increased stability for the femoral condyles, act as shock absorbers, and distribute synovial fluid to the underlying hyaline articular cartilage. The lateral meniscus has a C shape and is uniform in thickness and size throughout. The medial meniscus is slightly larger and less tightly curved, and the posterior horn is thicker and wider than the anterior horn. On sagittal images, the anterior and posterior horns of the lateral meniscus are equal in size, whereas the posterior horn of the medial meniscus is larger than that of the anterior horn (Figure 13-1). The entire periphery of the medial meniscus is attached to the joint capsule. In contrast, the anterior horn and body of the lateral meniscus are attached to the joint capsule, but the posterior horn is focally separated from the joint capsule, forming an obliquely running tunnel at the meniscocapsular junction, called the *popliteus hiatus*, through which runs the popliteus tendon (Figures 13-1 and 13-2). In addition to their capsular attachment, the menisci are attached to the tibial plateau by fibrous bands at the roots of their anterior and posterior horns. The anterior horns of the menisci are also connected to each other by the transverse meniscal ligament, and the attachment site of this ligament on the meniscus sometimes can mimic a meniscal tear (Figure 13-3). The meniscofemoral ligaments of Humphrey and Wrisberg are anatomically inconstant anatomic structures that run from the lateral aspect of the medial femoral condyle to the posterior horn of the lateral meniscus. The Humphrey ligament lies anterior to the posterior cruciate ligament, whereas the Wrisberg ligament is posterior to the posterior cruciate ligament (PCL) (Figure 13-4). These meniscofemoral ligaments, in concert with meniscal attachments from the popliteus tendon, help to control motion of

the posterior horn of the lateral meniscus during knee flexion. During knee flexion, there is mild rotation of the tibia relative to the femur. The flexion-extension motion occurs predominantly at the superior articular surface of the meniscus, whereas the rotatory motion occurs primarily at the inferior articular surface of the meniscus. The posterior horn of the medial meniscus has greater excursion than the lateral meniscus, a fact that is thought to be responsible in part for the higher incidence of tears of the medial than of the lateral meniscus.

Several ligaments help to bind the tibia and femur together and prevent abnormal motion of the two bones relative to each other. Within the knee joint itself are the anterior cruciate ligament (ACL) and PCL. These ligaments are intracapsular but extrasynovial, ie, the joint synovium reflects over the anterior surface of the ACL and over the posterior surface of the PCL. The ACL is located in the lateral aspect of the intercondylar notch and runs from the posterior aspect of the intercondylar roof to the anterior aspect of the base of the lateral tibial spine. It is composed of anteromedial and posterolateral bundles that twist upon themselves as they run their course, giving the ligament thickness and a typical striated appearance on magnetic resonance imaging (MRI). However, MRI does not resolve the composite structure into the two discrete bundles. The ligament should be straight, of intermediate signal intensity, and run a course parallel to or slightly steeper than the roof of the intercondylar notch (known as the *Blumensaat line* on plain radiographs; Figure 13-5). The purpose of the ACL is to prevent anterior subluxation of the tibia relative to the femur. The PCL lies in the medial aspect of the intercondylar notch, arising from the lateral aspect of the medial femoral condyle and running in a curved course to a small flange at the posterior aspect of the tibia, below the level of the articular tibial plateau. It also is composed of two bundles, but its collagen fibers are more tightly packed than that of the ACL, so it has a more uniformly low signal intensity appearance on MR images (see Fig. 13-4). Its primary function is to prevent posterior subluxation of the tibia.

The medial side of the knee is stabilized by the medial collateral ligament (MCL), which is the primary restraint against valgus stress of the knee. It is a band of fibrous tissue that originates at the superior aspect of the medial femoral condyle and courses inferiorly to attach to the medial aspect of the proximal tibial shaft. As it crosses the joint space, its deep fibers blend with the superficial fibers of the joint capsule of the medial side of the knee (Figure 13-6). Posterior to the MCL is the semimembranosus tendon that inserts on the posteromedial aspect of the

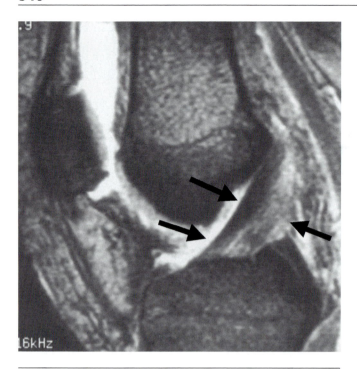

FIGURE 13-5. Sagittal gradient echo T$_2$-weighted image shows the normal anterior cruciate ligament (arrows). Note that it has intermediate signal intensity, a striated appearance, and is parallel to or slightly steeper than the dark line of the cortex of the roof of the intercondylar notch. The most anterior aspect of the anterior cruciate ligament tends to have darker signal intensity than the remainder of the ligament.

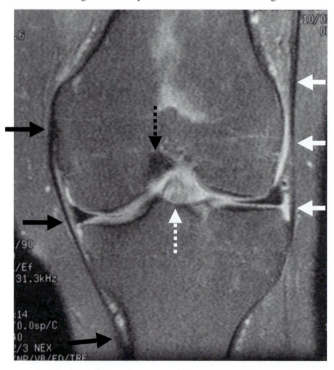

FIGURE 13-6. Coronal fat-suppressed T$_2$-weighted magnetic resonance image shows the normal medial collateral ligament (arrows) arising from the superior aspect of the medial femoral condyle and inserting on the proximal aspect of the medial side of the tibial shaft. It is normal to have focal areas of signal heterogeneity between the distal aspect of the medial collateral ligament and the tibia due to fat and vessels. Notice also the PCL (dashed black arrow), ACL (dashed white arrow), and iliotibial band (white arrows).

proximal tibia just below the plateau. Also located posteromedially are the three tendons that compromise the *pes anserinus* group, namely the sartorius, gracilis, and semitendinosus tendons. This group lies medially to the semimembranosus tendon and inserts as a conjoined tendon on the medial aspect of the proximal tibial shaft, between the insertions of the more proximal semimembranosus and the more distal MCL.

The lateral side of the knee is stabilized by several different tendinous and ligamentous structures. Posterolaterally, the tendon of the biceps femoris muscle inserts on the lateral aspect of the fibular head. This distal tendon attachment is joined by the fibular collateral or lateral collateral ligament, which extends from the superior aspect of the lateral femoral condyle to the lateral aspect of the fibular head (Figure 13-7). Slightly more anterior to these structures is the popliteus sulcus of the lateral femoral condyle, from which the popliteus tendon originates and runs in a posteroinferior fashion, behind the posterior horn of the lateral meniscus, to become the popliteus muscle, which attaches to the posteromedial aspect of the tibia (see Fig. 13-2). The popliteus muscle and tendon not only contribute to stabilization of the posterolateral aspect of the knee but also act to "unlock" the fully extended knee by causing mild internal rotation of the tibia relative to the femur, which then allows the extended knee to flex. The anterolateral aspect of the knee is stabilized by the iliotibial band, which is a fascial extension of the tensor fascia lata muscle of the hip, and which inserts on the bony prominence of the proximal tibia, known as *Gerdy tubercle* (Figure 13-8).

Anteriorly, the quadriceps tendon is a thick striated band of tissue that inserts on the superior pole of the patella. The most anterior fibers of this tendon, typically from the rectus femoris

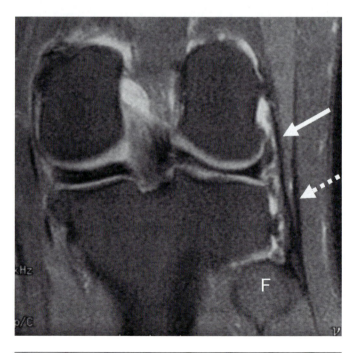

FIGURE 13-7. Coronal fat-suppressed proton density image shows the normal fibular collateral ligament (solid arrow) and distal biceps femoris tendon (dashed arrow) joining together to form a conjoined tendon that inserts on the lateral aspect of the fibular head. F = fibular head.

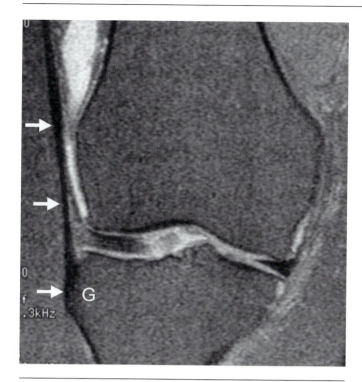

FIGURE 13-8. Coronal fat-suppressed proton density image shows a normal iliotibial band (arrows) projecting on the Gerdy tubercle. The high signal intensity between the iliotibial band and the femur represents normal joint fluid in the lateral recess of the joint. G = Gerdy tubercle.

muscle, continue along the anterior surface of the patella and become the patella tendon, extending from the inferior pole of the patella to the tibial tubercle (Figure 13-9). The quadriceps tendon, patella, and patellar tendon are known collectively as the *extensor mechanism*. The patella is the largest sesamoid bone in the body and acts to increase the mechanical advantage of the extensor mechanism.

Meniscal Injury

The menisci can tear as a result of a single acute traumatic event or as the result of chronic degeneration. The posterior horn of the medial meniscus is the most common site of tear. The two criteria that should be used for determining a meniscal tear are the presence of linear signal intensity within the meniscus which convincingly reaches the superior or inferior articular surface, and abnormal meniscal morphology. Early descriptions of abnormal signal within the meniscus used a grading system, in which grade 1 was globular signal within the meniscus, grade 2 was linear signal within the meniscus that did not reach an articular surface, and grade 3 was linear signal in the meniscus that did reach an articular surface. Grades 1 and 2 represent intrasubstance degeneration and grade 3 is a tear, but most musculoskeletal radiologists no longer use this system. Instead, it is preferable just to report that the meniscus is either normal, has intrasubstance degeneration, or is torn.

There are many different configurations and orientations of meniscal tear. Although early descriptions categorized acute traumatic tears as vertically oriented and chronic degenerative

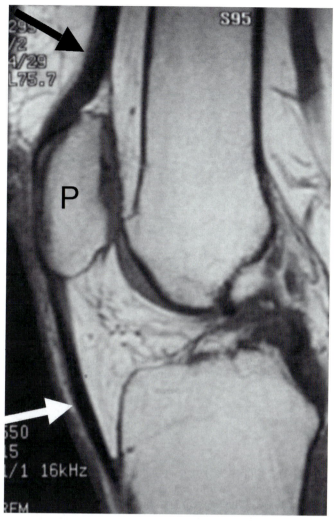

FIGURE 13-9. Sagittal T_1-weighted magnetic resonance image shows the normal extensor mechanism consisting of the quadriceps tendon (black arrow), the patella, and the patellar tendon (white arrow). Note that the patellar tendon is normally thinner than the quadriceps tendon. P = patella.

tears as horizontally oriented, the fact is most meniscal tears actually have an oblique orientation and most involve the inferior articular surface. The linear abnormal signal intensity should involve the articular surface of the meniscus on at least two consecutive images to have a high likelihood of being a true tear. Some tears can be diagnosed only by recognizing the abnormal morphology of the meniscus and not from the visualization of abnormal signal intensity within the meniscus.

Specific types of tears are the radial tear, the parrot-beak tear, the bucket-handle tear, and the flap tear. In the radial tear, the cleavage plane is perpendicular to the free edge of the meniscus. The normal wedge-shape meniscus may appear truncated or blunted when the image slice is directly in the plane of the tear (Figures 13-10 and 13-11). The parrot-beak tear is similar to a radial tear except that the plane of the tear is curved. In the bucket-handle tear, the tear runs longitudinally along the length of the meniscus, and the inner rim flips into the intercondylar notch while remaining attached to the anterior and posterior

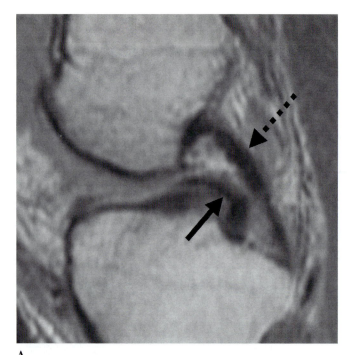

A

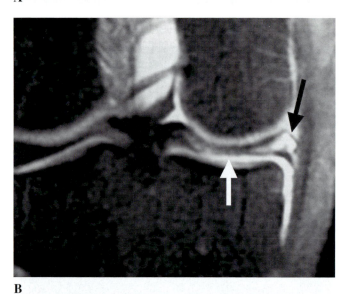

B

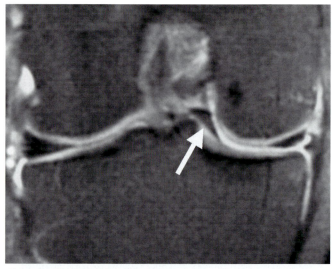

C

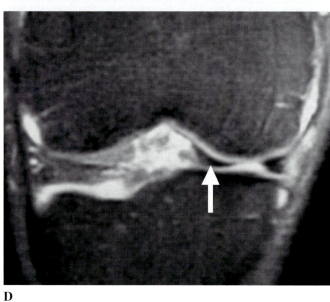

D

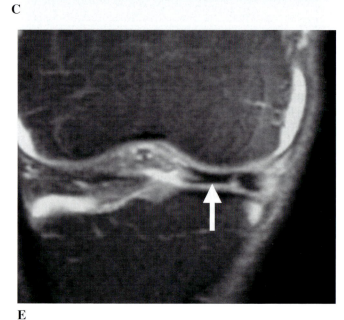

E

FIGURE 13-12. Bucket-handle tear. *(A)* Sagittal proton density image shows the displaced meniscal fragment (arrow) forming the "double PCL sign" with the more superficial and normal-appearing posterior cruciate ligament (dashed arrow). *(B)* Coronal fat-suppressed T$_2$-weighted image shows high signal intensity tearing in the periphery of the meniscus (black arrow) and thinning centrally (white arrow). *(C)* Slightly more anterior, the meniscal fragment is present in the notch (arrow). *(D)* More anterior, the anterior aspect of the displaced fragment (arrow) is starting to come back to the periphery. *(E)* A more anterior coronal image now shows the displaced fragment (arrow) reattaching to the periphery of the meniscus.

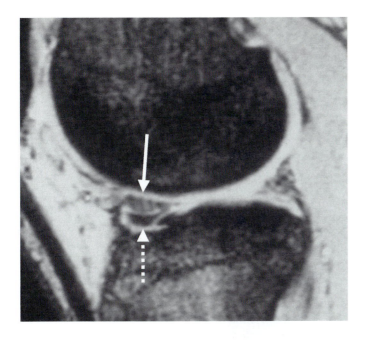

FIGURE 13-13. Flap tear of the lateral meniscus. Sagittal gradient echo image shows the displaced fragment (solid arrow) on top of the more normal underlying anterior horn (dashed arrow). Notice the abnormal truncation of the posterior horn.

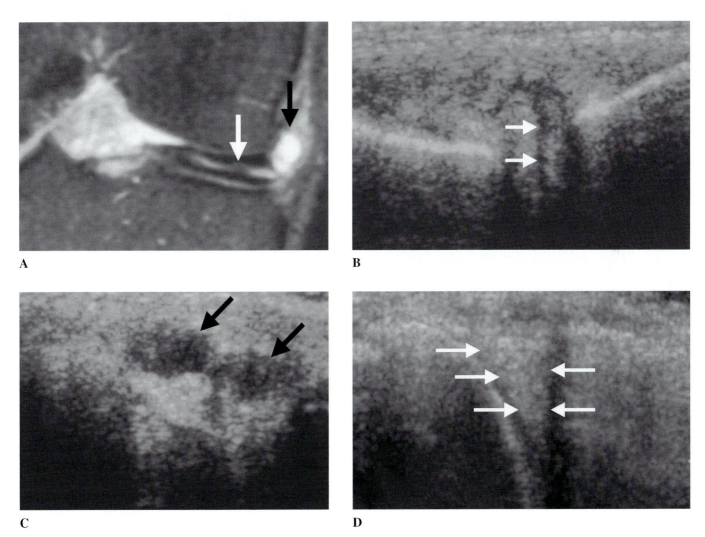

A

B

C

D

FIGURE 13-14. Meniscal tear and parameniscal cyst. *(A)* Coronal fat-suppressed T_2-weighted image shows a high signal intensity transverse tear through the anterior horn of the lateral meniscus (white arrow), with a small high signal intensity parameniscal cyst forming in the adjacent soft tissue (black arrow). *(B)* Corresponding sonogram shows the hypoechoic tear (arrows) in the meniscus. *(C)* Sonogram at a slightly different level now shows the hypoechoic cyst (arrows). *(D)* Corresponding normal meniscus for comparison shows a homogeneously echogenic wedge-shape meniscus (arrows).

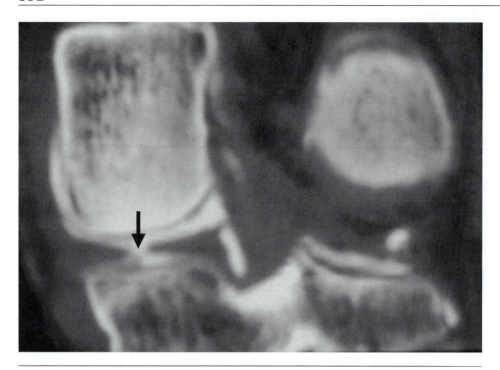

FIGURE 13-15. CT arthrogram of a tear of the medial meniscus. Reformatted coronal image shows the high density contrast filling a tear of the posterior horn of the medial meniscus (arrow).

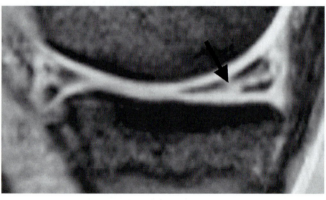

A

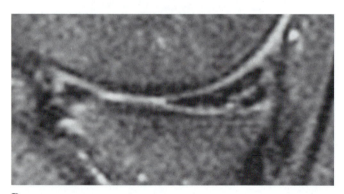

B

FIGURE 13-16. Persistence of signal in a healed tear. *(A)* Preoperative magnetic resonance gradient echo image shows high signal intensity tear (arrow) in the posterior horn of the medial meniscus. *(B)* Sagittal fat-suppressed T$_2$-weighted magnetic resonance image 8 months after surgical repair shows persistent high signal intensity. The patient had a normal physical examination, and the magnetic resonance examination was performed for symptoms elsewhere in the knee.

on every slice (Figure 13-17), whereas a normal meniscus will appear as a wedge in most slices. Because of its abnormal shape, a discoid meniscus is subject to greater shear forces than a normal meniscus and is therefore more prone to tear. These menisci usually present in children or young adults as pain due to tear or as knee stiffness.

Ligament Injury

CRUCIATE LIGAMENT INJURY.   Injury of the ACL is common and can occur due to a variety of mechanisms. Pure hyperextension or hyperflexion of the knee can cause tear of this ligament, but the most common mechanism of injury involves a rotational and/or valgus component, such as occurs during skiing, when the ski and tibia go in one direction and the femur and the rest of the body go in a different direction, or as a result of a clipping-type injury in football, when the knee is hit from the lateral side, causing it to go into valgus.

A ruptured ACL will appear on MRI as replacement of the normal linear striated appearance by an amorphous cloud-like appearance of high signal intensity or as a discrete discontinuity of the ligament with fibers that do not course parallel to the intercondylar roof (Figures 13-18 and 13-19). A large hemarthrosis usually accompanies an acute ACL rupture because of the well-vascularized nature of this ligament. Partial tears of the ACL may appear as focal loss of the normal striated appearance, which does not affect the entire diameter of this ligament, or as generalized swelling of the ligament. Sometimes, it can be difficult to distinguish partial tears from complete ruptures. Sonography is not as good as MRI for evaluating suspected ACL injury because the ACL cannot be visualized directly. Instead, indirect

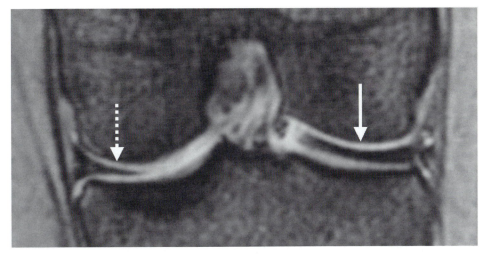

A

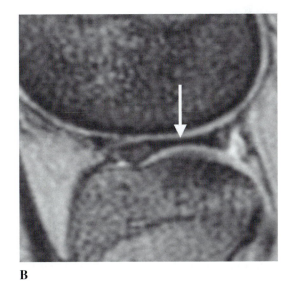

B

FIGURE 13-17. Discoid lateral meniscus. *(A)* Coronal gradient echo image shows the large slab-like meniscus (solid arrow). Compare this image with the normal wedge shape of the medial meniscus (dashed arrow). *(B)* Sagittal gradient echo magnetic resonance image shows the persistence of the slab (arrow). Normally on a sagittal image at this level of the knee, the anterior and posterior horns should be separate.

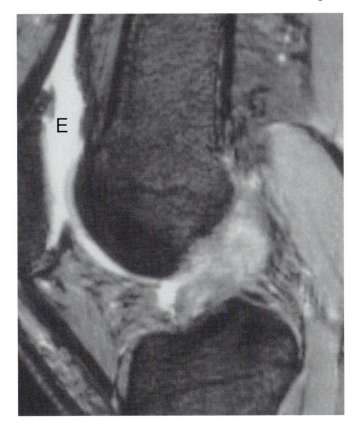

FIGURE 13-18. Sagittal gradient echo magnetic resonance image shows the high signal intensity "cloud-like" appearance of a rupture of the anterior cruciate ligament, with almost complete loss of the normal ligament architecture. Note the joint effusion. E = effusion.

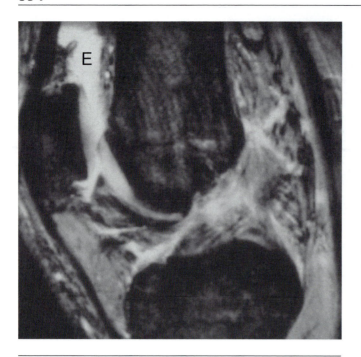

FIGURE 13-19. Sagittal gradient echo magnetic resonance image shows high signal intensity discontinuity of the anterior cruciate ligament. Note the joint effusion. E = effusion.

signs, such as the presence of a hemarthrosis or sonographic demonstration of anterior tibial subluxation, are used.

Other knee injuries often accompany ACL tear. A common constellation of injuries is the *O'Donoghue triad*, consisting of ACL rupture, MCL injury, and tear of the medial meniscus. This triad typically results from a clipping- or cutting-type injury in which there is external rotation of the femur relative to the tibia and valgus stress. The *Segond fracture*, a small vertically oriented avulsion fracture from the anterolateral aspect of the proximal tibia, at the site of insertion of the lateral joint capsule just below the plateau, is always associated with ACL rupture and often with tear of the medial or lateral meniscus (Figure 13-20). The Segond injury is due to internal rotation and varus stress, and, if the significance of the radiographic visualization of this fracture is not recognized, the patient can have chronic anterolateral instability of the knee. Similarly, a rotational injury can cause damage to the posterolateral corner of the knee, associated with ACL and/or PCL injury and tear of the fibular collateral ligament and other posterolateral stabilizing structures, leading to chronic posterolateral instability of the knee.

In addition to the Segond fracture, there are other typical sites of bone injury associated with ACL rupture. The most common involves the combination of bone bruises in the weight-bearing portion of the lateral femoral condyle and posterior aspect of the lateral tibial plateau (Figure 13-21). This offset pattern of lateral bone bruises occurs as a result of the internal rotation of the tibia and valgus angulation of the knee, thus allowing the posterolateral aspect of the tibial plateau to impact the weight-bearing portion of the lateral side of the lateral femoral condyle. "Kissing" bone bruises may occur in the anterior aspect of the tibial plateau and anterior aspects of the femoral condyles during a hyperextension injury, when the anterior aspects of the

tibia and femoral condyles impact each other. A less common site of bone injury is the posterior aspect of the medial tibial plateau, consisting of either bone bruise, impaction fracture, or small chip fracture due to avulsion of the semimembranosus tendon.

These bony injuries are not only clues to the existence of an ACL tear but are also comorbid causes of pain. Other secondary signs of ACL injury, although not injuries themselves, are anterior subluxation of the tibia relative to the femur, with resultant uncovering of the posterior horn of the lateral meniscus, and buckling of the PCL (Table 13-1 and Figure 13-22).

In skeletally immature patients, the tibial attachment of the ACL is weaker than the ligament itself, so ACL injuries occur as tibial avulsions of the ACL rather than as ruptures of the ligament. The avulsed fracture fragment, immediately anterior to the anterior tibial spine and sometimes involving it, can often be appreciated on radiographs, but CT with sagittally reformatted images may be requested by the orthopedic surgeon to better evaluate the amount of bony distraction (Figure 13-23).

A chronically ruptured ACL will be manifest as nonvisualization of the ligament, angulation of the ligament (instead of a straight course) due to scarring and tethering, or a shallow orientation instead of paralleling the intercondylar roof (Figure 13-24). The torn ACL may scar onto the PCL and parasitize a blood supply, accounting for this shallow orientation. The associated findings of acute ACL injury such as large hemarthrosis and bone bruises typically are not present with chronic ACL tear, although there may be anterior subluxation of the tibia and buckling of the PCL due to residual joint laxity. A deepened condylo-patellar sulcus on the lateral femoral condyle is another sign of chronic ACL insufficiency (see Fig. 13-24). Sometimes, a cyst forms within the ligament as a result of a prior partial tear (Figure 13-25).

A ruptured ACL can be surgically reconstructed, typically by using the patient's own patellar tendon. In this procedure, the

TABLE 13-1

Secondary Signs of ACL Tear

1. Offset bone bruises in the weight-bearing portion of the lateral femoral condyle and posterior aspect of the lateral tibial plateau
2. Anterior "kissing" bone bruises in the anterior aspect of the tibial plateau and anterior aspects of the femoral condyles
3. Bone bruise or fracture in the posterior aspect of the medial tibial plateau
4. Deepened condylo-patellar sulcus of the lateral femoral condyle (the "lateral femoral notch" sign—usually associated with chronic ACL tear)
5. Buckling of the PCL
6. PCL line sign: a line drawn along the curve of the PCL on sagittal images does not intersect the femur within 5 cm of the distal aspect of the femur
7. Anterior subluxation of the tibia: a line drawn vertically along the posterior aspects of the femoral condyles is farther than 5 mm from the posterior cortex of the tibial plateau
8. Uncovering of the posterior horn of the lateral meniscus: a line drawn vertically along the posterior cortex of the tibial plateau intersects the posterior horn of the lateral meniscus
9. Horizontal shearing tear of Hoffa fat pad.

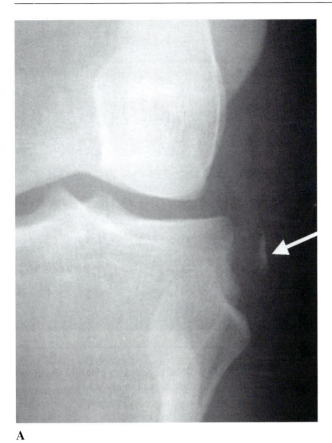

A

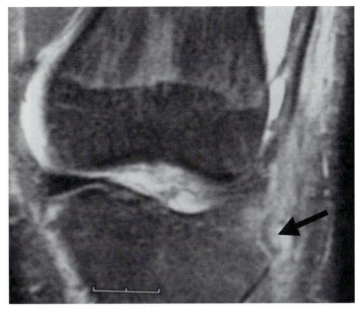

B

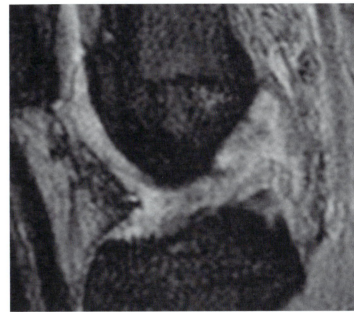

C

FIGURE 13-20. Segond fracture. *(A)* Anteroposterior radiograph shows a small, vertically oriented fragment of bone (arrow), indicating avulsion of the lateral joint capsule. *(B)* Coronal fat-suppressed fast spin echo T_2-weighted image of a different patient shows the displaced fragment (arrow) with surrounding soft tissue edema. *(C)* Corresponding sagittal gradient echo magnetic resonance image shows the ruptured anterior cruciate ligament.

central third of the patellar tendon with a small piece of bone from the patellar attachment and tibial attachment is harvested, tunnels are made in the distal femur and proximal tibia, and one end of the tendon graft is placed in the proximal tunnel and the other in the distal tunnel. The ends of the graft are held in the bone tunnel by "interference" screws whose sole role is to hold the bony ends of the graft in place until they fuse with the bone tunnel itself. The screws can be metal or made of bioabsorbable material. The dephasing artifact from the interference screws usually is not severe enough to preclude MRI of the reconstructed ligament or the menisci. The neo-ligament can have a variable appearance, such as being low, intermediate, or high signal intensity on T_2-weighted images and can be straight or

mildly bowed. Occasionally, scar tissue may form anteriorly to the entrance of the ligament into the tibial bone tunnel, constituting a "cyclops" lesion that can interfere with extension of the knee (Figure 13-26).

The PCL is two to four times stronger than the ACL and therefore is not often found as an isolated injury. Typical mechanisms of injury are similar to those of the ACL, namely hyperextension and hyperflexion, with or without rotational components. Injury of the PCL does not look the same as injury of the ACL. PCL ruptures tend to appear as generalized thickening of the ligament on MRI and sonography, with intermediate signal intensity on T_1-weighted sequences and heterogeneous high signal intensity on T_2-weighted MR sequences (Figure 13-27).

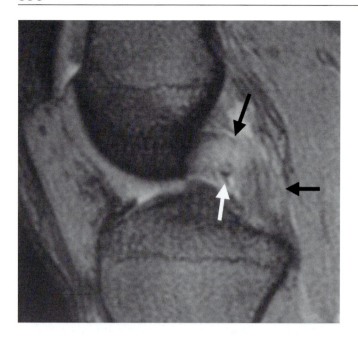

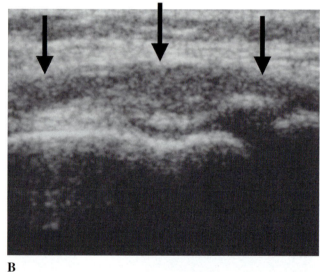

FIGURE 13-27.   Tear of the posterior cruciate ligament. Sagittal gradient echo image shows the swollen, high signal intensity ligament (black arrows). Note the small meniscofemoral ligament of Humphrey in cross section (white arrow).

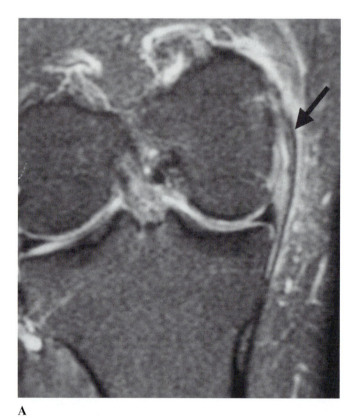

A

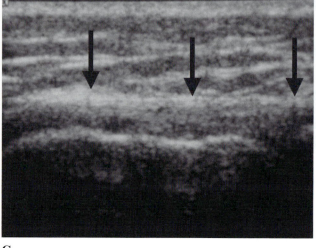

B

C

FIGURE 13-28.   Sprain of the medial collateral ligament. *(A)* Coronal fat-suppressed T$_2$-weighted magnetic resonance image shows thickening, internal signal heterogeneity, mild outward bulging of the proximal aspect of the ligament (arrow), and surrounding soft tissue edema. *(B)* Corresponding longitudinal sonogram shows the thickened and mildly outwardly bowed ligament (arrows). *(C)* Longitudinal sonogram of the patient's contralateral normal medial collateral ligament shows the normal-appearing ligament (arrows).

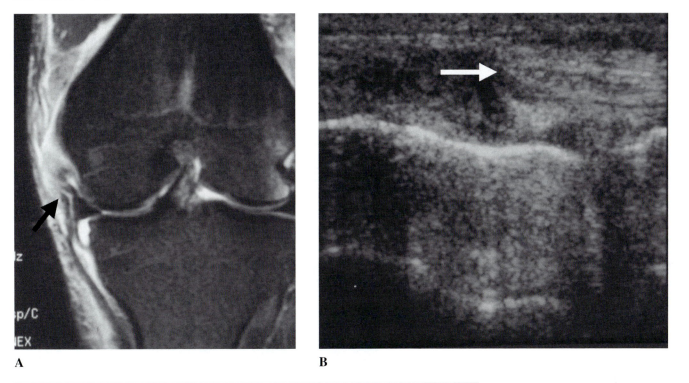

A

B

FIGURE 13-29. Rupture of the medial collateral ligament. *(A)* Coronal T$_2$-weighted fat-suppressed image shows rupture of the proximal aspect of the ligament (arrow). *(B)* Corresponding sonographic image shows the torn distal edge of the ligament (arrow) with proximal hypoechoic edema and hemorrhage.

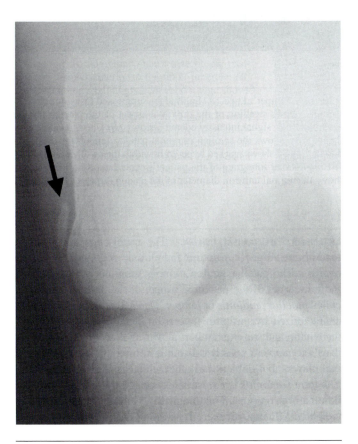

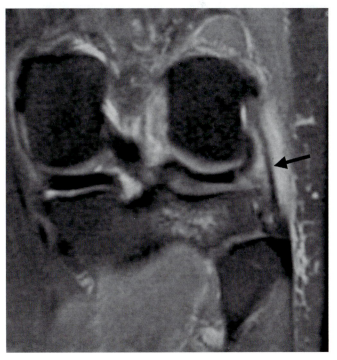

FIGURE 13-30. Anteroposterior radiograph shows a small focus of heterotopic ossification in the proximal aspect of the medial collateral ligament, indicating old trauma to the ligament.

FIGURE 13-31. Coronal fat-suppressed T$_2$-weighted magnetic resonance image shows sprain of the fibular collateral ligament (arrow) manifest by surrounding high signal intensity edema.

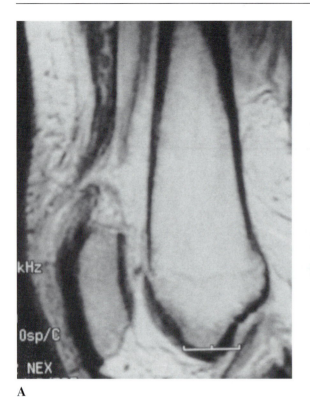

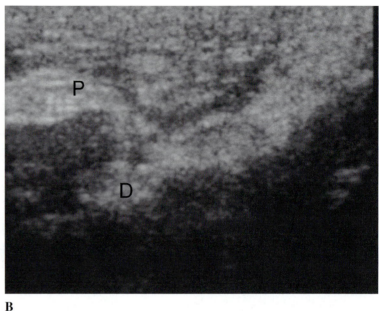

FIGURE 13-34. Quadriceps tendon rupture. *(A)* Sagittal T₁-weighted image shows a chronic rupture of the quadriceps tendon with separation of the tendon edges. *(B)* Corresponding longitudinal sonogram shows the torn proximal and distal tendon edges. D = distal tendon edge, P = proximal tendon edge.

contraction of the extensor mechanism as the knee tries to extend while being flexed by the weight of the stumbling person. The diagnosis usually is made clinically by weakness of extension and a palpable defect in the suprapatellar region, but it is not always easy to distinguish a partial tear, which might be treated conservatively, from a complete rupture, which might be treated

surgically if there is retraction of the torn tendon edge. In the case of quadriceps tendon tear, a lateral radiograph may show suprapatellar soft tissue swelling with blurring of the fat planes and a low lying patella, whereas a patellar tendon rupture will show a high-riding patella with infrapatellar soft tissue swelling and blurring of the fat planes. Sagittal T₂-weighted MR

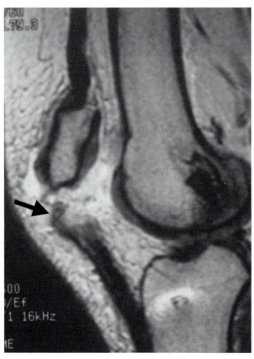

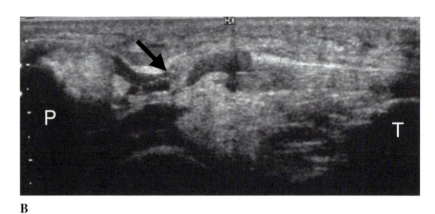

FIGURE 13-35. Acute patellar tendon rupture. *(A)* Sagittal fast spin echo T₂-weighted image shows the ruptured patellar tendon (arrow) with surrounding high signal intensity edema. The patella is elevated and tilted. *(B)* Corresponding longitudinal sonogram shows the patellar tendon (arrow) with hypoechoic edema and hemorrhage in the gap. P = patella, T = tibial tubercle.

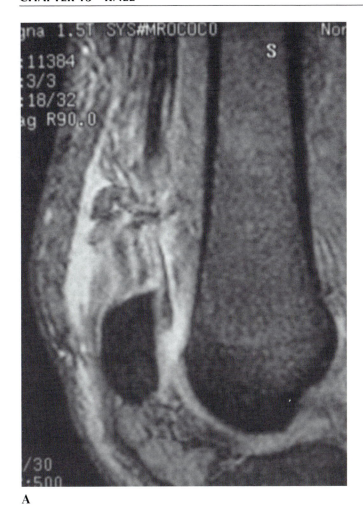

A

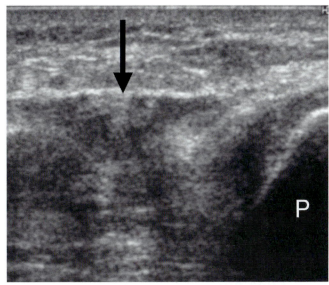

B

C

FIGURE 13-36. Acute quadriceps tendon rupture. *(A)* Sagittal gradient echo image shows close apposition of the disrupted quadriceps tendon. *(B)* Corresponding longitudinal sonogram in extension shows the defect in the anterior aspect of the tendon (arrow). The remainder of the tendon has the appearance of continuity. *(C)* Longitudinal sonogram with the knee flexed shows the hypoechoic gap between the tendon edges, thus confirming the full-thickness nature of this injury. P = patella.

images and longitudinal sonographic images can be used to assess the degree of tendon rupture and retraction. Rupture typically appears as a balled-up and mildly retracted tendon edge with surrounding soft tissue edema and edema or hemorrhage in the tendon gap (Figures 13-34 and 13-35). In cases of non-retracted rupture, it can be difficult to distinguish a non-retracted tendon rupture from a partial tear of the tendon; sonography can be helpful in such cases by imaging the patient in the extended and flexed positions and looking for separation or retraction of the torn tendon edge in the flexed position (Figure 13-36).

The patella can dislocate, usually laterally, as the result of a quick rotational mechanism of injury such as cutting while

running. The patella usually reduces spontaneously, leaving a painful and sore knee anteriorly. MRI is the optimum modality for evaluating this injury, particularly in the axial plane, and shows bone bruises in the medial aspect of the patella and the lateral aspect of the lateral femoral condyle, which occur as the patella relocates itself back into the sulcus of the femoral condyles. There may be associated tearing of the medial retinaculum, manifest as thickening and internal high signal intensity on T_2-weighted images, and associated tear of the distal aspect of the vastus medialis oblique muscle, manifest by feathery high signal intensity within this muscle on T_2-weighted sequences (Figure 13-37).

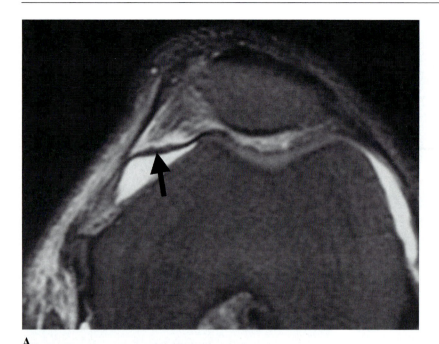

A

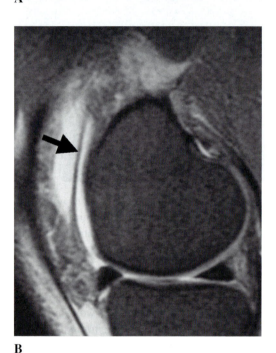

B

FIGURE 13-39. Complete medial plica. *(A)* Axial fat-suppressed T$_2$-weighted image shows the medial plica (arrow) extending from the medial aspect of the joint capsule to the intercondylar region, where it inserts on Hoffa fat pad. *(B)* Sagittal fat-suppressed fast spin echo T$_2$-weighted image of the same patient shows the plica (arrow) inserting on the fat pad.

effusion, or internal derangement of the knee, there is a baseline level of prevalence in the general population. This distended bursa is best appreciated in the axial MR plane or the transverse sonographic plane. With such orientation, the cyst will be comma-shaped, with its neck extending between the tendon of the medial gastrocnemius and the semimembranosus tendon (Figure 13-40). When large, the patient may complain of pain or tightness in the back of the knee. These cysts may become quite large and may track superiorly into the posterior aspect of the thigh or inferiorly into the calf, especially in patients with rheumatoid arthritis. The cysts may leak or rupture, thus exposing the surrounding tissue to irritative synovial fluid, and the patient will complain of severe pain and swelling which mimics

a deep venous thrombosis. These cysts also can cause deep venous thrombosis due to frank compression of the popliteal vein or to rupture or leakage because the irritative synovial fluid can cause a reactive thrombophlebitis.

Two other bursae that occur posteromedially are the pes anserinus and the semimembranosus-tibial collateral ligament bursae. The pes anserinus bursa is between the tendons of the pes anserinus and the distal aspect of the MCL. The semimembranosus-tibial collateral ligament bursa is located along the medial side of the distal aspect of the semimembranosus tendon and should be distinguished from the Baker cyst by the fact that it is medial to the semimembranosus tendon, whereas the Baker cyst is lateral to the semimembranosus

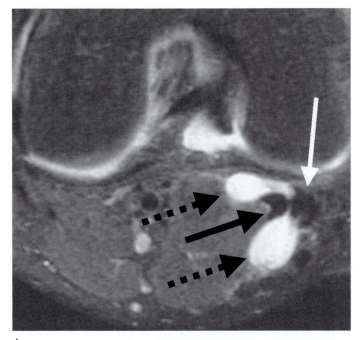

A

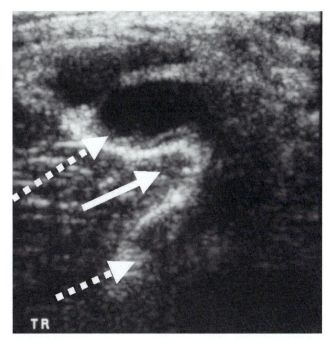

B

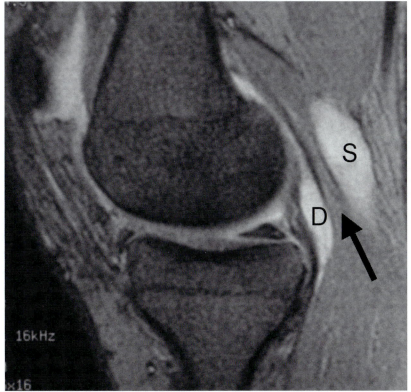

C

FIGURE 13-40. Baker cyst. *(A)* Axial fat-suppressed T_2-weighted magnetic resonance image shows the comma-shape bilobed cyst (dashed arrows) with its neck between the tendon of the medial gastrocnemius muscle (solid black arrow) and the semimembranosus tendon (white arrow). *(B)* Corresponding transverse sonographic image shows the comma-shape hypoechoic Baker cyst (dashed arrows). The tendon of the medial gastrocnemius muscle indents the neck (solid arrow). *(C)* Sagittal gradient echo magnetic resonance image shows the superficial and deep portions of the cyst as they wrap around the medial gastrocnemius tendon (arrow). D = deep cyst portion, S = superficial cyst portion.

tendon, and it should be distinguished from the pes anserinus bursa by the fact that the semimembranosus-tibial collateral ligament bursa is deep to the MCL (Figure 13-41). The Baker cyst, pes anserinus bursa, and semimembranosus-tibial collateral ligament bursa do not communicate with each other.

Two bursae of clinical concern in the anterior aspect of the knee are the prepatellar bursa and the superficial infrapatellar bursa. The prepatellar bursa is anterior to the patella, and

the superficial infrapatellar bursa is anterior to the tibial tubercle and the distal aspect of the patellar tendon. MRI demonstrates these bursae as low signal intensity on T_1-weighted sequences and high signal intensity on T_2-weighted sequences. Similarly, sonography demonstrates these processes as anechoic (Figure 13-42). The prepatellar bursa is also called *housemaid's knee* because, in the days when housemaids used to scrub a floor on their hands and knees, the irritation of the patella rubbing

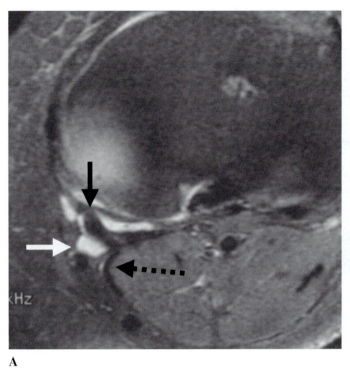

A

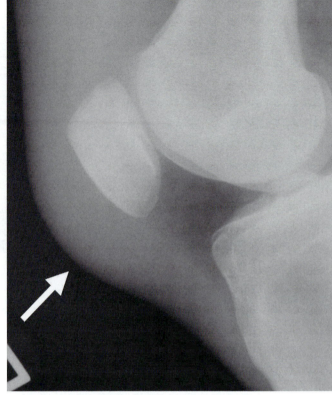

A

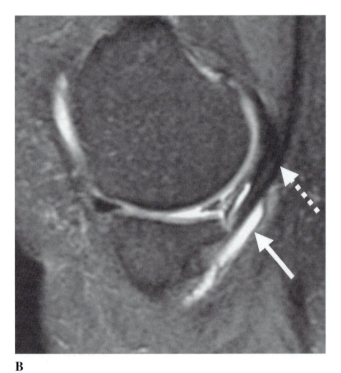

B

FIGURE 13-41. Semimembranosus-tibial collateral ligament bursitis. *(A)* Axial fat-suppressed T$_2$-weighted image shows horseshoe-shape fluid (white arrow) surrounding the semimembranosus tendon (solid black arrow). Note that this fluid is not between the semimembranosus and the tendon of the medial gastrocnemius muscle (dashed black arrow; compare with Figure 13-40). *(B)* Corresponding sagittal fat-suppressed fast spin echo T$_2$-weighted image shows the high signal intensity fluid (solid arrow) wrapping around the distal aspect of the semimembranosus tendon (dashed arrow). Note also the tear of the posterior horn of the medial meniscus.

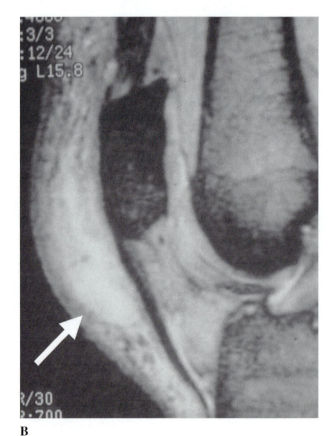

B

FIGURE 13-42. Prepatellar bursitis. *(A)* Lateral radiograph shows marked swelling anterior to the patella (arrow). *(B)* Sagittal gradient echo T$_2$-weighted image shows the high signal intensity inflamed bursa (arrow). *(Continued)*

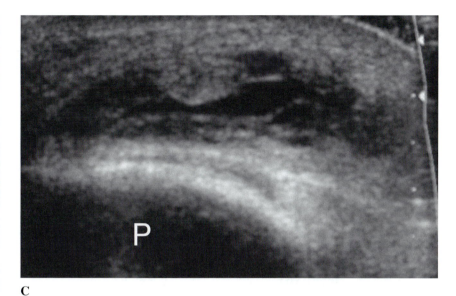

C

FIGURE 13-42. *(continued)* *(C)* Corresponding longitudinal sonogram shows the hypoechoic fluid within the bursa. P = patella.

against the hard surface of the floor would cause inflammation and distention of this bursa. The symptomatic superficial infrapatellar bursa is called *preacher's knee* because this bursa is compressed between the tibial tubercle and the wooden bench on which the preacher kneels.

SUGGESTED READINGS

Bencardino JT, Rosenberg ZS, Brown RR, et al. Traumatic musculotendinous injuries of the knee: diagnosis with MR imaging. *Radiographics*. 2000;20:S103–S120.

Brandsner EA, Riley MA, Berbaum KS, et al. MR imaging of anterior cruciate ligament injury: independent value of primary and secondary signs. *AJR*. 1996;167:121–126.

Chan KK, Resnick, D, Goodwin D, et al. Posteromedial tibial plateau injury including avulsion fracture of the semimembranous tendon insertion site: ancillary sign of anterior cruciate ligament tear at MR imaging. *Radiology*. 1999;211:754–758.

Davis KW, Tuite MJ. MR imaging of the postoperative meniscus of the knee. *Semin Musculoskelet Radiol*. 2002;Mar;6:35–45. Review.

Haims AH, Katz LD, Ruwe PA. MR arthrography of the knee. *Semin Musculoskelet Radiol*. 1998;2:385–396.

Hayes CW, Brigido MK, Jamadar DA, Propeck T. Mechanism-based pattern approach to classification of complex injuries of the knee depicted at MR imaging. *Radiographics*. 2000;20:S121–S134.

Lance E, Deutsch AL, Mink JH. Prior lateral patellar dislocation: MR imaging findings. *Radiology*. 1993;189:905–907.

Lim PS, Schweitzer ME, Bhatia M, et al. Repeat tear of postoperative meniscus: potential MR imaging signs. *Radiology*. 1999;210:183–188.

Magee T, Shapiro M, Rodriguez J, Williams D. MR arthrography of postoperative knee: for which patients is it useful? *Radiology*. 2003;229:159–163.

Miller TT. Sonography of injury of the posterior cruciate ligament of the knee. *Skeletal Radiol*. 2002;31:149–154.

Miller TT, Gladden P, Staron RB, Henry JH, Feldman F. Posterolateral stabilizers of the knee: anatomy and injuries assessed with MR imaging. *AJR*. 1997;169:1641–1647.

Miller TT, Staron RB, Koenigsberg T, Levin TL, Feldman F. MR imaging of Baker cysts: association with internal derangement, effusion, and degenerative arthropathy. *Radiology*. 1996;201:247–250.

Miller TT, Staron RB, Feldman F. Patellar height on sagittal MR imaging of the knee. *AJR*. 1996;167:339–341.

Miller TT, Stein BE, Staron RB, Feldman F. Relationship of the meniscofemoral ligaments of the knee to lateral meniscus tears: magnetic resonance imaging evaluation. *Am J Orthop*. 1998;27:729–732.

Mutschter C, Vande Berg BC, Lecouvet FE, et al. Postoperative meniscus: assessment at dual-detector row spiral CT arthrography of the knee. *Radiology*. 2003;228:635–641.

Pao DG. The lateral femoral notch sign. *Radiology*. 2001;219:800–801.

Recht MP, Kramer J. MR imaging of the postoperative knee: a pictorial essay. *Radiographics*. 2002;22:765–774. Review.

Recondo JA, Salvador E, Villanua JA, et al. Lateral stabilizing structures of the knee: functional anatomy and injuries assessed with MR imaging. *Radiographics*. 2000;20:S91–S102.

Robertson PL, Schweitzer ME, Bartolozzi AR, et al. Anterior cruciate ligament tears: evaluation of multiple signs with MR imaging. *Radiology*. 1994;193:829–834.

Rose PM, Demlow TA, Szumowski J, et al. Chondromalacia patellae: fat-suppressed MR imaging. *Radiology*. 1994;193:437–440.

Sanders TG, Medynski MA, Feller JF, et al. Bone contusion patterns of the knee at mr imaging: footprint of the mechanism of injury. *Radiographics*. 2000;20:S135–S151.

Sciulli RL, Boutin RD, Brown RR, et al. Evaluation of the postoperative meniscus of the knee: a study comparing conventional arthrography, conventional MR imaging, MR arthrography with iodinated contrast material, and MR arthrography with gadolinium-based contrast material. *Skeletal Radiol*. 1999;28:508–514.

Singson RD, Feldman F, Staron RB, et al. MR imaging of displaced bucket-handle tear of the medial meniscus. *AJR*. 1991;156:121–124.

Staron RB, Haramati N, Feldman F, et al. O'Donoghue's triad: magnetic resonance imaging evidence. *Skeletal Radiol*. 1994;23:633–636.

Tuckman GA, Miller WJ, Remo JW, et al. Radial tears of the menisci: MR findings. *AJR*. 1994;163:395–400.

Weber WN, Neumann CH, Barakos JA, et al. Lateral tibial rim (Segond) fractures: MR imaging characteristics. *Radiology*. 1991;180:731–734.

Yu JS, Petersilge C, Sartoris DJ, et al. MR imaging of injuries of the extensor mechanism of the knee. *Radiology*. 1994;14:541–552.

CHAPTER 14

ANKLE AND FOOT

MARK E. SCHWEITZER

Foot and ankle pain is a common indication for imaging and can be due to acute injury or chronic overuse and degeneration of any of the numerous tendons and ligaments about the ankle and hindfoot and to osseous injuries.

ANATOMY

There are four sets of tendons and three sets of ligaments about the ankle.

Tendons

The Achilles tendon is the strongest tendon and the second longest tendon on the body, after the plantaris. The Achilles is made up of the tendons of the two heads of the gastrocnemius muscle, and it inserts on the posteromedial aspect of the calcaneus. The anterior and posterior surfaces of the tendon should be flat, and the tendon should gently taper distally; on sagittal magnetic resonance (MR) images, the tendon is uniformly low signal intensity on all pulse sequences and has a fibrillar echogenic appearance on longitudinal sonographic images (Figure 14-1). The retrocalcaneal bursa, not usually visible unless it is swollen, is located between the Achilles tendon and the posterior tuberosity of the calcaneus and acts to protect the deep surface of the Achilles from irritation by the posterior tuberosity. The Achilles tendon lacks a surrounding sheath but does have a thin paratenon. The tendon of the soleus muscle, which is deep to the gastrocnemii, inserts onto the Achilles at its musculotendinous junction.

The flexor tendon group is located medially and is comprised of the posterior tibial tendon (PTT), the flexor digitorum longus tendon, and the flexor hallucis longus tendon (Figure 14-2). The posterior tibial tendon is the most anterior of the three and is normally about twice as large as the immediately adjacent flexor digitorum longus tendon. All three tendons have their own sheaths.

The two peroneal tendons are located laterally and are flexors and everters of the foot (see Fig. 14-2). The peroneus longus and brevis tendons share a common tendon sheath proximally and then are invested in their own sheaths at the level of the calcaneus, at which level they divide, with the brevis continuing on the lateral side to insert on the base of the fifth metatarsal bone and the longus turning medially under the cuboid bone to insert on the first metatarsal shaft.

The extensor tendon group contains the counterparts to the flexors, namely the anterior tibial, extensor hallucis longus, and extensor digitorum tendons (see Fig. 14-2).

Ligaments

Three sets of ligaments stabilize the ankle joint: the syndesmotic ligaments, lateral ligament complex, and the deltoid ligament. Although there are many of them and the names sound confusing, the ligaments are simply named for their bony attachments and whether they are anterior or posterior.

The syndesmotic ligaments bind the distal tibia and fibula together, so that these two bones form a sturdy socket into which sits the talus. There is an anterior tibiofibular ligament, which is thin and short, and a thicker and longer posterior tibiofibular ligament (Figure 14-3). The interosseous membrane also ties the tibia and fibula together, but its distal edge ends about 6 cm proximal to the ankle joint.

The lateral ligament complex is comprised of the anterior and posterior talofibular ligaments and the intervening calcaneofibular ligament (Figure 14-4). The anterior and posterior talofibular ligaments are usually well seen on routine axial MR images, but the calcaneofibular ligament is the thinnest of the three and has an oblique course and is therefore sometimes not routinely seen.

The deltoid ligament is located medially and is actually comprised of four separate components: the anterior and posterior tibiotalar ligaments, which are deep, and the tibiocalcaneal and tibionavicular ligaments, which are superficial. There also may be a thin ligamentous connection between the tibia and the spring ligament, which some people consider part of the deltoid complex. The tibiotalar and tibiocalcaneal components are usually well seen on routine coronal MR images (Figure 14-5).

Injury

ACHILLES TENDON. Achilles tendon disorders are the most common running injury, and overuse is the mechanism of pathology. Such pathology typically involves the Achilles 3 to 5 cm from its calcaneal insertion, and can be thought of as a sequence of abnormalities that build on each other. As with most tendons anywhere in the body, first there are micro-tears of its collagen fibrils due to overuse. The tendon tries to heal these micro-tears but cannot make new collagen. Instead, it heals itself with any of

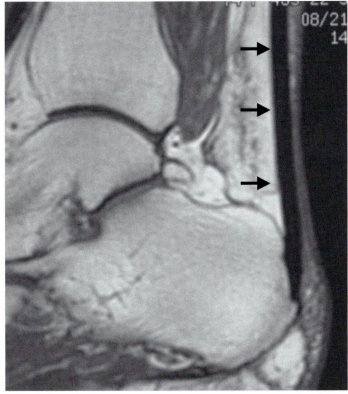

A

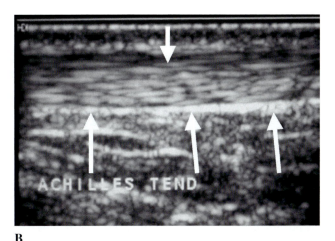

B

FIGURE 14-1. Normal Achilles tendon. *(A)* Sagittal T$_1$-weighted magnetic resonance image shows a uniformly low signal intensity Achilles tendon (arrows) with uniform thickness. *(B)* Longitudinal sonogram shows the "snake-skin" appearance of the multiple echogenic interfaces of the collagen fibers. The tendon is uniformly thick (arrows).

several histologic changes that constitute degeneration and that may further weaken the tendon and predispose it to macro-tear.

There are four types of degeneration: hypoxic, mucoid, calcific or ossific, and lipoid. Hypoxic degeneration can alter the size and shape of the tendon, usually has normal signal intensity, is symptomatic, and may or may not lead to a tear. In mucoid degeneration, the signal intensity of the tendon is abnormal; it is often asymptomatic but can lead to tears. Lipoid is age related and does not lead to tears. Calcific or ossific degeneration may or may not alter the size and shape of the tendon, may or may not be symptomatic, but usually does not lead to tears. Although these histologic changes are degenerative and not inflammatory, they are often described clinically as *tendinitis*.

Chronic hypoxic Achilles tendonitis appears on sagittal MR images or longitudinal sonographic images as tendon thickening, with an outwardly bulging anterior margin or as fusiform thickening (Figure 14-6). This stage of chronic Achilles tendonitis, with a thickened distal tendon, can be mimicked by hypercholesterolemia and occasionally by rheumatologic conditions; in the latter two conditions, the thickening will be less focal and more dramatic.

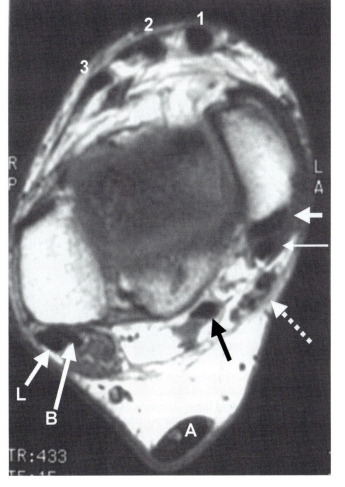

FIGURE 14-2. Normal anatomy. The flexor tendons are composed of the posterior tibial tendon (short white arrow), the flexor digitorum (thin long white arrow), and the flexor hallucis longus (black arrow). The posterior tibial artery nerve and veins are marked by the dashed white arrow. The peroneal tendons are composed of the longus laterally and the more medial brevis. The extensor tendons are composed of the anterior tibial tendon (1), the extensor hallucis longus (2), and the extensor digitorum longus tendon (3). The Achilles tendon is posterior. A = Achilles tendon, B = brevis, L = longus.

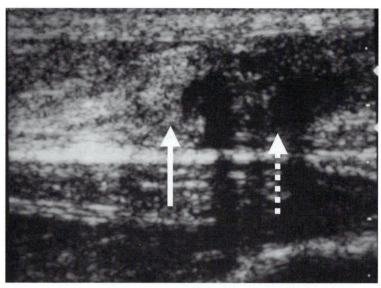

B

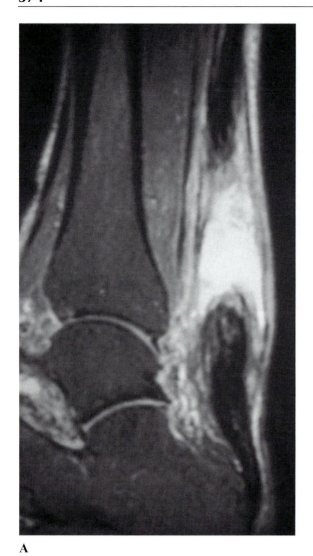

A

FIGURE 14-8.   Rupture of the Achilles tendon. *(A)* Sagittal fat-suppressed fast spin echo T$_2$-weighted image shows the torn and retracted edges, with high signal intensity edema and hemorrhage within the large gap. *(B)* Corresponding longitudinal sonogram shows the torn proximal tendon edge (solid arrow), with refractive shadowing of its edge, and heterogeneous hypoechoic edema and hemorrhage in the gap (dashed arrow).

but such rupture is unusual. Instead, the tendon usually is just severely thinned, with a thread of residual tendon present. More common than rupture is interstitial tearing longitudinally within the tendon (Figure 14-11).

Tendinosis and tenosynovitis are common findings in patients with clinical "tendinitis." The tendinosis is the same type of degeneration that occurs in the Achilles and other tendons. The PTT may be thickened and have internal signal heterogeneity on MRI and internal hypoechogenicity on sonography (Figure 14-12). The MR criterion for tenosynovitis of the PTT is synovial fluid extending to the tendon insertion on the navicular or measuring thicker than 1 mm at any location. The tenosynovitis also can be appreciated sonographically as anechoic fluid surrounding the tendon.

Associated secondary findings of PTT dysfunction are unroofing of the talus and plantar flexion of the talus. Unroofing the talus is appreciated on axial images when the top of the navicular covers less than 85% of the articular aspect of the talus. Plantar flexion of the talus is described on sagittal images by a line drawn along the long axis of the talus lying plantar to the navicular; clinically, the patient may exhibit a flat-foot deformity.

Normal anatomic variations of the navicular bone at the site of posterior tibial tendon insertion also may predispose to PTT

disorders due to altered insertional biomechanics and stress or development of adventitial bursitis. A hypertrophied medial navicular tubercle is termed a *cornuate*, or type III, navicular and can predispose to tendon tear or overlying adventitial bursitis. A type II accessory navicular is a large sesamoid connected to the navicular by a synchondrosis. The PTT inserts onto the accessory navicular, which may create stress across the synchondrosis, and is demonstrated on MR images as marrow edema in the navicular and accessory bones (Figure 14-13).

PERONEAL TENDONS

As with the PTT, peroneal tendinitis is uncommon, but, when it occurs, it usually affects the peroneus brevis rather than the longus. Patients with acute pain usually have tenosynovitis. Peroneal synovitis is usually mechanical in origin. Because of the shared tendon sheath, high signal intensity fluid on MRI or anechoic fluid on sonography is seen around both tendons.

Peroneal subluxation usually is a consequence of repetitive ankle sprains because the peroneal tendons are important lateral stabilizers of the ankle. Normally, the two tendons are located in the shallow peroneal groove of the posterior aspect of

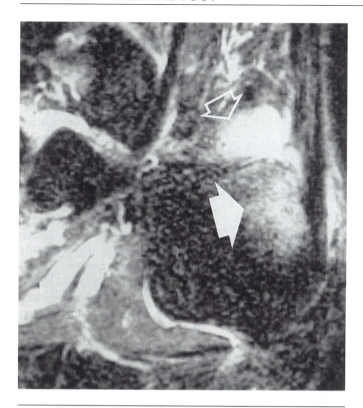

FIGURE 14-9. Haglund syndrome. Sagittal T$_2$-weighted fat-suppressed sequence shows an enlarged retrocalcaneal bursa (open arrow), a prominent posterior tuberosity of the calcaneus with internal marrow edema (solid arrow), thickening and heterogeneity of the distal Achilles tendon consistent with chronic degeneration with a superimposed partial tear of its deep surface, and high signal intensity posterior to the Achilles tendon representing adventitial retro-Achilles bursitis.

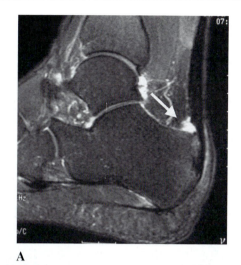

A

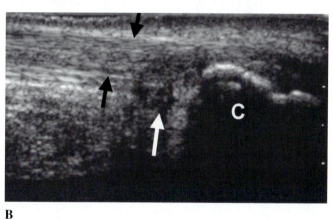

B

FIGURE 14-10. Insertional changes in a runner with pain. *(A)* Sagittal fat-suppressed T$_2$-weighted image shows a proximally thickened and distally thinned Achilles tendon. There is distention of the retrocalcaneal bursa (arrow). *(B)* Corresponding longitudinal sonogram shows the thickened distal Achilles tendon (black arrows), the heterogenous distended retrocalcaneal bursa (white arrow), and the calcaneal tuberosity. C = calcaneal tuberosity.

the lateral malleolus and are held in place by the peroneal retinaculum. Subluxation should be assessed on axial images at the level of the malleolus (Figure 14-14) because, proximally, the peroneal tendons are normally physiologically positioned somewhat laterally. Frank dislocation of the tendons often is related to calcaneal fracture. A subtle area of marrow edema may be seen at the lateral aspect of the distal fibula after dislocations, likely secondary to retinacular avulsion. Sonography can dynamically assess recurrent subluxation when using transverse scanning during plantar and dorsiflexion.

Repetitive peroneal subluxation will lead to *peroneal brevis splits syndrome*, in which the peroneal brevis develops a longitudinal tear that splits the brevis in half (Figure 14-15). Brevis splits syndrome is the most common type of peroneal tear. Other peroneal tears more commonly involve the longus rather than the brevis. These other tears characteristically occur at the level of the calcaneocuboid joint, where the longus changes direction.

Other Tendons

Flexor hallucis tendon abnormalities, excluding impingement by the os trigonum, are uncommon but can be seen in kicking athletes and ballet dancers. Anterior tibialis tendon disorders also are rare and usually do not present with much clinical

dysfunction. Synovitis of any extensor tendon should raise the possibility of rheumatoid arthritis, especially if combined with posterior tibial tendon abnormalities.

Ankle Sprains

A "twisted" ankle is the most common reason for orthopedic visits to emergency rooms, and 85% of these are inversion injuries. The anterior talofibular ligament is always affected, accompanied by injury of the calcaneofibular ligament in more severe twists and by injury of the posterior talofibular ligament in the most severe instances. The anterior talofibular ligament is best assessed on axial MR images or sonographic images oriented parallel to the expected course of the ligament. Acute severe ankle sprains show focal discontinuity or absence of the ligament, with edema in the gap (Figure 14-16), whereas milder sprains show edema around the margins of a dysmorphic ligament (Figure 14-17). In the setting of an acute inversion injury,

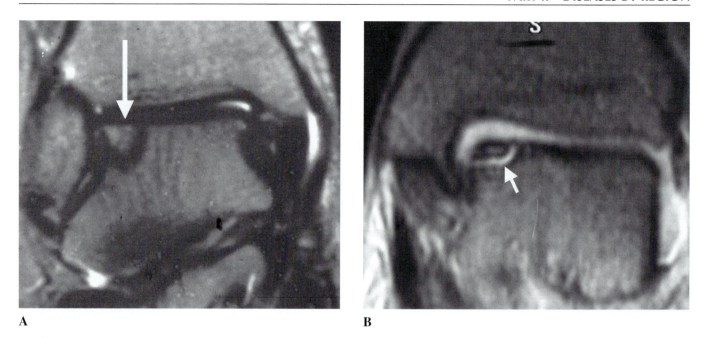

A   B

FIGURE 14-23.   Osteochondral injury of the talus. *(A)* Coronal fat-suppressed fast spin echo T_2-weighted sequence shows an osteochondral fragment (arrow). Low signal intensity surrounds it, indicating that this is a stable fracture. *(B)* Coronal fat-suppressed fast spin echo T_2-weighted sequence in a different patient shows an osteochondral fragment with high signal intensity fluid surrounding its base (arrow), indicating that it is unstable.

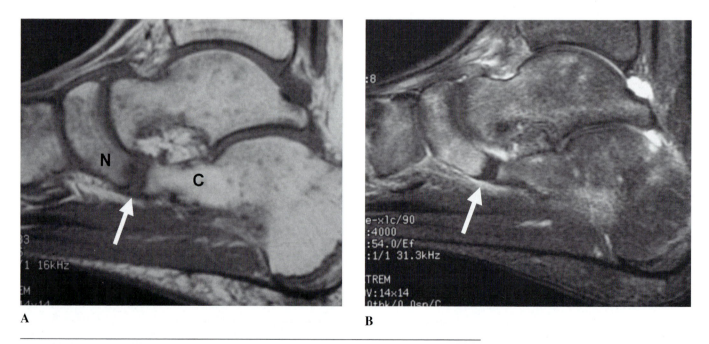

A   B

FIGURE 14-24.   Fibrous calcaneonavicular coalition. *(A)* Sagittal T_1-weighted magnetic resonance image and *(B)* corresponding fat-suppressed fast spin echo T_2-weighted magnetic resonance image show elongated processes of the calcaneus and navicular connected by a fibrous coalition that is low signal intensity on both pulse sequences (arrow). The surrounding high signal intensity soft tissue edema and navicular marrow edema on the fat-suppressed sequence suggests stress across this syndesmosis. C = calcaneus, N = navicular.

Fractures

Occult fractures are common in the ankle and most often involve the talus and navicular (Figure 14-22). Stress fractures also can be seen in the calcaneus, cuboid, talus, and the navicular, locations that are difficult to diagnose by conventional radiography. In particular, talar and navicular stress fractures are typically quite difficult to diagnose clinically.

Osteochondritis dissecans is discussed more fully in Chapter 2, but a few points specific to the ankle are in order. Medial talar dome injuries are more common than lateral ones and are associated more commonly with repetitive injuries, whereas lateral dome lesions usually are associated with an acute episode of trauma. The medial talar dome injuries tend to have a round shape, whereas lateral talar dome injuries are more flat ("wafer" shape). The medial lesions are posterior to the midline of the talus, whereas the lateral lesions occur about the midline of the talus or just anterior to it (Figure 14-23). The mechanism of lateral dome injury is inversion of the hindfoot with concurrent dorsiflexion of the foot, whereas that of medial dome injury is hindfoot inversion with plantar flexion.

Reflex Sympathetic Dystrophy

Reflex sympathetic dystrophy has many etiologic factors including myocardial infarction and cerebrovascular accidents but the most common is soft tissue or bone injury. The clinical

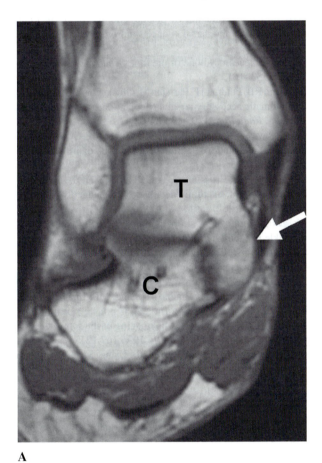

A

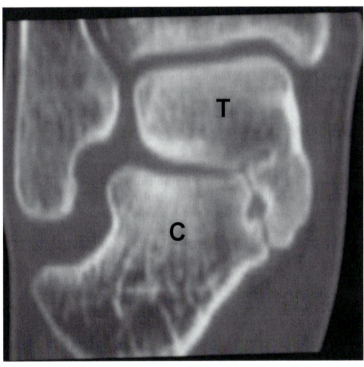

B

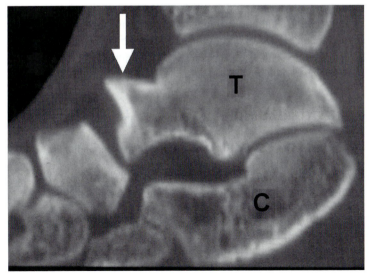

C

FIGURE 14-25. Subtalar coalition. *(A)* Coronal T_1-weighted magnetic resonance image shows a large bony bridge (arrow) connecting the talus to the calcaneus. There is a thin fibrous cleft between the calcaneus and the enlarged bony bridge. *(B)* Corresponding coronal reformatted CT image shows the large bony bridge and the intervening cleft. *(C)* Sagittally reformatted image of this same patient shows a large dorsal beak (arrow) arising from the neck of the talus. C = calcaneus, T = talus.

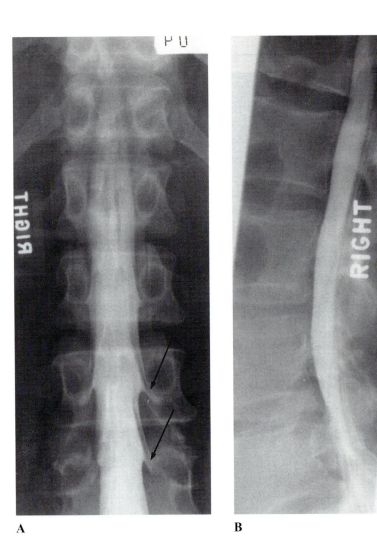

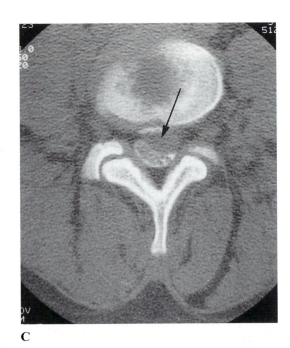

C

FIGURE 15-11. Conventional and computed tomographic myelography. *(A)* Anteroposterior view of a normal lumbar myelogram. The nerve roots appear as thin, linear filling defects within the contrast filled thecal sac. Arrows point to the root sleeves within the neural foramina. *(B)* Normal lateral myelogram. The ventral surface of the contrast-filled thecal sac has a smooth contour. *(C)* Axial computed tomographic myelogram of a different patient shows a herniated disc (arrow) indenting the left anterolateral aspect of the thecal sac.

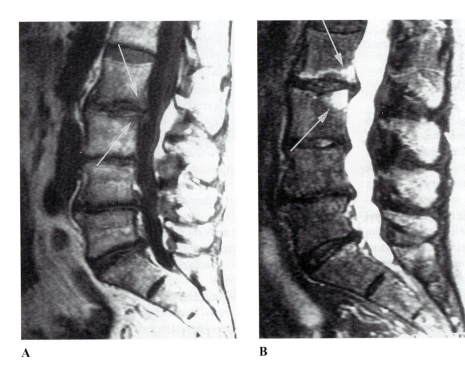

A   B

FIGURE 15-12. Modic type 1 changes. *(A)* Sagittal T_1-weighted magnetic resonance image shows decreased signal intensity in the inferior endplate of L_2 and superior endplate of L_3 (arrows). *(B)* Corresponding T_2-weighted magnetic resonance image shows high signal intensity (arrows). Also note the degenerated desiccated discs at all visible levels as demonstrated by loss of a normal high signal intensity.

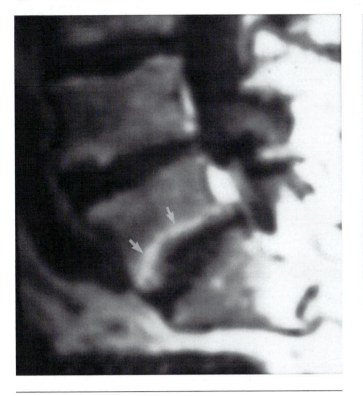

FIGURE 15-13. Sagittal T$_1$-weighted magnetic resonance image shows Modic type 2 fatty endplate change demonstrated as high signal intensity along the inferior endplate of L$_5$ (arrows).

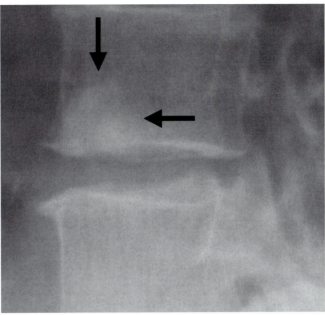

FIGURE 15-14. Lateral radiograph shows hemispherical discogenic sclerosis (arrows). Note that it abuts the inferior endplate and that there is degenerative osteophyte formation at this disc level.

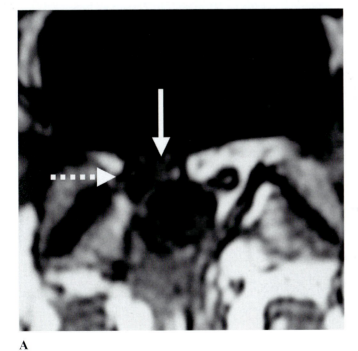

A

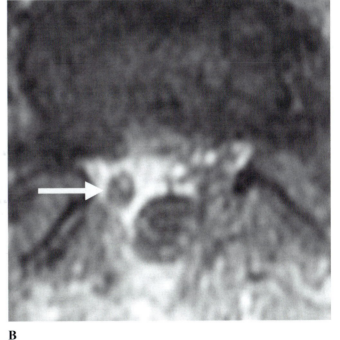

B

FIGURE 15-15. Postoperative scar. (A) Axial T$_1$-weighted magnetic resonance image shows low signal intensity material in the right paracentral region of the epidural space (solid arrow) abutting the nerve (dashed arrow). (B) Corresponding fat-suppressed T$_1$-weighted magnetic resonance image after intravenous administration of contrast shows uniform enhancement of the scar tissue. Note that it encases the nerve (arrow) rather than compressing or deforming it.

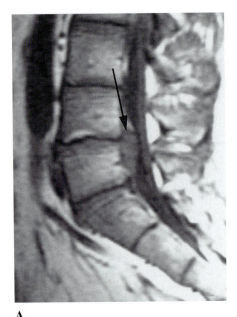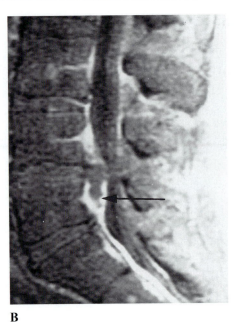

A　　　　　　　　　　　　　　B

FIGURE 15-16. Recurrent disc herniation. *(A)* Sagittal T_1-weighted magnetic resonance image. *(B)* Fat-suppressed T_1-weighted image after intravenous contrast shows circumferential peripheral enhancement of an extruded disc (arrows).

In contrast, a recurrent or residual disc herniation has mass effect, is typically focal, and has well-defined borders (Figure 15-16). It usually does not enhance, although, occasionally, the periphery may enhance due to invagination of small vessels along its surface. Further, if the disc fragment is small, the entire fragment may enhance, and such enhancement sometimes may be difficult to distinguish from focal scar.

INTRAVERTEBRAL DISC HERNIATIONS

Intravertebral disc herniations may result in a limbus vertebra, Schmorl nodes, and Scheuermann disease.

The limbus vertebra occurs before skeletal maturity and is caused by an intravertebral disc herniation, which separates a fragment of the ring apophysis from the rest of the vertebra. This remnant of the ring apophysis will continue to grow separately from the rest of the vertebral body. The limbus vertebra usually is found incidentally on lateral radiographs in adults and appears as a triangular piece of bone adjacent to the blunted corner of the vertebral body. The pieces often do not precisely fit together because they have been growing separately from each other (Figure 15-17). Most limbus vertebrae are asymptomatic and usually occur in the lumbar spine, especially at L_4.

Schmorl nodes are extrusions of nuclear material through the endplate into the vertebral body. They can occur at any time in life but typically occur before complete skeletal maturity.

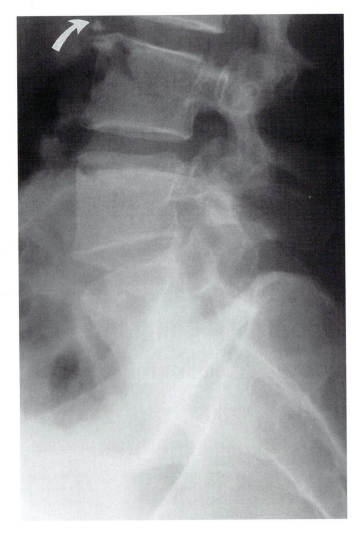

FIGURE 15-17. Lateral radiograph shows small limbus vertebra (arrow).

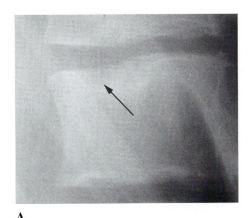

A

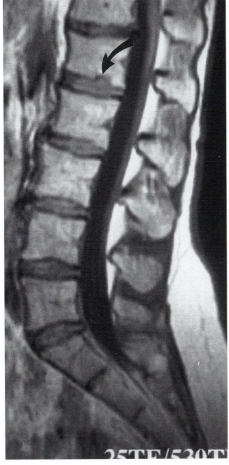

B

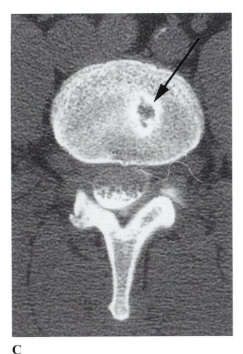

C

FIGURE 15-18. Schmorl node. *(A)* Lateral radiograph of the lumbar spine shows the small indentation in the superior endplate (arrow). *(B)* Sagittal T_1-weighted magnetic resonance image of a different patient demonstrates the central herniation of disc material through the inferior endplate of L_1 (curved arrow). *(C)* Axial computed tomographic image demonstrates Schmorl node (arrow) with a surrounding sclerotic rim.

changes also can occur in the surrounding bone but are chronic findings.

Scheuermann disease (*juvenile kyphosis* or *multiple Schmorl nodes*) is the most frequent cause of kyphosis in adolescents and teenagers, being present in 4 to 10% of the population. Patients with Scheuermann disease may complain of intermittent low back pain that may radiate into the lower extremities. This pain is increased with activity and ameliorated by rest.

Scheuermann disease is diagnosed on erect lateral radiographs, and the criteria are the presence of 3 or more adjacent vertebral bodies, with each wedged 5°, and a thoracic kyphosis of greater than 40° (see Chapter 2). There also is irregularity of the vertebral endplates and multiple Schmorl node formation. Scheuermann disease is likely due to genetic weakness of the vertebral endplates, which predisposes to disc invagination, but overuse and mechanical factors may contribute.

Scheuermann disease is divided into thoracic and lumbar types. Thoracic Scheuermann disease is more common, and the apex of the kyphosis is between T_7 and T_9. Lumbar Scheuermann disease is less common; it has similar radiographic manifestations but is localized between T_{10} and L_4.

NEUROPATHIC SPINE

Neuropathic spine, also known as *Charcot spine*, is a destructive process that predominantly affects the intervertebral disc spaces, but the adjoining vertebral bodies and facet joints are also affected to a lesser degree. Although neuropathic disease is much more common in the extremities than in the spine, it is not infrequent in the spine and may mimic infection radiographically and clinically. It is seen most commonly in the fifth and sixth decades, and most patients with neuropathic spine do not have neuropathy elsewhere. The most common causes are traumatic paralysis and diabetes, but syringomyelia and tabes dorsalis may lead to it. Because the condition may be painless, it may not be clinically apparent until radiographs demonstrate marked disc destruction.

Schmorl nodes also may be seen associated with any process that weakens the endplates such as hyperparathyroidism, osteoporosis, infection, focal trauma, or neoplasms. The most common cause in adults in osteoporosis.

Schmorl nodes occur mostly in the thoracic and lumbar spine, and are quite common. They are usually asymptomatic and may be seen on lateral radiographs but are best appreciated on sagittal MR images due to the tomographic nature of the modality (Figure 15-18). Marrow edema around the Schmorl node suggests an acute herniation; Modic-type

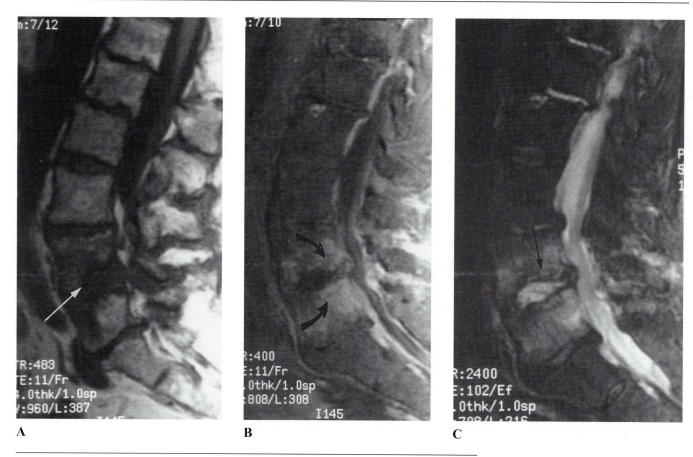

FIGURE 15-19.   Neuropathic spine. *(A)* Sagittal T_1-weighted magnetic resonance image shows decreased signal intensity at L_4-L_5 (arrow). *(B)* This region demonstrates enhancement (curved arrows) after contrast administration on this fat-suppressed T_1-weighted image. Note the lack of enhancement of the intervertebral disc. *(C)* Corresponding T_2-weighted magnetic resonance image shows increased signal intensity in the vertebral bodies and in the intervertebral disc (straight arrow). Note that this appearance is nearly identical to that of infection, but the lack of contrast enhancement of the disc mitigates against infection.

The disease usually is limited to one vertebral segment, but sometimes up to three segments can be involved. The appearance is that of "osteoarthritis with a vengeance," with large hypertrophic spur formation and extensive lysis of the adjacent disc spaces. On cross-sectional modalities, there is often the appearance of a completely disorganized spinal segment, which may look like a chronic or partly treated infection. A large fluid collection or pseudoabscess is often present in the paradoxically widened disc space, making the differentiation from infection even more difficult. However, when low signal intensity is present on T_2 images, infection can be excluded (Figure 15-19).

Vacuum phenomena are frequent in the neuropathic spine and are the most helpful differentiator of neuropathic spine from infection (the inflammatory edema and exudate of infection fill any gas-occupied space in the disc). Facet involvement is another discriminator, being relatively more common in neuropathic disease. Marked destruction or disorganization of the spinal segment also is unusual for infection and suggests neuropathic change.

SPONDYLOLISTHESIS AND SPONDYLOLYSIS

Spondylolisthesis is translation or "slippage" of one vertebral body with respect to the subjacent vertebra anteriorly, termed *anterolisthesis*, or posteriorly, termed *retrolisthesis*. The two most common types are *degenerative*, due mostly to facet joint degeneration, and *isthmic*, due to lysis of the pars interarticularis bilaterally. The amount of listhesis is graded by quartile percentages of the AP diameter of the vertebral body: grade I is up to 25% of the diameter, grade II is up to 50%, grade III is up to 75%, and grade IV is greater than 75%. Degenerative listhesis usually is not greater than grade II, whereas isthmic listhesis may allow complete translocation of the vertebra, but the lysis must be bilateral for any listhesis to occur. Complete translocation is rare, but the L_5 vertebra is affected most often and gives rise to the "Napoleon's hat" sign on AP radiographs because the displaced L_5 vertebra tilts into the x-ray beam and looks like the French emperor's hat (Figure 15-20).

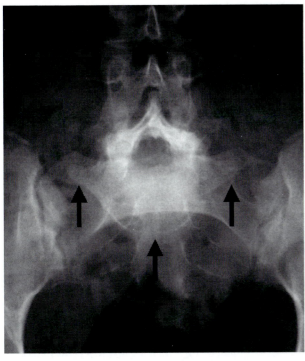

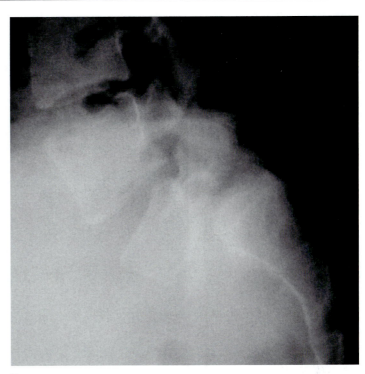

A   B

FIGURE 15-20. Napoleon's hat sign. *(A)* Anteroposterior radiograph shows the 3-cornered hat configuration of the slipped and tilted L_5 vertebral body (arrows). *(B)* Lateral radiograph shows grade IV spondylolisthesis.

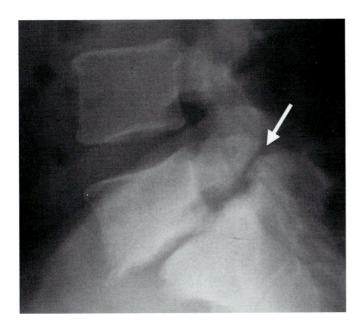

FIGURE 15-21. Lateral radiograph shows bilateral spondylolysis manifest as lucency in the region of the pars (arrow). There is an associated grade II spondylolisthesis.

Spondylolysis (the so-called pars defect) is an overuse stress fracture of the pars interarticularis of the lumbar spine, typically at L_5 or L_4. The usual clinical scenario is the teenage football player or gymnast with focal low back pain because the chronic hyperextension performed during these sports puts stress across the pars. Pars defects are not present at birth, although there is genetic predisposition to their development in certain populations, such as Eskimos. Much less commonly, the pars defect can occur in conditions of bone weakening such as Paget disease or osteogenesis imperfecta. Rarely, the pars is dysplastic; although there is no defect, there is spondylolisthesis because of the abnormal morphology.

Bilateral pars defects can be seen on routine lateral radiographs as radiolucency (Figure 15-21), but a unilateral pars defect may not be appreciated on this view due to overlap by the contralateral intact side. To assess for unilateral lysis, oblique views are used, and the posterior elements have been likened to a "scotty dog" on oblique radiographs, with the transverse process being the nose, the pedicle being the face, the superior articular facet being the ears, the pars being the neck, the inferior facet being the legs, and the lamina being the body. Lysis appears as a linear lucency across the neck of the scotty dog (Figure 15-22). Radiographs have two disadvantages: they do not demonstrate an abnormality until there is frank lysis and cannot determine whether the stress is ongoing even with radiographic evidence of lysis.

MRI is the modality of choice for evaluating suspected pars injury and is best appreciated in the sagittal plane although

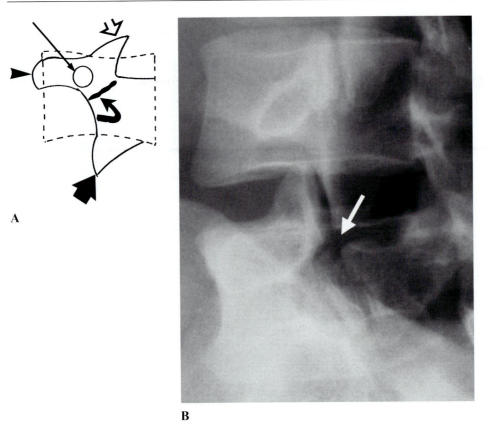

A

B

it is sometimes subtle. Stress reaction without frank fracture is demonstrated as marrow edema in the pars on fat-suppressed T_2-weighted imaging (Figure 15-23), whereas frank lysis shows an actual break across the pars. Persistent marrow edema across the lysis in a symptomatic patient suggests ongoing stress and instability in that region, whereas a well-corticated lysis without associated edema is chronic and asymptomatic (Figure 15-24). MRI is preferable to bone scan for the evaluation of these injuries because it provides the anatomic resolution to differentiate stress reaction from frank lysis that bone scan cannot. Similarly, MRI is preferable to CT, because CT can demonstrate the lysis but cannot demonstrate the symptomatic stress reaction that occurs before lysis (Figure 15-25).

FIGURE 15-22.   Spondylolysis. *(A)* Diagrammatic representation of a right posterior oblique view of a lumbar vertebra demonstrating the "scotty dog" appearance. The "scotty dog" is formed by the posterior elements of the side to which the patient is obliqued, ie, a right posterior oblique view demonstrates the right posterior elements. The break in the pars interarticularis corresponds to the dog's collar (curved black arrow), the inferior articular facet corresponds to the front leg (short solid arrow), the superior articular facet is represented by the ear (open arrow), the pedicle corresponds to the eye (long thin arrow), and the transverse process corresponds to the nose (arrowhead). *[A] modified with permission from Alam F, Moss GG, Schweitzer ME. Imaging of degenerative disc disease of the lumbar spine and related conditions. Semin Spine Surg. 1999;2:76–96). (B)* Right posterior oblique view shows the lucent lysis (arrow). Note the normal "scotty dog" at the level above.

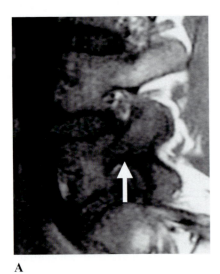

A

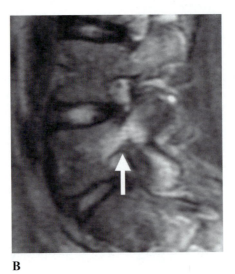

B

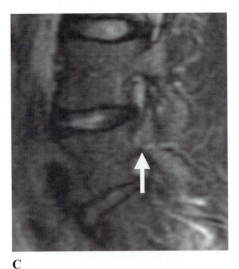

C

FIGURE 15-23.   Stress reaction across the pars. *(A)* Sagittal T_1-weighted magnetic resonance image shows low signal intensity edema (arrow) in the pedicle and intact pars. *(B)* Sagittal fat-suppressed T_2-weighted magnetic resonance image of the same patient shows high signal marrow edema (arrow) in the pedicle and pars. *(C)* Sagittal fat-suppressed T_2-weighted magnetic resonance image of the asymptomatic contralateral side of the same patient shows normal marrow signal (arrow).

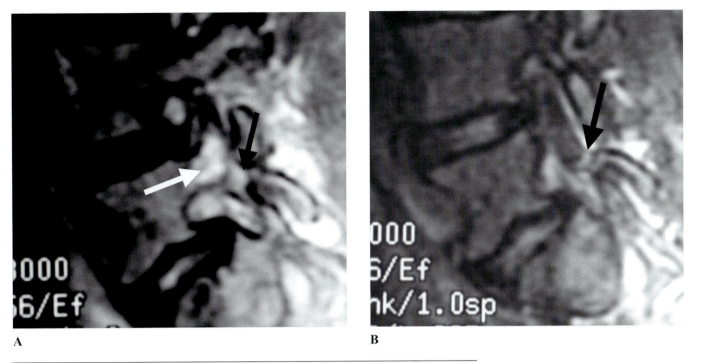

A B

FIGURE 15-24. Acute and chronic spondylolyses. *(A)* Sagittal fat-suppressed T$_2$-weighted magnetic resonance image shows a frank lysis (black arrow) with surrounding marrow edema (white arrow), indicating that it is an acute process. *(B)* Sagittal fat-suppressed T$_2$-weighted magnetic resonance image of a different patient shows the lysis (arrow) but without surrounding marrow edema, indicating that it is a chronic process.

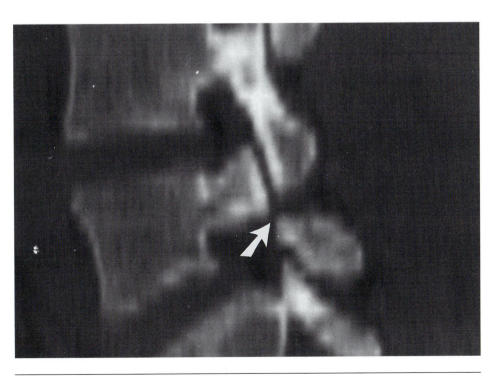

FIGURE 15-25. Sagittal reconstructed computed tomographic image shows the pars defect (arrow). *(Modified with permission from Alam F, Moss GG, Schweitzer ME. Imaging of degenerative disc disease of the lumbar spine and related conditions. Semin Spine Surg. 1999;2:76–96).*

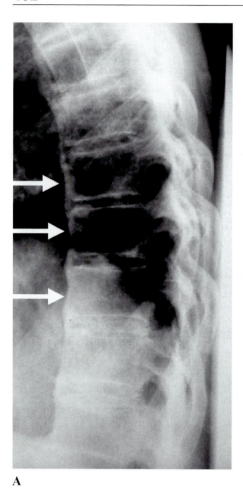

A

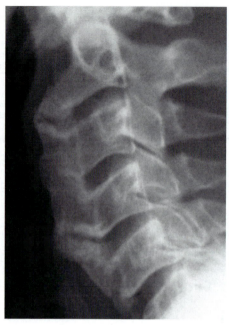

B

FIGURE 15-26.   Two patients with diffuse idiopathic skeletal hyperostosis of the spine. *(A)* Lateral radiograph of the thoracic spine shows flowing ossification of the anterior longitudinal ligament (arrow), which bridges more than 4 disc spaces. Note the lucency between the ossified ligament and the endplates. Note also that the disc spaces are preserved. *(B)* Lateral radiograph of the cervical spine of a different patient shows marked thickening of the anterior longitudinal ligament. The disc spaces are normal, and four vertebrae are involved, excluding degenerative disc disease. This patient complained of dysphagia, which was caused by the ossified ligament compressing the hypopharynx.

LIGAMENT OSSIFICATION

Diffuse Idiopathic Skeletal Hyperostosis

Diffuse idiopathic skeletal hyperostosis (DISH; or *Forestier disease*) is a bone-forming enthesopathy in which there is ossification of ligamentous and tendinous attachments, most often involving the spine and pelvis. It is present in approximately 8% of men and 4% of women, typically in middle to old age.

In the spine, DISH usually affects the anterior longitudinal ligament, most commonly in the cervical region, followed by the thoracic and lumbar regions. The affected anterior longitudinal ligament has the appearance of thick, flowing ossification along the anterior aspect of the spine and crossing the disc spaces. Occasionally, a lucency may be seen between the ossified ligament and the corners of the vertebral bodies, reflecting the fact that the anterior longitudinal ligament attaches to the central portion of the vertebral body and not to the endplates. Involvement is predominantly on the right side, possibly because aortic

pulsation inhibits formation along the left side. Patients with DISH have normal mineralization of the bones.

The criteria for DISH, based on lateral radiographs, are *(a)* the presence of flowing ossification anteriorly involving at least four contiguous vertebral bodies (this excludes spondylosis deformans as a mimicker), *(b)* the preservation of disc space height and the lack of degenerative disc disease (this excludes intervertebral osteochondrosis as a mimicker), and *(c)* the absence of apophyseal joint or sacroiliac joint ankylosis (this excludes patients with ankylosing spondylitis as a mimicker) (Figure 15-26). In addition, patients with DISH lack the squaring of the vertebral bodies and "shiny corners" at the edges of the vertebral bodies commonly seen in patients with ankylosing spondylitis, and ankylosing spondylitis is an ascending process (the lumbar region is always involved), whereas DISH affects random spinal regions.

Radiographs of the pelvis are useful for evaluating suspected DISH because they demonstrate the sacroiliac joints (which should be normal) and may reveal enthesophytes along the

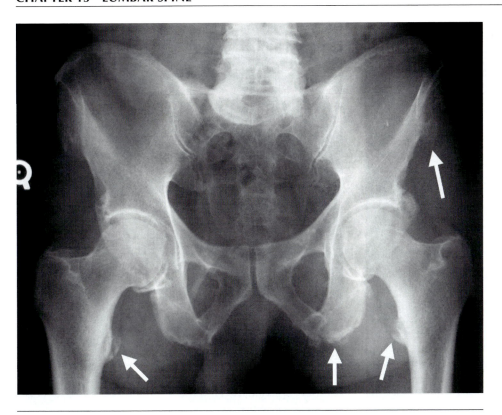

FIGURE 15-27.   Anteroposterior radiograph of the pelvis of a patient with diffuse idiopathic skeletal hyperostosis shows the enthesophytes (arrows).

iliac crests, the ischial tuberosities, and the greater and lesser trochanters (Figure 15-27).

Osteophytes versus Syndesmophytes versus Paravertebral Ossification

Osteophytes are seen at the endplates of vertebral bodies and are traction phenomena due to the pull of Sharpey fibers from a degenerated bulging anulus. They are more common anteriorly than posteriorly because pulsation of the cerebrospinal fluid is thought to inhibit their development. They may be small or large, horizontal or claw-like, and may bridge the disc space.

Syndesmophytes are associated with ankylosing spondylitis and represent ossification of Sharpey fibers. They are thin and vertically oriented and are visible on frontal and lateral radiographs paralleling the edges of the vertebral bodies but do not extend past the vertebral endplates (in contrast to the ossified anterior longitudinal ligament in DISH; Figure 15-28).

Paravertebral ossification is associated with Reiter syndrome and psoriasis and resembles osteophytes (see Chapter 3). Paravertebral ossification is asymmetric and occurs predominantly at the thoracolumbar junction.

Ossification of the Posterior Longitudinal Ligament

This disorder of ossification is more frequent in men than in women and usually occurs in the seventh decade. Although ossification of the posterior longitudinal ligament (OPLL) may be associated with DISH, in most patients the ossification is isolated to the posterior longitudinal ligament or involves the posterior longitudinal ligament and the ligamentum flavum. Symptoms are directly related to the thickness of the ossification; the thicker the ossification, the more likely there is to be central stenosis. Symptoms may be acutely exacerbated by trauma, with patients presenting with an acute central cord syndrome typically after some type of hyperextension injury.

Radiographically, there is ossification just posterior to the vertebral bodies and intervertebral discs. OPLL typically is seen in the midcervical region (Figure 15-29) but can occur in the lumbar or thoracic spine. On CT, the ossification is posterior to the vertebral body along the course of the posterior longitudinal ligament. OPLL is low signal intensity on T_1- and T_2-weighted MR images, which sometimes makes it difficult to appreciate, and it almost never has visible marrow within it.

SCOLIOSIS

Scoliosis refers to lateral curvature of the spine and, as with many other conditions, can be acquired, congenital, or idiopathic. Acquired causes include tumor, radiation therapy, infection, neuromuscular conditions, metabolic abnormalities, and trauma. Congenital scoliosis is secondary to abnormal development of a vertebral body or bodies, most commonly a hemivertebra in which part or all of one side of a vertebra is absent. As a result, curvature develops at the level of the malformed body and may be complex if multiple levels are involved. Other congenital endplate of the superior end vertebra and the inferior endplate of the inferior end vertebra. A line parallel to a line connecting the pedicles may be used if the endplates are not well visualized. The angle at which these lines intersect is the *angle of curvature* (Figure 15-30). This angle also can be determined by the intersection of lines drawn perpendicular to the superior and inferior end vertebra endplate lines. If the superior and inferior end vertebrae are not readily apparent, several measurements using different vertebrae can be made, and the largest measurement should be used. Once the superior and inferior end vertebrae are chosen, these should be used consistently for all follow-up studies so that a true comparison can be made without introducing a confounding factor. Therefore, in addition to reporting the degree of curvature, the levels chosen for measuring the curve must be included in a report.

Spinal curvatures of less than 25° usually are treated with a brace aimed at preventing progression of the curvature; more severe cases require surgery. There are many different forms of instrumentation, but, in general, surgery is performed with the use of metal rods, laminar hooks, and interspinous wires. Attached to each end of a metal rod is a laminar hook that wraps around the superior or inferior aspect of the lamina of the vertebra, depending on whether compression or distraction is needed, respectively. Rods and laminar hooks are used to create compression on the convex side of the curvature and to distract the concave side. The interspinous wires connect the spinous processes to the metal rods and provide additional stability.

An anterior or posterior curve often is superimposed on the lateral curvature of the spine. If the apex is directed posteriorly, it is called *kyphosis*; if the apex is directed anteriorly, it is called *lordosis*. Lordotic and kyphotic curvatures are measured the same way as scoliotic curvatures. Frequently, a rotational component is superimposed on a scoliotic curve.

SUGGESTED READINGS

Alvarez AJ, Hardy HR. Lumbar spine stenosis: a common cause of back and leg pain. *Am Fam Phys.* 1998;57:1825–1834.

Bradford DS, Moe J, Montalvo FJ, et al. Scheuermann's kyphosis and roundback deformity. *J Bone Joint Surg.* 1974;56A:740–758.

Bundschuh CV, Stein L, Slusser JH, et al. Distinguishing between scar and recurrent herniated disc in postoperative patients: value of contrast-enhanced CT and MR imaging. *AJNR.* 1990;11:949–958.

Doyle AJ, Merrilees M. Synovial cysts of the lumbar facet joints in a symptomatic population: prevalence on magnetic resonance imaging. *Spine* 2004;29:874–878.

Fardon DF, Milette PC. Nomenclature and classification of lumbar disc pathology. Recommendations of the Combined Task Forces of the North American Spine Society, American Society of Spine Radiology, and American Society of Neuroradiology. *Spine.* 2001;5:E93–E113.

Goldman AB, Ghelman B, Doherty J. Posterior limbus vertebrae: a cause of radiating back pain in adolescents and young adults. *Skeletal Radiol.* 1990;19:501–507.

Hamanishi C, Kawabata T, Yosii T, et al. Schmorl's nodes on magnetic resonance imaging, their incidence and clinical relevance. *Spine.* 1994;19:450–453.

Jayson M, Herbert C, Bark SJ. Intervertebral disc: nuclear morphology and bursting pressures. *Ann Rheum Dis.* 1973;32:308–315.

Kapila A, Line M. Neuropathic spine arthropathy: CT and MR findings. *J Comput Assist Tomogr.* 1987;11:736–739.

Law JD, Lehman RAW, Kirsch WM. Reoperation after lumbar intervertebral disc surgery. *J Neusurg.* 1978;48:259–263.

Lowe GT. Current concept review Scheuermann's disease. *J Bone Joint Surg.* 1990;72A:940–945.

Modic MT, Steinberg PM, Ross JT, Masaryk TJ, Carter JR. Degenerative disc disease: assessment of changes in vertebral body marrow with MR imaging. *Radiology.* 1988;166:193–199.

Osti LO, Robert VB, Fraser DR. Anulus tears and intervertebral disc degeneration, an experimental study using an animal model. *Spine.* 1990;15:762–767.

Pfirmann CWA, Resnick D. Schmorl nodes of the thoracic and lumbar spine: radiographic-pathologic study of prevalence characterization, and correlation with degenerative changes of 1,650 spinal levels in 100 cadavers. *Radiology.* 2001;219:368–374.

Resnick D, ed. *Diagnosis of Bone and Joint Disorders.* Philadelphia: WB Saunders, 1995.

Resnick D, Niwayama G. Intervertebral disc herniations: cartilaginous (Schmorl's) nodes. *Radiology.* 1978;126:57–65.

Schweitzer ME, Ei-Noueam KI. Vacuum disc: frequency of high signal intensity on T2-weighted MR images. *Skeletal Soc.* 1998;27:83–86.

Weishaupt D, Broxheimer L. Magnetic resonance imaging of the weight-bearing spine. *Semin Musculoskel Radiol.* 2003;7:277–287.

Yu SW, Sether LA, Ho PS, et al. Tears of the anulus fibrosus: correlation between MR and pathologic findings in cadavers. *Am J Neuroradiol.* 1998;9:367–370.

CHAPTER 16

TEMPOROMANDIBULAR JOINT

JAMES V. MANZIONE / RICHARD W. KATZBERG

ANATOMY, PHYSIOLOGY, AND PATHOPHYSIOLOGY

The bony structures of the temporomandibular joint consist of the mandibular condyle and the glenoid fossa and articular eminence of the temporal bone. The intraarticular soft tissues include the meniscus (or disc), its attachments, and the bilaminar zone. The meniscus is a biconcave structure composed predominantly of fibrous tissue, located between the surface of the condyle and the articulating portion of the temporal bone. It is attached posteriorly by the bilaminar zone or posterior attachment, which consists of loose fibroelastic tissue. The meniscus is firmly attached to the neck of the condyle medially and laterally. The meniscus attaches anteriorly to the joint capsule and anteromedially to the upper belly of the lateral pterygoid muscle. The meniscus separates the upper and lower joint spaces, which are lined by synovial tissue. The lower belly of the lateral pterygoid muscle attaches to the neck of the condyle. The joint itself is surrounded by a fibrous capsule. External to the capsule is a lateral ligament that strongly reinforces the lateral wall of the capsule.

Mouth opening requires coordinated movement of the condyle, muscles of mastication, and the meniscus. In the normal state, the meniscus and condyle move anteriorly in a synchronized fashion, with the meniscus always maintaining its position on the condylar surface. During mouth closure, the meniscus continues to maintain its position on the surface of the condyle due to a coordinated and balanced activity among the muscles of mastication, condyle, meniscus, pterygoid muscles, and the posterior attachment (Figure 16-1). Temporomandibular joint (TMJ) dysfunction or symptoms result when any of the conditions that affect the TMJ cause an imbalance of the complex coordinated function of the joint components.

Radiographic imaging modalities are used to determine whether TMJ dysfunction in a given patient is due to an extra- or an intraarticular abnormality or a combination of the two. Although there are different extraarticular causes of TMJ dysfunction such as a tumor, congenital and growth abnormalities, trauma, abnormalities within the infratemporal fossa, and masticatory muscle dysfunction, most of these extraarticular etiologies are relatively uncommon. Certain investigators believe that masticatory muscle dysfunction is a major cause of TMJ dysfunction. Some believe the muscle dysfunction is secondary to occlusal abnormalities, whereas others believe that it is due primarily to psychologic stress.

The more common intraarticular abnormalities are internal meniscal derangement and degenerative arthritis. These two conditions usually are linked to each other. The most common form of internal derangement is an anteriorly displaced meniscus. In this situation, when the mouth is closed, the meniscus, instead of maintaining a position on the condylar surface, moves anteriorly to the condyle and sits in an angle created by the anterior surface of the articular eminence. When the meniscus is displaced anteriorly, it fills the space normally occupied by the lateral pterygoid fat pad.

In some patients, an anteriorly displaced meniscus slips back into normal position over the condyle during mouth opening, thus creating an opening click or popping sound that also may be palpated. During mouth closure, the meniscus once again slips anteriorly off the surface of the condyle, resulting in a closing (reciprocal) click or joint noise. This type of internal derangement is referred to as *meniscus displacement with reduction* (Figure 16-2). In addition to opening and closing clicking, there is deviation of the mandible to the affected side before the opening click. Once the click has occurred and the meniscus has moved onto the surface of the condyle, the mandible returns to the midline.

In some patients, the meniscus remains anterior to the condyle regardless of the degree of condylar translation achieved. Translation is usually limited and there is persistent deviation of the mandible to the side of the abnormal joint. Patients in this setting are categorized as having *meniscus displacement without reduction* (Figure 16-3).

It is important to keep in mind that not all patients who have audible or palpable joint noises have a displaced, reducing meniscus. Studies have shown that some clicking patients have no intraarticular meniscal abnormality, whereas others have a displaced but non-reducing meniscus. Moreover, not all patients with limited translation have an intraarticular abnormality. Various extraarticular abnormalities such as muscle dysfunction, coronoid hyperplasia, and trauma can cause limitation of condylar motion.

IMAGING MODALITIES

Radiographs

Radiographs of the TMJ evaluate the osseous structures of the joint but provide no direct information regarding the intra- and

Katzberg RW, Bessette RW, Tallents RH, et al. Normal and abnormal temporomandibular joint: MR imaging with surface coil. *Radiology.* 1986;113:398–402.

Katzberg RW, Keith DA, Guralnick WC, Manzione JV, Ten Eick WR. Internal derangements of the temporomandibular joint and arthritis. *Radiology.* 1983;146:107.

Katzberg RW, Westesson P-L, Tallents RH, et al. Temporomandibular joint: MR assessment of rotational and sideways disk displacements. *Radiology.* 1988;169:741–748.

Laskin DM. Etiology of the pain-dysfunction syndrome. *J Am Dent Assoc.* 1969;79:147–153.

Manzione JV, Katzberg RW, Tallents RH, et al. Magnetic resonance imaging of the temporomandibular joint. *J Am Dent Assoc.* 1986;113:398–402.

McNamara JA Jr. The independent function of the two heads of the lateral pterygoid muscle. *Am J Anat.* 1973;138:197.

Merrill V. *Atlas of Roentgenographic Positions and Standard Radiologic Procedures.* Vol 2. 4th ed. St Louis: CV Mosby, 1975.

Miller TL, Katzberg RW, Tallents RH, Bessette RW, Hayakawa K. Temporomandibular joint clicking with non-reducing anterior displacement of the meniscus. *Radiology.* 1985;154:121–124.

Nrrgaard F. *Temporomandibular Arthrography* [thesis]. Copenhagen: Munksgard, 1947.

Oguteen-Toller M, Tasakaya-Yilmaz N, Yilmaz F. The evaluation of temporomandibular joint disc position in TMJ disorders using MRI. *Int J Oral Maxillofac Surg.* 2002;31:603–607.

Scapino RP. Histopathology associated with malposition of the human temporomandibular joint disc. *Oral Surg.* 1982;145:719–722.

Sicher H. Functional anatomy of the temporomandibular joint. In: Sarnat BG (ed), *The Temporomandibular Joint.* Springfield, IL: CC Thomas, 1951.

Stallard RE. Relation of occlusion to temporomandibular joint dysfunction: the periodontic viewpoint. *J Am Dent Assoc.* 1969;79:142–144.

Styles C, Whyte A. MRI in the assessment of internal derangement and pain within the temporomandibular joint: a pictorial essay. *Br J Oral Maxillofac Surg.* 2002;40:220–28.

Taskaya-Yylmaz N, Oguteen-Toller M. Clinical correlation of MRI findings of internal derangements of the temporomandibular joints. *Br J Oral Maxillofac Surg.* 2002;40:317–321.

Updegrave WJ. Visualizing the mandibular ramus in panoramic radiographic. *Oral Surg.* 1971;31:422.

Uysal S, Kansu H, Akhan O, Kansu O. Comparison of ultrasonography with magnetic resonance imaging in the diagnosis of temporomandibular joint internal derangements: a preliminary investigation. *Oral Surg Oral Med Oral Pathol Oral Radiol Endod.* 2002;94:115–121.

Weinberg LA. An evaluation of occlusal factors in TMJ dysfunction—pain syndrome. *J Prosthet Dent.* 1979;41:198–208.

Weinberg LA. Correlation of temporomandibular dysfunction with radiographic findings. *J Prosthet Dent.* 1972;28:519.

Weinberg LA. Role of condylar position in TMJ dysfunction-pain syndrome. *J Prosthet Dent.* 1979;41:636.

PART III

MISCELLANEOUS TOPICS

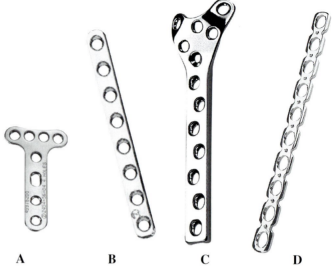

FIGURE 17-2. Cortical plates: *(A)* T-type stabilization plate, *(B)* straight neutralization plate, *(C)* buttress plate, and *(D)* reconstruction plate. *(Hardware courtesy of Zimmer Orthopedics.)*

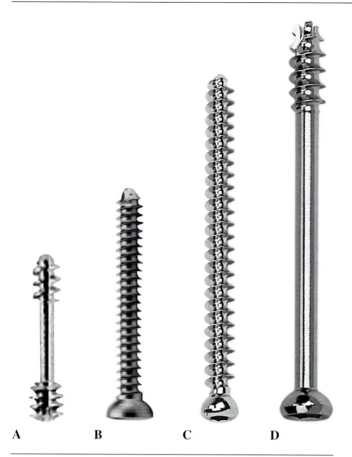

FIGURE 17-1. Fixation screws: *(A)* Herbert screw, *(B)* cortical screw, *(C)* cancellous screw, and *(D)* cancellous lag screw. *(Hardware courtesy of Zimmer Orthopedics.)*

Plates

Plates differ in size, shape, screw hole configuration and number, composition, and biomechanical purpose (Figure 17-2). Neutralization plates provide static stabilization of bone and serve to counter stresses on the fracture. Reconstruction plates are designed to be contoured to conform to the underlying osseous surface and are particularly useful in the fixation of bones with complex shapes.

Buttress plates typically are designed for the stabilization and fixation of metaphyseal or epiphyseal fractures that may be unstable with compressive or axial loading.

Compression plates are applied and fixed during the application of compression across a fracture or are specially configured to provide compression via specially designed holes and eccentrically placed screws that cause axial compression parallel to the plate as the screws are tightened.

Pins and Wires

Straight wires are used clinically for a variety of purposes including temporary stabilization of fracture fragments intraoperatively, as guides for placement of cannulated screws, and for the fixation of small bones and small osseous fragments. Cerclage wiring, in which wires are placed circumferentially in single or multiple strands around a bone, typically is used to hold fracture fragments in place. Wires also may be used as tension bands, in combination with straight wires or screws, to provide dynamic compression across specific anatomic fractures such as fractures of the olecranon and patella. With such fixation, a figure-of-eight wire is placed across the fracture on the tension side of the bone, thereby preventing distraction of fracture fragments and transmitting compressive forces across the fracture planes.

Pins and wires also are used for external fixation. In many cases of fracture reduction, stabilization is provided by the manipulation of externally projecting pins and wires, inserted through fracture fragments, and typically secured on either side of the limb by external rods and/or frames. Fixation of this type is particularly useful in circumstances such as open fractures unsuitable for internal fixation, treatment of infected fractures or infected nonunions, or treatment of closed comminuted fractures at the end of bony segments such as the distal radius to hold the bone to its normal length.

Rods and Nails

Rods and nails generally are used for intramedullary fixation of long bones. Intramedullary fixation devices differ in size, shape, and appearance. Biomechanically, they serve as internal splints or may internally bridge morphologically unstable fractures. Proximal and distal "locking" of an intramedullary device using transverse screws provides angular and rotational stability and maintains the length of the limb. Advantages of locked intramedullary fixation include the increased biomechanical strength of rods and nails relative to plates and screws and the ability to stabilize the fracture without exposure of the fracture site and the associated surgical damage to the surrounding soft tissue. A potential disadvantage is that the fracture fragments may be held at fixed distances from each other instead of being directly apposed. If healing of the femur or tibia does not occur within the expected time course, the distal interlocking screws may be removed to allow the distal fracture fragment to more closely appose the proximal fragment as the patient walks, a process called *dynamization*.

BONE AND JOINT ENDOPROSTHESES

Endoprostheses are devices designed for and used in the reconstruction of joints or bony structures. Joint replacement (arthroplasty) is most common in the large joints including the knee, hip, and shoulder. The design and structure of arthroplasty components have evolved over the past 40 to 50 years, with most current joint arthroplasties constructed of metal alloy with polymer or plastic components. Joint reconstruction may involve replacement of the entire joint (total joint arthroplasty) or just one side of it (hemiarthroplasty). The most commonly replaced joint in the body is the hip; total joint arthroplasty is performed for arthritis because the femoral head and acetabulum are affected by the disease, whereas hemiarthroplasty is the treatment for high grade subcapital fractures because the acetabulum is usually normal in these patients. A *unipolar* hemiarthroplasty involves only the femoral side of the joint. A *bipolar* hemiarthroplasty has both the femoral component and a cup that is placed into the acetabulum with which the prosthetic femoral head articulates; this is not a total arthroplasty because the acetabulum is not reamed out or prepared in any way for the cup, nor is the cup fixed in any way to the acetabulum. The cup is there merely to protect the native acetabular cartilage from being worn down by the prosthetic femoral head, but eventually even the cup itself will cause wear of the acetabular cartilage.

Endoprosthetic reconstruction of long bones is typically performed for treatment of neoplastic disease, often involving the end of a bone. Such reconstruction procedures often involve some type of joint replacement and typically use custom-designed modular endoprostheses.

COMPLICATIONS OF ORTHOPEDIC HARDWARE

The follow-up of patients with fixation devices and prostheses is geared toward the documentation and progression of normal osseous and soft tissue healing responses, assessment of residual or recurrent disease, and the exclusion or evaluation of possible complications related to the initial injury, disease, or the hardware itself. Complications depend on the anatomic region, procedure, and hardware used: delayed union, malunion, and nonunion of fractures (Figure 17-3; see Chapter 6); hardware malpositioning (Figure 17-4) and migration; hardware failure (loosening or fracture; Figures 17-5 and 17-6); perioperative or late osseous fracture; infection (Figure 17-7; see Chapter 1); heterotopic bone formation; and foreign body inflammatory reaction (granulomatosis).

Inadequate stabilization of a fracture can lead to nonunion or malunion due to fracture motion (see Fig. 17-3). Conversely, too

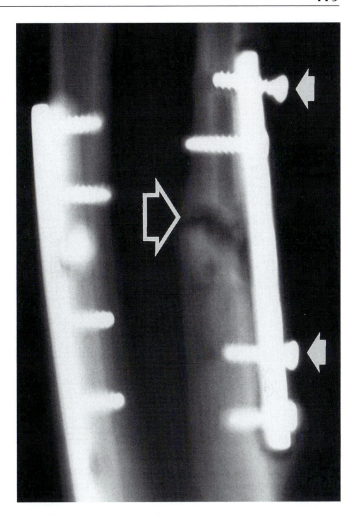

FIGURE 17-3. Nonunion: conventional tomography. Conventional coronal tomogram through the forearm, 9 months after open reduction and internal fixation, depicts stabilization plates and cortical screws for fixation of fractures of the diaphyses of the ulna and radius. A persistent lucent cleft is seen through the radial diaphysis with sclerotic margins, compatible with nonunion at the fracture site (open arrow). "Backing out" of several of the cortical screws (solid arrows) fixing the radial stabilization plate is seen, and lucency is visible along the interface of the plate and the underlying bone, all of which indicates loosening of the fixation hardware.

much stabilization may cause nonunion if the fracture fragments are held apart from each other; eg, a tibial fracture fixed with an intramedullary rod with proximally and distally locking screws may not heal until the rod is "dynamized" by removing one or both of the locking screws and allowing the fracture ends to be compressed.

Hardware loosening most commonly results from insufficient purchase or fixation of hardware within bone or as a result of inadequate stabilization of a fracture or reconstruction interface. Persistent motion at bone-hardware interfaces results in fibrous tissue proliferation and osseous resorption around the implant, leading to further loosening and migration of the instrumentation. Inadequate purchase or positioning of screws may result in their "cutting out" of bone into the adjacent joint or soft tissues or "backing out" of their intended points of fixation. Radiolucency

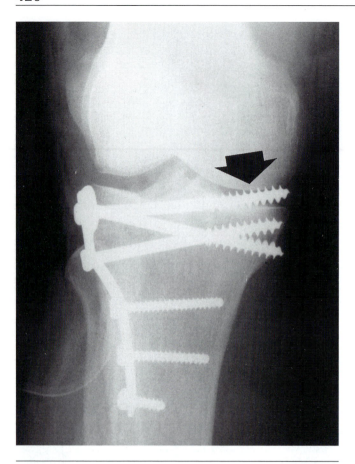

FIGURE 17-4. Suboptimal hardware placement. An immediate postoperative anteroposterior radiograph shows the right knee after open reduction and internal fixation of a lateral tibial plateau fracture. A lateral buttress plate and multiple cancellous screws are seen in place. The most proximal fixation screw (arrow) is seen extending through the articular surface of the medial tibial plateau into the medial compartment of the knee joint.

around screws and separation of a plate from the cortex are radiographic appearances of loosening. Intramedullary fixation devices or prostheses may shift within the bony canal due to hardware loosening or merely due to normal settling of the fracture and/or instrumentation.

Metal is stiffer than bone and may become fatigued by the biomechanical stress placed on it at the fracture site. Hardware failure due to loosening or metal fracture is inevitable if osseous union does not occur (see Figs. 17-5 and 17-6). Fracture of the metal also may occur after fracture healing due to the greater elasticity of bone, but the breakage in this setting is usually inconsequential unless the metal piece is intraarticular or painful.

Conversely, bones may fracture as a result of orthopedic fixation. Intraoperative fractures may occur during the manipulation and insertion of hardware. For example, accidental longitudinal split fractures of the shaft of the bone may occur during the intramedullary insertion of a prostheses or intramedullary nail, as may cortical penetration by the prosthetic stem, nail, or pin. In addition, differences between the stiffness of the hardware and the adjacent bone creates a *stress riser* at the proximal and distal tips of the metal, thus predisposing the bone to fracture at these

locations. For example, periprosthetic fractures frequently occur in the femur at or just distal to the prosthetic femoral stem. Screw holes also result in stress risers, further weakening the underlying bone and predisposing it to fracture at the hole. Atrophic changes and disuse osteopenia of a bone fixed with orthopedic hardware may also occur, predisposing the bone to fracture after the fixation device is removed.

The incidence of musculoskeletal infection postoperatively depends on multiple factors including the integrity of the overlying skin (eg, open vs closed fracture), the degree of soft tissue devitalization and/or contamination, and the method of fixation or reconstruction. Postoperative musculoskeletal infections may be superficial or involve deep soft tissues and bone and may manifest acutely in the early postoperative period or may smolder as late as a year or more postoperatively. Externally projecting pins in patients with external fixation provide a route of spread for contamination. The risk of pin tract infections with external fixation may be minimized by the insertion of strong pins through minimal soft tissue sleeves, better fixation at the bone-pin interface, and meticulous pin tract care. Pin tract infection, as with other hardware-associated infections, may result in osseous resorption at the bone-hardware interface, adjacent periosteal reaction, and possible sequestra formation.

Inflammatory foreign body reactions may occur secondary to foreign materials and particulate debris related to fixation or, more commonly, reconstruction hardware. The inflammatory reaction is a histiocytic response to some stimulus resulting in inflammatory osteolysis along an implant-osseous interface or synovitis within the adjacent joint. Debris accounting for such inflammatory responses may originate from silastic, polyethylene, metal, or methylmethacrylate (bone cement) and, hence, has been called many names such as "silicone synovitis," "cement disease," and "small particle disease."

Postoperative heterotopic bone formation is seen most commonly surrounding the hip after arthroplasty. An increased incidence of heterotopic ossification also occurs in paralyzed patients for unknown reasons and in patients with a predisposition to bone formation, including those with diffuse idiopathic skeletal hyperostosis, hypertrophic osteoarthritis, ankylosing spondylitis, and a history of prior postoperative heterotopic bone formation. A minority of patients with heterotopic ossification present with symptoms such as limited motion and/or pain. Prophylactic treatment of high risk patients includes perioperative nonsteroidal antiinflammatory medication or low level radiation therapy.

DIAGNOSTIC IMAGING OF ORTHOPEDIC HARDWARE

Conventional Radiography

Conventional radiography remains the single most important diagnostic imaging test in the evaluation of orthopedic hardware and the underlying bone. Radiographs are well established as a routine component of the perioperative and follow-up postoperative assessments of patients. Radiographs are readily accessible,

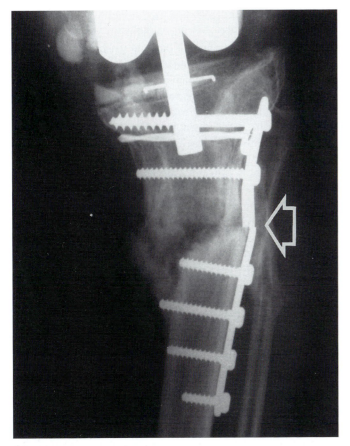

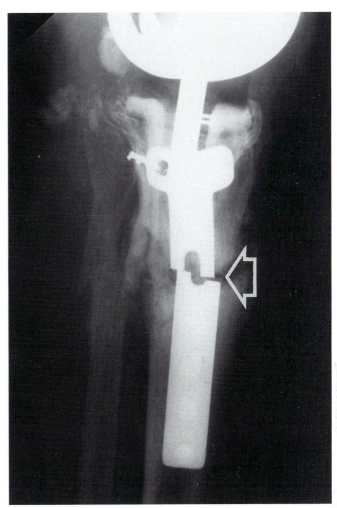

A   B

FIGURE 17-5.   Hardware fracture. *(A)* Anteroposterior and *(B)* lateral radiographs of the proximal tibia demonstrate a fracture of the proximal tibial diaphysis with an associated fracture of the lateral buttress plate that had been placed at the time of revision knee arthroplasty. The plate fracture (arrows) can be seen extending through a proximal screw hole of the plate, a site of biomechanical weakness and potential failure of the plate construct.

inexpensive, reproducible, and well suited to the evaluation of bone and metal hardware. Sequential radiographic studies are particularly important in the assessment of many bony and hardware-related complications. Radiographic appearances of loosening include a change in position of the hardware or fixated bone and radiolucency surrounding the metal appliance.

Because metallic orthopedic hardware may obscure the adjacent underlying bone, fluoroscopic examination can be helpful, particularly in the evaluation of hardware-osseous interfaces, which are not always seen tangentially with radiographs.

Radiographs are performed specifically to evaluate the painful prosthesis. *Total joint arthroplasty* refers to replacement of both sides of the joint, and the hip is the most commonly replaced joint in the United States. The components may be cemented or noncemented (press-fit or ingrowth). A common combination is a cemented femoral stem and noncemented acetabular cup. A high density polyethylene liner is present in the acetabular cup,

with which the metal femoral head articulates. A cemented stem may have a thin radiolucency with an adjacent thin sclerotic line representing a fibrous pseudocapsule formed during the marked exothermic curing of the cement. An ingrowth stem usually is coated with tiny beads to increase its surface area and promote ingrowth of bone onto its surface; the beads may give the prosthesis a fuzzy edge. The well-fixed ingrowth component shows bony sclerosis extending onto the prosthesis.

Radiographic appearances of loosening of the prosthesis are outlined in Table 17-1. Often, however, the question is not whether the prosthesis is loose, but what has caused the loosening. The most common cause is mechanical stress, but infection and small particle disease can look similar. The imaging evaluation of the infected hip arthroplasty is discussed in Chapter 1. Particle disease is suggested radiographically by large but focal, well-defined radiolucencies around the acetabular or femoral components.

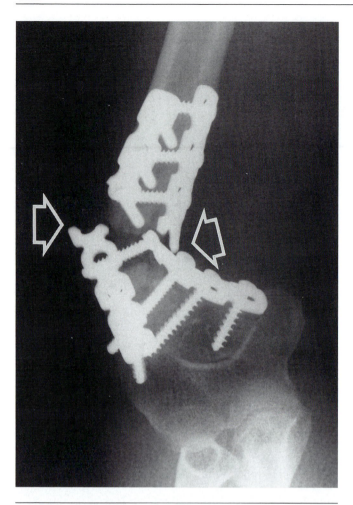

FIGURE 17-6.   Hardware failure: reconstruction plate fracture. Anteroposterior radiograph of the distal humerus shows medial and lateral reconstruction plates and screws in place for fixation of a prior distal metadiaphyseal fracture. Repeat trauma to the upper extremity resulted in fracture of the medial and lateral plates (arrows) with posttraumatic varus angulation of the distal humerus across the fracture line.

TABLE 17-1

Radiographic Signs of Loosening of a Total HIP Replacement

Cemented stem
    Lucency at the cement-bone interface >2 mm surrounding the
       component
    Development or widening of the lucency at the cement-bone interface
    Fracture of cement mantle
    Migration of component or change in alignment
    Fracture of component
    Component motion with stress views
Noncemented (ie, ingrowth) stem
    Lucency at the metal-bone interface >2 mm surrounding the
       component
    Development or widening of the lucency at the metal-bone interface
    Shedding of surface beads
    Migration of component or change in alignment
    Fracture of component
    Component motion with stress views

Aspiration Arthrography

Aspiration arthrography is an important modality in the evaluation of symptomatic joint arthroplasties, most commonly of the hip and knee, to distinguish infection from mechanical loosening. With these procedures, fluoroscopic guidance typically is used to optimize positioning of the joint structures and to guide needle advancement into the articulation.

After intraarticular placement of a needle, a joint aspirate can be performed and sent for microbiologic analysis. If no fluid is obtained, non-bacteriostatic saline can be injected into and recovered from the joint and sent for laboratory assessment. However, frequent false-negative results may be seen with aspiration in the diagnosis of arthroplasty infection, particularly if saline irrigation is required. Injection of contrast material after aspiration is performed for the documentation and confirmation of intraarticular positioning of the needle and in some cases to assess the integrity of the prosthetic fixation interface, particularly in the case of cemented arthroplasty prostheses. Contrast material is injected into the articulation until lymphatic filling is seen, contrast is visualized extending along the entire prosthetic fixation interface, or until the patient experiences discomfort. Contrast material extending along the prosthesis-cement or bone-cement interface indicates loosening of the cemented femoral component of a total hip arthroplasty (see Fig. 17-7) but may not always be abnormal around an acetabular component. Conventional tomography may assist in the differentiation of contrast material from radiopaque bone cement and make the distribution of injected contrast material easier to define. False-negative examinations may occur if debris or granulation tissue in the interface blocks the insinuation of contrast. Some institutions use arthroscintigraphy, in which technetium methylene diphosphonate (Tc MDP) is injected directly into the joint, and the patient ambulates and is then scanned with a gamma camera looking for radiotracer around the prosthesis. This technique is more involved than conventional contrast arthrography but may be more sensitive for loosening.

Nuclear Medicine

Tc MDP-, gallium-, and indium-labeled leukocyte scanning techniques are used routinely in the diagnostic evaluation of a wide variety of musculoskeletal disorders. In postoperative patients with orthopaedic hardware, these same radiopharmaceutical studies have proven to be valuable diagnostic modalities.

In patients with joint prostheses, Tc MDP bone scans normally may show increased activity surrounding the arthroplasty components in the early postoperative period as a result of increased bone turnover secondary to surgery. The degree of such increased activity generally depends on multiple factors including the patient's age and the type of arthroplasty performed (cemented vs ingrowth). For example, in a symptomatic patient with a cemented femoral component, increased activity at the inferior tip of the femoral component or surrounding it may indicate loosening and/or infection and other complications such as fracture or heterotopic bone formation. In a patient with an

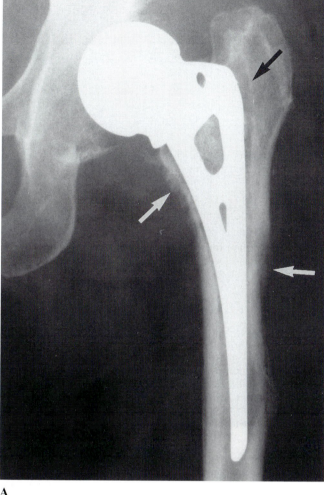

A

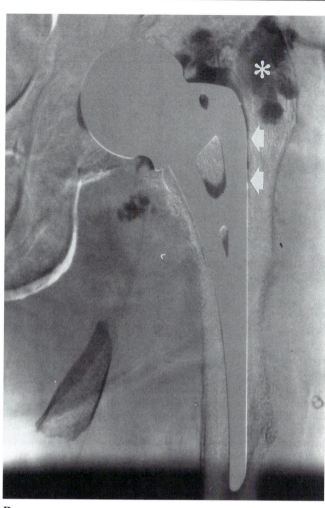

B

FIGURE 17-7.   Aspiration/arthrography: infection with prosthetic loosening. *(A)* Anteroposterior radiograph of the left hip shows a unipolar femoral hemiarthroplasty in place. Irregular periosteal reaction is visible along the medial and lateral aspects of the proximal femoral shaft (white arrows), and there is a lucency along the superior lateral aspect of the prosthesis-bone interface (black arrow). *(B)* Conventional subtraction image of the arthroplasty after aspiration of the joint and the injection of contrast material demonstrates contrast extending along the superior-lateral aspect of the bone-prosthesis interface (arrows) of the femoral prosthesis. Contrast is also seen extending into irregular lobulated periarticular collections (asterisk), representative of abscess cavities, in this patient with an infected femoral hemiarthroplasty and prosthetic loosening.

ingrowth type of femoral component, uptake surrounding the stem may merely reflect the desired bony incorporation of the prosthesis.

Tc MDP bone scanning combined with gallium or labeled white blood cell studies are valuable in the assessment of infection around prostheses and other orthopedic hardware. Increased gallium activity discordant to Tc MDP bone scan activity is suggestive of osteomyelitis. As with gallium, indium-labeled leukocytes may accumulate in sites of infection. However, displacement and changes of marrow elements after arthroplasty or intramedullary fixation surgery typically cause irregularities in the normal distribution of indium-labeled white blood cells. Combined sulfur colloid scanning (to assess marrow distribution) and indium-labeled leukocyte examinations have been used

to diagnose infection after orthopedic implant surgery. Increased indium-labeled leukocyte activity spatially incongruent to colloid accumulation has been shown to be highly accurate in the diagnosis of infection. The lack of increased gallium or labeled white blood cell activity at a corresponding site of increased Tc MDP uptake also helps to exclude infection (Figure 17-8).

Ultrasonography

High resolution real-time ultrasound scanning has been used to monitor the process of new bone formation and healing after certain orthopedic procedures including intramedullary nailing and limb lengthening. The identification of early callus formation by

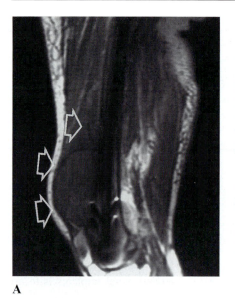

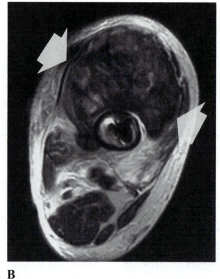

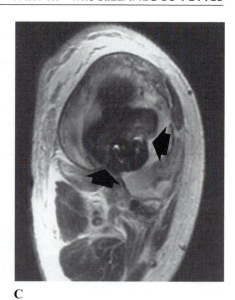

A   **B**   **C**

FIGURE 17-10.   Staging of neoplastic disease: magnetic resonance imaging after internal fixation. Sagittal fast spin echo T_1-weighted (repetition time, 500 milliseconds; echo time, 10 milliseconds; echo train length, 4) and axial fast spin echo T_2-weighted (repetition time, 4000 milliseconds; echo time, 95 milliseconds; echo train length, 8) images show an intramedullary nail within the femur placed for stabilization of an "impending" pathologic fracture. *(A)* Sagittal T_1-weighted image demonstrates a lobulated soft tissue mass (open arrows) abutting the anterior cortex of the distal femoral diaphysis. *(B)* Axial fast spin echo T_2-weighted imaging through the mass shows the large size of the lesion (arrows) in the extensor compartment of the thigh encircling the anterior two thirds of the femoral shaft. *(C)* Axial fast spin echo T_2-weighted image obtained more distally depicts destruction of the femoral cortex (black arrows) and medullary invasion of the distal femur in this patient with an aggressive soft tissue angiosarcoma.

Modifications to MRI parameters may reduce artifacts created by metal implants (Table 17-3). Misregistration artifacts result in signal variations related to implant shape and orientation. Resultant artifacts, seen in the frequency encoding direction, are inversely proportional to the applied frequency encoding gradient strength and thus may be minimized with the use of an increased frequency encoding gradient. Because increasing the frequency encoding gradient while maintaining a constant field of view is equivalent to widening of the receive bandwidth, increasing or widening the receive bandwidth on the MRI console results in a proportional decrease in misregistration artifact. Misregistration artifacts related to hardware also may be diminished with orientation of metal implants longitudinally within the magnetic field. Therefore, patients should be positioned, if possible, to have their metallic implants oriented along the long axis of the main magnetic field (Bo). Because misregistration artifacts are present only in the frequency encoding direction, selective orientation of the frequency and phase encoding directions may be helpful in the diagnostic evaluation of structures adjacent to metallic implants. By selectively changing the frequency and phase encoding directions, the direction of associated misregistration artifacts can be directed away from areas of possible clinical abnormality (Figure 17-12). Three-dimensional imaging techniques may be beneficial in MRI in the vicinity of metallic hardware to reduce the effects of slice thickness variation;

however, such sequences in general tend to be time consuming to perform.

Fast spin echo (FSE) pulse sequences with minimal interecho spacing may help reduce diffusion-related signal loss in the vicinity of metallic hardware compared to spin echo or gradient echo imaging. FSE imaging accomplishes this by using multiple refocusing 180° pulses within a single repetition time, thus minimizing the time for spin-spin diffusion and related signal loss to take place. Dephasing artifact also can be reduced by using a large matrix size and thin slices. Gradient echo imaging is extremely vulnerable to susceptibility and dephasing artifacts related to metallic hardware because it lacks the 180° refocusing pulse; this sequence generally should be avoided on high field strength magnets if hardware is present.

Fat suppression via inversion recovery provides more homogeneous fat saturation than the frequency selective fat saturation technique commonly used with FSE T_2-weighted imaging. This is due to the fact that inversion recovery sequences are less vulnerable to magnetic field inhomogeneities, such as in the vicinity of metallic structures.

The geometry and composition of specific orthopedic hardware devices may dictate the degree of artifact encountered. For example, susceptibility artifacts induced by hardware composed of titanium are typically less marked than those associated with steel or other metal alloys used in orthopedic hardware

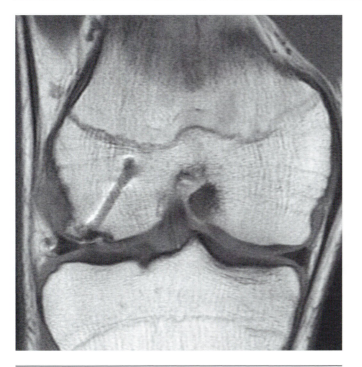

FIGURE 17-11.   Magnetic resonance image post open reduction and internal fixation of an osteochondral fracture of the knee. Coronal fast spin echo image (repetition time, 4000 milliseconds; echo time, 30 milliseconds; echo train length, 8; 4thk/0spc; field of view, 14; matrix, 512 × 512; BW, 64 kHz; NEX, 3) of the knee in a patient with prior open reduction and internal fixation of an osteochondral fracture of the lateral femoral condyle with a Herbert fixation screw. thk = slice thickness, SPC = interslice gap, BW = bandwidth, NEX = number of excitations.

TABLE 17-3

Strategies for Magnetic Resonance Imaging of Metal

Try to align the hardware with the external magnetic field

Use a large bandwidth (>32 kHz; increase the number of excitations to compensate for decreased signal-to-noise ratio)

Selectively choose the frequency and phase encoding directions (to shift the artifact away from the area of interest)

Use fast spin echo imaging with short echo train length

Use a large frequency encoding matrix (eg, 512)

Use short tau inversion recovery fat suppression instead of frequency selective fat saturation

construction. In addition, artifacts produced by hardware with complex geometric interfaces tend to be greater than those with simple geometric constructs.

Another strategy for MRI around metal implants is to use low to midfield strength magnets (0.2 to 0.5 T) as opposed to high field strength MR units. This technique commensurately reduces geometric distortion artifact with the same frequency encoding gradient strengths, but at the cost of decreased signal to noise for the same acquisition period.

The presence of anterior plates and screws in the cervical spine or posterior lumbar instrumentation and pedicle screws is not a contraindication to MRI of these locations, and useful clinical information can be obtained with regard to disc disease and canal stenosis. MRI of joint replacements is in its infancy and its role has yet to be defined. Although it cannot demonstrate the joint space due to artifact, it can demonstrate the surrounding soft tissue, which may be helpful for evaluation of abscess in

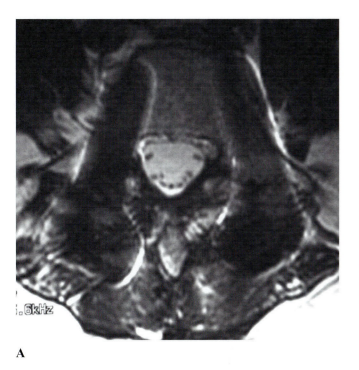

A

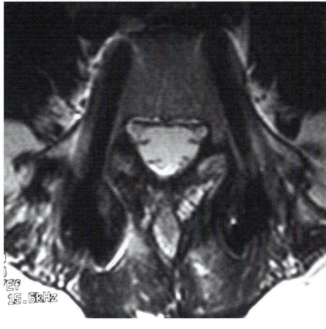

B

FIGURE 17-12.   Effect of frequency encoding direction on artifact. By changing the direction of the frequency encoding phase in (A), the misregistration artifact in (B) is directed along the length of the pedicle screws and not to their sides, thus allowing better visualization of the lateral recess of the vertebra.

cases of infection, and can show adjacent bone, which may be helpful for locating radiographically occult sites of early particle disease.

SUGGESTED READINGS

Czerny C, Krestan C, Imhof H, Trattnig S. Magnetic resonance imaging of the postoperative hip. *Topics Magn Reson Imaging.* 1999;10:214–20.

Kaplan PA, Montesi SA, Jardon OM, Gregory PR. Bone-ingrowth hip prostheses in asymptomatic patients: radiographic features. *Radiology.* 1988;169:221–227.

Keogh CF, Munk PL, Gee R, Chan LP, Marchinkow LO. Pictorial essay: imaging of the painful hip arthroplasty. *AJR.* 2003;180:115–120.

Manaster BJ. From the RSNA refresher courses. Total hip arthroplasty: radiographic evaluation. *Radiographics.* 1996;16:645–660.

Olsen RV, Munk PL, Lee MJ, et al. Metal artifact reduction sequence: early clinical applications. *Radiographics.* 2000;20:699–712.

Sofka CM, Potter HG. MR imaging of joint arthroplasty. *Semin Musculoskel Radiol.* 2002;6:79–85.

Tigges S, Stiles RG, Roberson JR. Appearance of septic hip prostheses on plain radiographs. *AJR.* 1994;163:377–380.

Tigges S, Stiles RG, Roberson JR. Pictorial essay: complications of hip arthroplasty causing periprosthetic radiolucency on plain radiographs. *AJR.* 1994;162:1387–1391.

White LM, Buckwalter KA. Technical considerations: CT and MR imaging in the postoperative orthopedic patient. *Semin Musculoskel Radiol.* 2002;6:5–17.

White LM, Kim JK, Metha M, et al. Complications of total hip arthroplasty: MR imaging—initial experience. *Radiology.* 2000;215:254–261.

CHAPTER 18

BONE DENSITOMETRY

RONALD B. STARON / THEODORE T. MILLER

The most common metabolic bone disease is osteoporosis, a systemic bone disease characterized by low bone mass with microarchitectural deterioration of bone, leading to increased risk of fracture. Almost 30 million Americans have osteoporosis or are at high risk of developing it.

Osteoporosis is clinically important because of fractures that result from it. Colles fractures and vertebral compression fractures carry significant morbidity, and hip fractures carry considerable mortality: up to 20% of individuals with hip fracture die within 1 year, and more than 50% of survivors will be incapacitated, often permanently.

Osteoporosis is most common in estrogen-deficient, postmenopausal women but can be related to environmental factors such as calcium deficiency, malnutrition, and alcoholism, to hormonal abnormalities, or to certain chronic diseases. Osteoporosis also can occur in men. Medical treatment includes bisphosphonate compounds and selective estrogen receptor modulators, but treatment can be instituted only if the diagnosis is established.

Conventional radiographs are inaccurate for diagnosing osteoporosis. The diagnosis can be suggested, but rarely is there sufficient loss of bone mineral for the diagnosis to be established. A 30 to 60% loss of bone mass must occur before the loss becomes radiographically visible. Moreover, the amount of bone cannot be quantitated, and differences in radiographic exposure techniques and in patient body habitus make radiography inconsistent from patient to patient and even for serial radiographs of the same patient.

During the past half-century, the shortcomings of radiographs have led to the development of numerous quantitative methods to assess bone mineral density (BMD). By the 1950s, such methods included radiogrammetry, the measurement of long bone cortical thicknesses, and photodensitometry (also called radiographic absorptiometry), in which visible bone density is compared with the density of an aluminum (or other metal) standard. In the 1960s and 1970s, the nuclear medicine technologies of single and dual photon absorptiometry were developed and popularized. Quantitative computed tomography (QCT) also was developed. Even today, the search for new methods continues, including ultrasonic and magnetic resonance methods. Nonetheless, the gold standard of diagnosis is dual x-ray absorptiometry (DXA), a technique introduced in the late 1980s.

DXA uses an x-ray source to produce photons of two different energies that pass through the patient. DXA machines cause only tiny amounts of scatter radiation and do not need lead-lined radiography rooms. The differential absorption of the photons of different energies by bone, and calibration against their absorption in soft tissues, allow the densitometric computer to calculate the bone mineral content (BMC) in grams. The machine also calculates the area measured (cm^2). BMC per unit area equals the bone mineral density (BMD) in (g/cm^2).

BMD becomes clinically useful when it is compared with the BMD of that same body part in hundreds of young, sex-matched, normal control subjects with peak bone mass. When the BMD is compared with the mean value of that normal population, the result is expressed as the T score. The T score is the number of standard deviations between the measured BMD and the mean BMD of the young normal population. If the measured BMD is greater than the young normal mean value, the T score has a positive value; if the measured BMD is less than the normal mean, it has a negative value (Figure 18-1A). Another use of BMD is comparison with an age-matched normal population, called the Z score, which also is expressed as the number of standard deviations from the normal mean (see Fig. 18-1B).

The significance of the T score is that it estimates fracture risk, and the risk of fracture increases with increasingly negative T-score values, even if the Z score is near its age-matched controls.

The World Health Organization developed criteria for osteoporosis based on the T score. If the T score is positive or is less negative than -1 (eg, -0.98), the BMD is considered normal, and there is no increased risk of fracture. If the T score is between -1 and -2.5, the BMD is diagnosed as demonstrating *osteopenia* or *low bone mass*, and the patient is considered at risk for the future development of osteoporosis. If the T score is more negative than -2.5, that bone is diagnosed as *osteoporotic*, and the person is at risk of fracture. There is a fourth category, *severe osteoporosis* or *established osteoporosis*, in which the T score satisfies the criterion for osteoporosis and the patient already has one or more fragility fractures.

Bone densitometry often may show osteoporosis of one body part but only osteopenia, or even normality, of another. Although this may seem inconsistent, such differing values of different body parts do have clinical significance: a specific bone with a lower T score is more likely to fracture. For example, if the femoral neck T score is -3.5, a normal forearm value does not imply a low probability of hip fracture. Thus, even though the BMDs of other bones do bear some statistical relation to the overall risk of fracture in a particular bone (which is why BMD measurement of the calcaneus has clinical value for overall assessment of fracture risk), the most accurate indication of the fracture risk of a specific bone is the BMD measurement of that

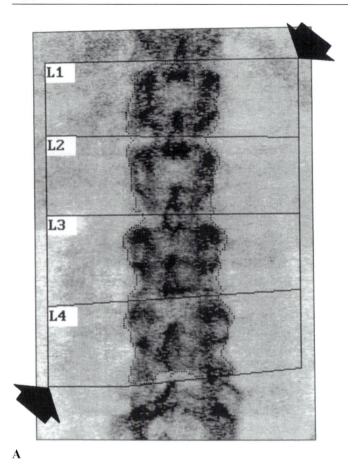

A

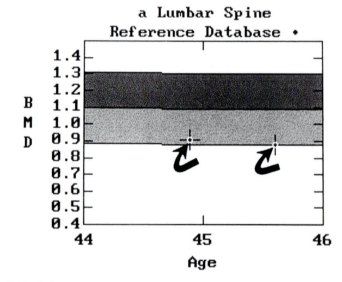

a Lumbar Spine
Reference Database •

BMD(L2-L4) = 0.875 g/cm^2

Region	BMD	T(30.0)		Z	
L1	0.821	−1.70	81%	−1.50	83%
L2	0.823	−2.47	75%	−2.24	77%
L3	0.928	−1.59	84%	−1.37	86%
L4	0.866	−2.54	76%	−2.30	77%
L2−L4	0.875	−2.18	78%	−1.95	80%

B

a Lumbar Spine
Reference Database •

L2−L4

	04/23/97
01/08/98	−3.0%*

C

FIGURE 18-1.   *(A)* Posteroanterior DXA digital radiograph obtained during densitometry of the lumbar spine in a 45-year-old woman. The outer lines mark the external limits of the analysis region (arrowheads); the horizontal lines mark the levels of the disc spaces. *(B)* Computerized BMD analysis of the spine shown in A. For L$_2$–L$_4$, the BMD is 0.875 g/cm^2 (arrowhead), the *T* score is −2.18 (arrow), and the *Z* score is −1.95 (curved arrow). The *T* score of 2.18 indicates that the spine's BMD is 2.18 standard deviations below the mean BMD of a young normal female population. *(C)* Computerized BMD comparison (for the region of L$_2$–L$_4$) between the latest study and the previous (baseline) study shows a decrease of 3.0% (slanted arrow). The asterisk beside the percent sign (arrowhead) indicates that this change is statistically significant. The graph shows the BMD for the age of the patient at each time of measurement (curved arrows). The horizontal bars represent BMD values from 2 standard deviations above the mean of the age-matched female population to 2 standard deviations below that mean. Both measurements in this patient are nearly 2 standard deviations below that mean value.

particular bone itself. This is the reason BMD is frequently measured in the spine, the hip, and the forearm: such measurements give a good indication of the patient's risk of fracturing each of those areas.

Measurements at these three sites also give a good indication of what is happening to the medullary bone and cortical bone. Vertebral body measurements (L_1–L_4 or L_2–L_4) give the BMD of areas with predominantly medullary bone. In contrast, the distal radius evaluates cortical bone (which can be lost with hyperparathyroidism). The femoral neck is a combination of the two.

Different sites can be evaluated within each anatomic region. For example, within the hip, one can evaluate the femoral neck, Ward triangle, or the total hip; in the spine, one can evaluate one vertebra or several vertebrae. Most bone densitometers have the capability of whole-body imaging, and each institution should establish its own standard protocols based on the needs of the referring physicians and the regional standards of care. One widely used approach is to measure only axial skeletal sites such as the hip and spine because of the significant morbidity and mortality associated with vertebral compression fractures and hip fractures.

Figure 18-1A shows a lumbar spine posteroanterior digital radiograph used for BMD calculation. The radiograph was obtained with the patient supine and legs raised on a pad (supplied by the manufacturer) to minimize lumbar lordosis. The technologist ensured that the total size of the region of interest was correct, that the horizontal analysis lines passed through the disc spaces, and that the vertebrae were properly numbered.

Figure 18-1B shows the resulting analysis, with BMD, T scores, and Z scores for each vertebra, and combined values for L_2–L_4. It is this combined value that is included in the final result. However, if there were a severe compression fracture of one vertebra, the analysis would be changed by the technologist to exclude that vertebra and include L_1 in its place.

Figure 18-1C shows comparison of the final result with the results of a previous, baseline scan. In this case, there was a 3% decrease of BMD compared with the earlier scan. The study was repeated at an 8-month interval because this patient was scanned as part of a research protocol; normally, repeated scans would be at longer intervals. For example, if a screening bone densitometric scan diagnosed low bone mass or osteoporosis and treatment was instituted, an interval of 1 year before the next scan would be reasonable for checking the efficacy of treatment. If no osteopenia were found on a first screening examination, it would be reasonable to wait 3 to 5 years before the next scan, in part because the statistical power of a scan series increases with increasing time between scans.

The asterisk next to the percentage change of −3.0 (see Fig. 18-1C) labels the change as statistically significant. It is important to remember that statistical significance and clinical significance are not always identical. A series of scans can show a statistically significant increase, followed by a significant loss, followed by another significant increase—with no overall change from the original baseline scan. Hence, in reporting such a series, the change from the previous scan plus the change from the baseline scan is reported. This report gives the referring physician a better picture of the overall trend in the results.

Figure 18-2A shows the hip analysis region of the nondominant hip in a 61-year-old woman. The computer analyzes the femoral neck and other areas near the hip, but only the total hip BMD is included in the final report. The results of that measurement are seen in Figure 18-2B. The resulting T score is −2.00, indicating osteopenia or low bone mass according to World Health Organization criteria. Figure 18-2C shows that the BMD represents a decrease of BMD at a rate of 0.0351 g/cm^2 per year as compared with the baseline study performed 10 months previously, representing a rate of decrease of 4.83% per year. This reporting of change per year represents an alternate reporting strategy from that previously demonstrated with the lumbar spine, where comparisons with the baseline scan and previous scan were reported; either type of report yields information valuable to the referring physician.

No matter which scanning regimens are used, the radiologist must remember that bone densitometry exposes the patient to radiation. Proper quality control scanning must be performed and adequate documentation must be kept. If the machine function is within acceptable limits, patient examinations for the day can begin; otherwise, machine maintenance must be performed. After all, patients must not be irradiated unless meaningful results can be obtained. Proper quality control and maintenance are absolutely necessary, and all technical considerations must be monitored carefully by the supervising radiologist. Two quality control terms that should be understood are *accuracy* and *precision*. Accuracy is the ability of the scanner to correctly measure BMC, and precision is the percentage of variability of such measurements over time. A scan that cannot accurately detect osteoporosis is useless, and improvement or worsening of osteoporosis in a patient on therapy cannot be appreciated if the scanner has poor precision. The radiologist should look at each anatomic image to ensure that the technologist has properly positioned the different analysis regions.

In addition to DXA, other methodologies exist for bone mass measurement. QCT is used frequently for obtaining spinal bone mass measurements because it can easily separate the mass of the medullary bone from the confounding effects of nearby osteophytes or sclerotic facet joints, which are frequently found in the spines of postmenopausal women. QCT can be adapted to measure other bones, for which it yields good results. The usefulness of QCT is limited, however, because of its higher cost and radiation dose as compared with DXA. Third-party sources of payment, such as the government, which are willing to finance DXA, are not willing to invest in the future of QCT. In light of the large numbers of people who will be screened for osteoporosis, QCT has almost no role in routine screening for osteoporosis because of its cost and radiation exposure.

Other devices for measuring peripheral bone mass, such as small densitometers to measure the wrist or calcaneus, or quantitative ultrasound machines to measure the calcaneus, also are being used for screening. Such devices are lightweight and portable, and ultrasound machines avoid radiation, thereby bypassing many regulatory requirements and technologist training issues. Calcaneal ultrasound devices measure broadband ultrasound attenuation or speed of transmission of sound, or a ratio of the two, rather than actual BMD. Such measurements give an indication of the quality of the bone, not just its quantity.

ARTHROGRAPHY

Arthrography continues to play an important role in the diagnosis of joint disorders. The number of conventional contrast arthrograms performed in recent years has decreased due to the wide availability of MRI, but MR arthrography of the shoulder and hip is increasing and one should know how to inject the joint. In addition, evaluation for prosthetic loosening or the presence of joint infection remains a common reason for performing contrast arthrography in the hip, and wrist arthrography continues to be a fairly commonly requested procedure for the diagnosis of intrinsic intercarpal ligament tears. Moreover, these same arthrographic techniques can be used for the therapeutic injection of steroid and long-acting anesthetic.

Shoulder arthrography is performed most commonly in preparation for an MR arthrogram to evaluate suspected labral tear and to evaluate suspected rotator cuff tear in patients with contraindications to MRI (although sonography should be the preferred alternative method for cuff tear). When performing shoulder arthrography, the patient is supine on the radiography table, with the designated shoulder closest to the physician. The shoulder is placed in neutral rotation by positioning the arm at the side with the thumb up. A slightly more tangential view of the joint may be obtained by placing a small amount of padding under the contralateral shoulder. If the glenohumeral joint is completely tangential, the fibrocartilaginous labrum of the glenoid may obstruct the needle path into the joint. A mark is placed on the skin at the level of the junction of the middle third of the glenoid, with the inferior third overlying the space between the glenoid and humeral head (Figure 19-1). Sterile preparation of the skin and draping of the area is performed. A 25-gauge needle and 5-mL syringe is used to raise a skin wheal with 1% lidocaine. The pain of the lidocaine injection itself can be avoided by adding a small amount of 7.5% or 8.4% sodium bicarbonate to buffer the lidocaine hydrochloride (1 part bicarbonate to 4 or 5 parts lidocaine). The local anesthetic is then infiltrated into the deeper tissues with a vertically oriented needle placed at the site of the skin wheal. The needle is then removed. The physician inserts a 22-gauge 3^1/$_2$-in spinal needle vertically until it intercepts bone. At this point, the position of the needle tip can be checked fluoroscopically and repositioned, if indicated. A 10-mL syringe and contrast-filled tubing are then connected to the needle, and, under fluoroscopic visualization, a test injection of radiographic contrast is performed. If the needle tip is extraarticular, the contrast will pool around the needle tip. An intraarticular position is indicated by the rapid flow of contrast away from the needle tip forming a crescent around the humeral head or of contrast extending across the humeral neck. Alternatively, shoulder arthrography may be performed under sonographic or CT guidance or even by palpation alone, depending on the expertise of the radiologist. The needle may be advanced into the joint through an anterior or a posterior approach.

If a conventional double contrast arthrogram is being performed, 3 to 4 mL of Conray 60 is instilled into the joint followed by 10 to 12 mL of room air. Postinjection radiographs are often obtained with the patient upright and holding an approximately 5-lb weight (2 cassettes) with internal and external rotation of the shoulder. Axillary and bicipital groove views also

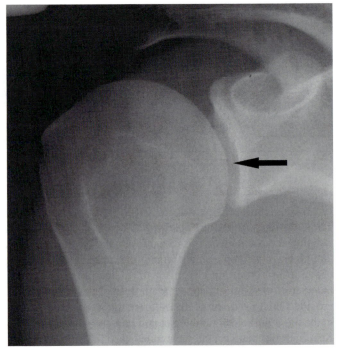

A

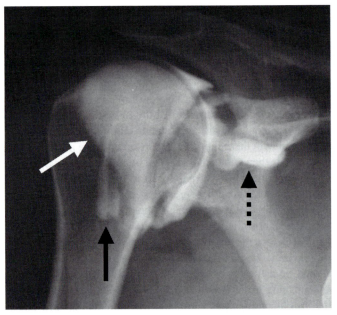

B

FIGURE 19-1. Shoulder arthrography. *(A)* Anteroposterior scout view of the shoulder shows the point of needle insertion (arrow) between the humeral head and glenoid. *(B)* Normal arthrographic image shows the lateral extent of the joint capsule (white arrow). A small amount of contrast extends into the subcoracoid recess (dashed black arrow) and into the bicipital groove (solid black arrow).

are performed. If no pathology is detected after review of these 4 radiographs, the patient is asked to exercise the joint. The patient may move the joint in a circular motion several times. The upright radiographs in internal and external rotation are then repeated after minimal exercise.

The entry of air or contrast into the subacromial or subdeltoid bursa indicates a full-thickness rotator cuff tear (see Chapter 9).

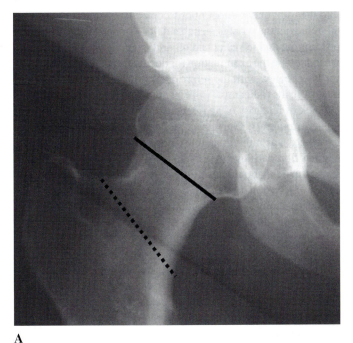

A

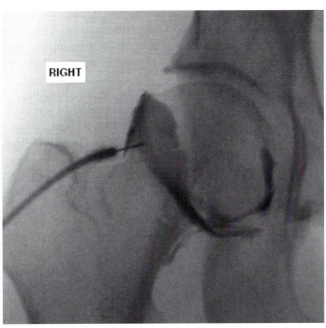

B

FIGURE 19-2. Hip arthrography. *(A)* Anteroposterior view. The needle can be placed into the subcapital recess (anywhere along the solid line) or into the intertrochanteric recess (anywhere along the dashed line). *(B)* Fluoroscopic spot view during injection shows the needle in a subcapital location and normal filling of the joint.

The size of the defect normally can be assessed. Labral pathology can be identified on the axillary view. The bicipital groove view is used to evaluate the integrity of the bicipital tendon and whether or not it is located within the groove. A complete rupture is diagnosed radiographically by failure to visualize the shadow of the tendon within the capsule or sheath or by distortion of the sheath.

If the shoulder arthrogram is being performed for MR arthrography, only 1 mL of iodinated contrast is instilled to confirm the intraarticular position of the needle tip. Then, 10 to 14 mL of a 1:200 dilution of an MR contrast agent is instilled into the joint (1 mL of gadolinium diethylene triamine pentacetic acid (DTPA) diluted in 200 mL of normal saline). The patient is then escorted from the fluoroscopy suite to the MR suite. If delay in MR scanning is anticipated, 1 mL of 1:1000 epinephrine may be added to the contrast solution to decrease joint resorption.

Hip joint puncture can be performed to aspirate a suspected joint infection, evaluate prosthetic loosening, inject anesthetic or steroids into a painful degenerated hip, or as part of MR arthrography to evaluate the acetabular labrum. For hip aspiration or arthrography, the patient is placed in a supine position on the fluoroscopy table. A small cushion placed under the knee is useful for the patient's comfort and relaxes the joint capsule. A sand bag may be placed along the outer border of the foot or the feet may be taped together to prevent external rotation of the femur. External rotation of the femur causes lateral displacement of the femoral vessels, which places them in jeopardy of accidental puncture during needle placement. The femoral pulse should be palpated, and its course marked to avoid needle puncture. If there is excessive abdominal pannus, the patient may be requested to manually lift it out of the way or it may be taped. Using fluoroscopy, the skin is marked at the level of the proxi-

mal femoral neck slightly to the medial side (Figure 19-2). After sterile skin preparation and draping and infiltration of the area with local anesthetic, a 22-gauge 3½-in spinal needle is inserted into the joint. This can be done in a number of ways. The needle can be inserted vertically. However, a more lateral and inferior point of needle insertion, with slanting of the needle superiorly and medially, may be needed to avoid the femoral vessels and nerve. During needle insertion, the position of the tip can be identified with intermittent fluoroscopy. When the needle strikes the femoral neck, aspiration of synovial fluid can be attempted. If only a small amount of fluid is present, it may lie in a recess at the very medial margin of the neck. The needle tip may be "walked" along the neck to the medial edge until successful aspiration of fluid for Gram stain, culture, and sensitivity is accomplished. If the patient has a hip prosthesis, the needle may be difficult to visualize fluoroscopically, but it is directed to the medial aspect of the metallic femoral neck near its junction with the prosthetic head. If synovial fluid cannot be aspirated, a small amount of contrast may be injected. Pooling of contrast around the tip indicates an extraarticular position. If an intraarticular position is confirmed but no synovial fluid can be aspirated after needle repositioning, the joint may be lavaged with 10 mL of non-bacteriostatic sterile saline. After joint lavage, the return aspirate can be sent for culture, although this is not as optimal as obtaining native fluid.

Injection of iodinated contrast, with a volume of up to 15 mL, may be performed through sterile tubing so it can be viewed fluoroscopically. When evaluating for prosthetic loosening, very careful comparison must be made between the preliminary radiographs and those obtained after contrast administration. The presence of a small amount of contrast at the bone-cement needed before causing symptoms. Occasionally, a disc is so degenerated and the anulus so incompetent that not enough pressure can be generated in the disc to provoke symptoms and contrast extravasates into the paravertebral or epidural spaces. If the injection causes pain, it is important to ask the patient about its type, severity, distribution, and similarity to the patient's usual symptoms. The more closely the contrast injection into a specific disc matches the patient's usual pain, the more likely the cause of symptoms resides in the injected disc.

Discograms are performed with local anesthesia with or without conscious sedation. Conscious sedation must be titrated carefully. The patient should not be so heavily sedated as to be unable to respond coherently at the time of disc injection or so anesthetized that the pain response is deadened.

At the end of the discogram, plain radiographs of the injected discs are obtained, followed by CT scan. The CT images demonstrate anular tears, disc bulges, and herniations. A sequestered fragment that has lost contact with the disc of origin may not be demonstrated with discography. An anular tear may result in contrast extravasating from the disc into the epidural space.

Discograms can be performed in the cervical spine. This is done with the patient supine, the shoulders elevated to extend the cervical spine, using biplane or C-arm fluoroscopy, local anesthesia, and proper aseptic technique. The sternocleidomastoid muscle is palpated and compressed until the discographer feels the side of the cervical spine. A 22-gauge spinal needle is advanced into the anterolateral surface of the disc, contrast is injected, and the patient's response is observed. Of particular concern in cervical discography is the esophagus because it cannot be displaced from its anatomic position in front of the spine. For this reason, antibiotic prophylaxis is used routinely when performing cervical discography.

The final report of the procedure must identify whether the patient's pain syndrome was re-created, the level or levels this occurred, the configuration of the disc, including any mass effect it is exerting, and the appearance of the facet joints and neural foramina.

Therapeutic Injections

Low back pain is one of the most common problems facing a physician. The etiology of the pain is often multifactorial, making diagnosis and treatment complex. Traditionally, conservative therapy included bed rest, traction, antiinflammatory medications, and physical therapy. If these treatment measures failed, surgical invention often was the next step. An injection of anesthetics and steroids into selected sites of the spine offers a new approach. This section discusses the indications, techniques, and expected results of these injections.

PATIENT SELECTION. Low back and radicular pain usually are multifactorial in origin. In general, however, radicular pain is due to direct compression of a nerve (often by a herniated disc), low back pain is due to abnormalities in the apophyseal joints, and a combination of radicular pain and low back pain is often due to spinal stenosis. Other causes for pain are neoplastic disease (primary or metastatic) and infection, when pain is due to bone

involvement and/or abnormal soft tissue masses. Radicular pain can be due to abnormalities at sites removed from the spine such as compression of the sciatic nerve as it courses by the piriformis muscle. Other diseases such as metabolic conditions can cause pain of spinal origin. These differential diagnoses always should be entertained when the decision to treat with pain control is made.

The physical examination of the patient should include a neurologic evaluation. The purpose of the neurologic evaluation is twofold. The current functional status of the patient is assessed. It is also used to determine which nerve root, apophyseal joint, or section of the spine is most likely to be the cause of the patient's symptoms.

MRI and CT of the spine should be obtained and carefully evaluated by someone familiar with these imaging modalities. The quality of the scans should be critically assessed. Significant findings may be overlooked with less than optimal images, and studies should be repeated, if necessary. In general, MRI scans are better for evaluation of soft tissue masses (herniated discs, abscesses, or neoplastic masses). CT scans are better for imaging the abnormal changes in the apophyseal joints and osteophytes. Both studies are useful in the assessment of spinal stenosis. Other imaging tests such as plain radiographs, tomograms, and radionuclide bone scans can be helpful.

The patient should be informed of the purpose of the injection, which can be diagnostic (only anesthetics are injected) or therapeutic (steroids are also injected). The site to be injected (nerve root, apophyseal joint, or epidural space) also should be explained to the patient.

INJECTIONS. Fluoroscopic or CT guidance may be used, depending on availability and the training and experience of the radiologist. When using CT guidance, the patient is placed prone on the CT table, and axial images, 3 mm thick, are obtained through the area of interest. The axial image that offers the best approach is selected, and markers are placed on the skin so that a point can be selected for introduction of the needle. The procedure is performed under local anesthesia and with proper aseptic technique.

The skin is infiltrated with local anesthetic by using a short 25-gauge needle, followed by introduction of a 20-gauge spinal needle that is directed by serial CT images toward the chosen target. Once the spinal needle is close to the target (2 to 3 cm away), a 25-gauge needle, 5 or 6 in long, is advanced through the 20-gauge needle. Pain is often described, especially if a nerve root is the target. The pain usually feels like an electric shock. More important than the type of pain is its distribution because it may confirm that the particular nerve root is or is not the cause of the patient's symptoms. A small amount of contrast agent (nonionic and low osmolality) is injected through the 25-gauge needle. The contrast material should be located around the nerve root, in the epidural apace, or in a facet, depending on the type of injection being performed. If contrast is demonstrated in the thecal sac, the 25-gauge and possibly also the 20-gauge needle should be repositioned because steroids in the crystalline form should not be introduced into the subarachnoid space. After injection of contrast, if the CT images fail to demonstrate it, the contrast most likely is in the thecal sac and the contrast has moved toward the most dependent portion of the spine, which is usually the thoracolumbar junction when the patient is prone. Long-acting steroids (eg, 80 mg of methylprednisolone acetate [Depo-Medrol]) and a small amount of 1% lidocaine are injected when the needle is correctly positioned. Larger amounts of anesthetic should not be used because it can cause significant weakness of the lower extremities for several hours. If the purpose of the injection is purely diagnostic, a small amount of long-acting anesthetic (methylparaben-free bupivacaine) can be used. The patient should be watched for at least 30 minutes and should be accompanied by a family member or a friend. Motor weakness can occur, and the patient should be advised of this possibility.

The apophyseal joint is approached through its most posterior surface and should be penetrated by a thin needle, usual 25 or 22 gauge. The 25-gauge needle is difficult to control, so a coaxial system with a 20-gauge needle is recommended.

The nerve root usually is approached from the posterolateral surface of the spine. The needles are angled close to 45° in relation to the sagittal plane. At times, especially in older individuals, osteophytes prevent access with this approach. The same situation exists in the postoperative patient, when hardware and bone fusion masses can block access to the spine. In these situations, the injection can be performed through the spinal canal. The 20-gauge spinal needle is aimed toward the nerve root along a line that crosses the spinal canal as close as possible to its bony walls while trying to avoid the thecal sac. The 20-gauge needle is advanced into the most posterior aspect of the spinal canal, and the 25-gauge needle is then introduced and placed close to the nerve root in question. Contrast agent should be injected to confirm the extrathecal location of the needle. The same trans-spinal approach can be used for injections and possible aspirations of synovial cysts of the apophyseal joints. Depending on the location and size of the cyst, a combination of a 6-in 22-gauge needle and an 18-gauge needle (instead of the usual 25- and 20-gauge combination) can be used if one is attempting to aspirate fluid from the cyst.

Epidural injections are performed with the needle placed into the posterior aspect of the spinal canal adjacent to the thecal sac. The injections often can be performed with just the 20-gauge spinal needle. Epidural injections are used most often for cases of spinal stenosis. The stenosis can be multilevel. In general, compression of the thecal sac and nerves results in edema in the area of stenosis and distal to it; therefore, in most cases, one should introduce the epidural medication proximal to the level of stenosis. Osteophytes, bone ridges, and telescoping of vertebrae can make advancing the needle into the abnormal section of the spine impossible. In these cases, one can try a proximal injection cephalad to the area of stenosis. If the injected contrast agent fails to opacify the epidural space distal to the stenosis, it is unlikely the steroid will reach that section of the spine; in these cases, the hope for relief of the spinal pain is limited.

Another access to the epidural space is transforaminal. The spine is approached as if for a nerve root block, but the needle is advanced farther through the foramen into the spinal canal. In this situation, the needle is placed anterior to the thecal sac. During nerve root injections, injected contrast is seen at times to opacify the epidural space even though the needle has not been advanced through the neural foramen. The disc may be penetrated through the transforaminal approach, and, in this case, minimal superficial displacement of the needle will suffice to place it in the proper location.

INJECTIONS OF THE CERVICAL SPINE. The same principles of injections into the lumbar spine can be used for injections into the cervical spine, but there are important differences. The use of local anesthetic in the cervical spine should be limited because of the obvious risk of the anesthetic reaching the thecal sac or even the epidural space. As a rule, the deeper a needle targeted to a cervical nerve root or cervical epidural space is introduced, the less local anesthetic should be injected. Contrast must be injected once the needle is in position; if there is no opacification of the subarachnoid space, long-acting steroid is then injected. The apophyseal joints of the cervical spine correspond to the space between the lateral masses of cervical vertebrae. Injections can be performed not only in the cervical apophyseal joints but also between the condyles of the occiput and the lateral masses of C_1, usually in patients with headache, which is occipital in distribution.

The injection of the cervical spine usually is done with the patient in a lateral decubitus position, with the affected side uppermost. The patient's head should be kept slightly tilted toward the CT table to open the intervertebral foramina and apophyseal joints. Most cervical injections are performed with a 22-gauge pediatric spinal needle. The vertebral artery courses anteriorly to the intervertebral foramina from C_6 to C_1; the foramen transversarium should be avoided.

INJECTIONS OF THE THORACIC SPINE. Most rarely, these injections are performed in the thoracic spine, usually in patients with scoliosis. These patients tend to be older individuals with previous surgery (bone fusion with or without hardware), many of them with underlying neurologic conditions such as poliomyelitis or traumatic injuries. The principles for injections are the same as those described for the lumbar spine. The patient is placed prone on the CT table.

INJECTIONS IN A SPINE WITH HARDWARE. The presence of rods, plates, pedicle screws, and apophyseal joint screws can limit accessibility to the spine for injections to control pain. In most cases, one is able to introduce the medication at the targeted site or close to it. In some instances, local injection of anesthetic is used to demonstrate whether a broken piece of hardware is the culprit in postoperative pain.

RESULTS. It is often the case that it is difficult to measure in precise numbers the success of different treatments for pain of spinal origin. In some patients, an injection once a year is enough to control pain; in others, the injections have no effect whatsoever. The type of pain, the age of the patient, the duration of symptoms, the neurologic evaluation, and the appearance of the spine in the various imaging tests are usually of no help in predicting the outcome of these injections. The patient should be informed of the limitations. Many physicians will try at least three successive injections before changing the treatment. The injections should be at least 1 month apart after the first encounter with the patient. If the injections become the treatment modality in a given patient, these should not be performed more often than every 3 months.

A patient who undergoes a therapeutic injection should be informed that the injected local anesthetic has effect for only a few hours and that it may take 2 to 3 days before the steroid starts producing pain relief.

COMPLICATIONS. The long-acting steroid relies on its crystalline form for its delayed effect. The presence of crystals in the subarachnoid space may induce a foreign body reaction, leading to arachnoiditis and disastrous consequences. This is the main reason to try as much as possible to avoid introducing slow-releasing steroids into the thecal sac.

Anesthetics in the subarachnoid space can cause significant but temporary anesthesia. If anesthesia is introduced into the lumbar thecal sac, the patient very quickly describes loss of sensation and motor power in the lower half of the body. The patient should be placed in the sitting position because the various anesthetics tend to be heavier than cerebrospinal fluid. The patient should be transferred immediately to an acute postanesthesia care environment and watched closely for possible cephalad migration of the level of anesthesia. Rarely, bleeding can result from these spinal injections; in rare cases, the bleeding can involve the subarachnoid space. A patient complaining of headaches, stiff neck, or new onset of complaints after these injections should be reexamined, preferably by the neurologist, and appropriate tests, usually CT and/or MRI, should be obtained. Damage to the spinal cord is avoided by making sure that the needle does not penetrate the cervical or thoracic spinal canal.

In our experience, there is no documented case of injury to a nerve root with the 25-gauge needle used as described in this text; however, this possibility cannot be ignored. If severe radicular pain is described at the time of needle placement, the needle should be repositioned. Careful neurologic evaluation before and after the test will allow a judgment as to whether the nerve has been injured.

VERTEBROPLASTY AND KYPHOPLASTY

Vertebroplasty is a relatively new technique that was first performed in 1984 in France for the stabilization of a C_2 vertebra with a hemangioma. Vertebroplasty is the stabilization of a compressed vertebral body through the percutaneous injection of radiopaque cement. The procedure can be used to treat compression fractures resulting from metastatic disease, multiple myeloma, and benign bone tumors such as painful hemangioma, but it is used far more commonly to treat painful osteoporotic compression fractures.

Candidates for the procedure should have significant pain from the fracture, usually causing alteration of lifestyle. Potential patients require a careful physical examination and usually MRI and/or bone scan in addition to plain radiographs. Palpation of the spinous process(es) of the affected vertebrae should elicit the pain complained of by the patient. However, this is accurate only within 1 to 2 levels of the fracture. MRI is helpful

in excluding other causes such as spinal stenosis, disc herniation, or infection as the source of the patient's pain. Patients with the best response to vertebroplasty generally have fractures that are less than 1 year old. These fractures will demonstrate a pattern of marrow edema on MRI. In patients with multiple compression fractures, treatment of those levels with a bone marrow edema pattern is more likely to lead to a favorable outcome. Sometimes, even compression fractures with normal marrow signal on fluid-sensitive sequences such as fat-suppressed fast spin echo T_2-weighted images or short tau inversion recovery will show increased uptake on bone scan. Treatment of these fractures also may lead to a favorable clinical response.

The procedure should not be performed in patients with infection, fever, or elevated white blood cell counts.

The procedure is done most commonly in a biplane fluoroscopy suite. Single-plane fluoroscopy suites can be used but generally lead to longer procedure times. Conscious sedation is necessary for the procedure. Very careful attention to sterile technique is critical for all personnel present in the fluoroscopy suite. With the patient lying prone, the level to be treated is identified. The x-ray tube is angled until the pedicle at the desired level is centered between the vertebral endplates or is located slightly toward the upper endplate. Adjusting the position of the patient may be necessary to achieve this. A true lateral view of the desired level is very important, with the pedicles directly superimposed and the posterior cortex viewed in profile. After the administration of local anesthetic, the beveled vertebroplasty needle is advanced carefully through the pedicle into the vertebral body, and the needle position is checked in AP and lateral planes. In general, the starting point of the needle is in the upper outer aspect of the pedicle. The needle tip is placed into the anterior third of the vertebral body, and, typically, injections are made through both pedicles to achieve maximal vertebral filling; however, as the radiologist gains experience in the procedure, it is often possible to angle the needle so the tip crosses the midline of the vertebra, and in this way the vertebra can be stabilized with a single cement injection rather than injections through both pedicles (Figure 19-5). Once correct needle position is achieved, a contrast vertebrogram may be performed to evaluate the venous drainage pattern of the vertebra. This serves to alert the radiologist to the possibility of cement extravasation and the need for repositioning the needle if there is immediate venous drainage, but some people do not perform the vertebrogram.

The polymethylmethacrylate cement powder is opacified with sterile barium powder. Antibiotic (eg, tobramycin) should be added to the cement-barium mixture. Liquid monomer is added to this mixture to activate the cement until the desired consistency is achieved. Delivery of the cement into the vertebral body is performed in a very controlled manner. The lateral view is used to view the injection to ensure that there is no extravasation of cement into the epidural space. The AP view is checked periodically to ensure that there is no extravasation of cement laterally. While injecting, the needle usually is pulled back into the mid and posterior thirds of the vertebral body to optimize cement filling. Stabilization of the load-bearing anterior third of the vertebral body is probably the most important region to be filled.

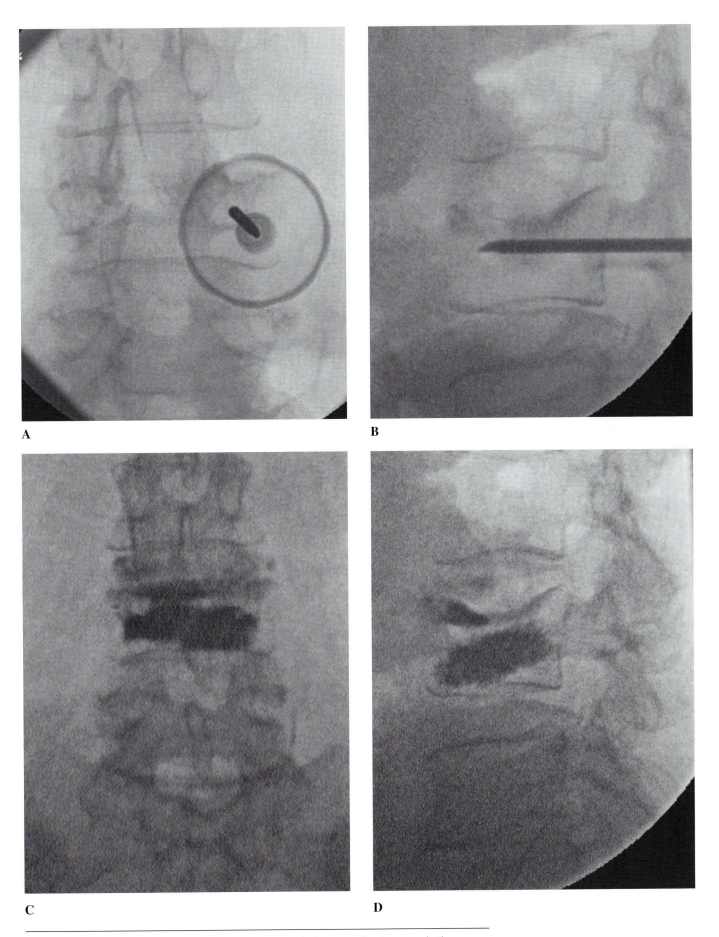

FIGURE 19-5. Vertebroplasty. *(A)* Frontal spot radiograph shows needle placement in the supero-lateral aspect of the pedicle. *(B)* Lateral spot radiograph shows proper positioning of the needle tip in the anterior third of the vertebral body. *(C)* Frontal and *(D)* lateral spot views after cement injection show the radiopaque cement filling the vertebral body. There is no extravertebral extravasation.

It is possible to stabilize more than 1 level in a session, but most radiologists choose to treat no more than 2 or 3 levels per session. Patients are normally observed for approximately 4 hours post procedure.

In experienced hands, vertebroplasty has a very low complication rate. Specific risks of the procedure include infection, bleeding, contrast reaction, pulmonary embolism from deep venous thrombosis or cement embolization, nerve root pain, or new neurologic deficit.

Vertebroplasty has become a widely performed technique for the treatment of osteoporotic compression fractures and often is very rewarding because patients usually experience significant pain relief and often can attain their prefracture activity level.

Kyphoplasty is a similar technique that involves the percutaneous placement of an expandable balloon into the compressed vertebral body, with the goal of restoring the height of the affected vertebral body before stabilizing it with opacified cement. Indications for kyphoplasty and vertebroplasty often overlap. Usually, a compression fracture must be less than 6 months old to respond to kyphoplasty. Kyphoplasty may not be indicated unless there is greater than 40% loss of anterior height of the involved vertebra.

SUGGESTED READINGS

Bellaiche L, Hamze B, Parlier-Cuav C, Laredo J. Percutaneous biopsy of musculoskeletal lesions. *Semin Musculoskel Radiol.* 1997;1:177–187.

Cotten A, Boutry N, Cortet B, et al. Percutaneous vertebroplasty: state of the art. *Radiographics.* 1998;18:311–320.

Gangi A, Guth S, Dietemann J, et al. Interventional musculoskeletal procedures. *Radiographics.* 2001;21:E1.

Newberg A. Anesthetic and corticosteroid joint injections: a primer. *Semin Musculoskel Radiol.* 1998;2:415–420.

Resnick D. Needle biopsy of bone and soft tissue. In: Resnick D, Niwayama G, eds. *Diagnosis of Bone and Joint Disorders.* 4th ed. Philadelphia: WB Saunders; 2002:425–437.

Sarazin L, Chevrot A, Pessis E, et al. Lumbar facet joint arthrography with the posterior approach. *Radiographics.* 1999;19:93–104.

INDEX

3